Role of Probiotics in Animals

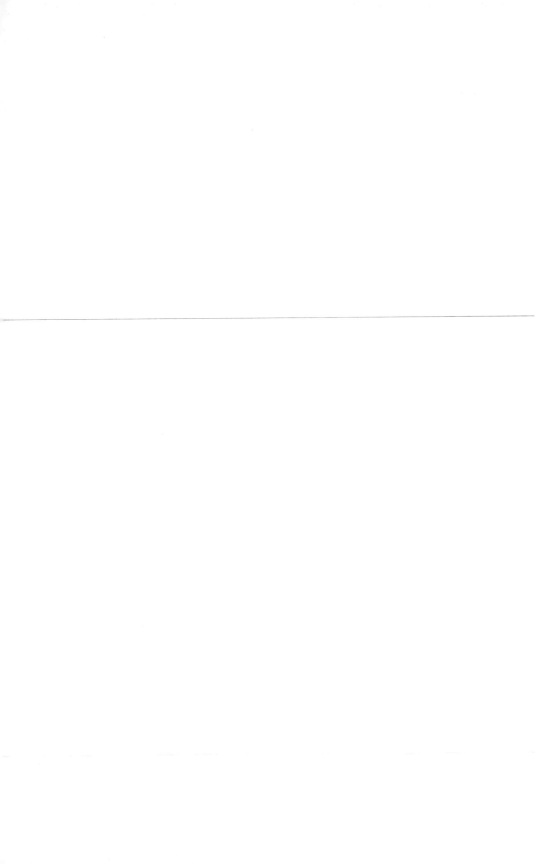

Role of Probiotics in Animals

Edited by **Shawn Kiser**

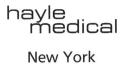

New York

Published by Hayle Medical,
30 West, 37th Street, Suite 612,
New York, NY 10018, USA
www.haylemedical.com

Role of Probiotics in Animals
Edited by Shawn Kiser

International Standard Book Number: 978-1-63241-345-1 (Hardback)

Printed in the United States of America.

Contents

Preface

Every book is initially just a concept; it takes months of research and hard work to give it the final shape in which the readers receive it. In its early stages, this book also went through rigorous reviewing. The notable contributions made by experts from across the globe were first molded into patterned chapters and then arranged in a sensibly sequential manner to bring out the best results.

This book provides essential information on the various roles of probiotics in animals. Over the past few decades, the prevalence of analysis regarding probiotic strains has significantly grown in most regions of the world. The use of probiotic strains in animal production may decrease numerous complications caused by growth promoter, antibiotics therapy and problems from improper management. Probiotics are particular strains of microorganisms, which when served to animals or humans in suitable amounts, have an advantageous impact, enhancing health or decreasing the risk of getting sick. The book would serve as an important source of reference to a wide range of readers.

It has been my immense pleasure to be a part of this project and to contribute my years of learning in such a meaningful form. I would like to take this opportunity to thank all the people who have been associated with the completion of this book at any step.

Editor

Probiotic Meat Products

Renata Ernlund Freitas de Macedo, Sérgio Bertelli Pflanzer
and Carolina Lugnani Gomes

Additional information is available at the end of the chapter

1. Introduction

The growing concern of consumers regarding the food health and safety issues has led to the development of products that promote health and well-being beyond its nutritional effect [1]. Functional foods are those which promote beneficial effects to human´s health beyond nutrition. Their effects are due to the addition of active ingredients, the removal or the replacement of undesirable compounds in its composition [2].

The marketing of food for health benefits began in 1960s. In 1970s the trend was to eliminate or reduce the harmful constituents like sugars and fats from food. In 1980s, the trend continued with the reduction or elimination of food additives, which led to the induction and addition of useful components like vitamins, minerals and probiotics in 1990s [1, 3].

Among the different types of functional food, probiotics represent a large share of the functional food market, being used mainly in dairy beverages, cereal products, infant feeding formulas, fruit juices and ice cream [4-7].

In meat industry, the demand for new products has greatly influenced its development, especially for sausage type products. However, lately, those meat products are considered unhealthy by a part of population because of their fat content and the use of additives and spices in their formulation. Therefore, the addition of probiotics to the fermented sausages could promote the health benefits associated with lactic acid bacteria and contribute to the increase in the consumption of such products [7, 8].

The use of probiotics seems more promising in raw fermented meat products like salami as they are made with raw meat and consumed without prior heating, which would kill the probiotic bacteria [9, 10]. However, the incorporation of probiotic bacteria to these products also represents a technological challenge because of the known sensitivity of probiotic to curing salts, spices and other ingredients used in the formulation of the fermented sausages [11]. Furthermore, this addition requires the use of microorganisms that are resistant to the fermentation process and that remain in a minimal viable number of cells to survive the stomach pH and exert beneficial effects in the intestines [8].

Additionally, the processing of probiotic meat products implies taking into account the appropriateness of the probiotic culture to the target consumer, the intestinal functionality expected for the probiotic species, the rate of survival of probiotic during food processing and the need of maintenance in the probiotic product of the same sensory attributes that characterize the regular product [8, 10, 12].

This chapter presents the potential applications of probiotics in fermented meat products, focusing on the technological challenges, the functional effects of probiotics and on the researches that address the addition of probiotics in fermented meat products.

2. Fermented meat as a probiotic product

2.1. Fermented sausages

Fermented sausages are defined as a mixture of ground lean meat and minced fat, curing salts, sugar and spices, which are embedded into a casing and subjected to fermentation and drying [6, 13, 14].

The quality of fermented sausages is closely related to the ripening process that gives color, flavor, aroma, and firmness to the product which are developed by a complex interaction of chemical and physical reactions associated with the fermentative action of the microbiological flora present in the sausage. In handmade production processes of fermented sausages, fermentation occurs spontaneously by the action of *in nature* bacteria present on meat. In industrial processes the microbiological flora, responsible for the fermentation process, is known as starter culture [6]. Starter cultures are defined as preparations containing live microorganisms capable of developing desirable metabolic activity in meat. They are used to increase the microbiological safety, to maintain stability by inhibiting the growth of undesirable microorganisms and to improve the sensory characteristics of fermented sausages [1].

Starter cultures are formed by mixing of different types of microorganisms, where each one has a specific function. Lactic bacteria are used in order to generate controlled and intense acidification which inhibits the development of undesirable microorganisms, and provides increased safety and stability to the product. On the other hand, coccus catalase positive type bacteria, as *Staphylococccus* and *Kocuria*, yeasts as *Debaryomyces*, and molds as *Penicillium* usually provide desirable sensory characteristics to the product [1, 2, 8].

Table 1 shows the microorganism species most commonly used as starter cultures to fermented meat products.

Microorganism	Genus and Species
Lactic acid bacteria	*Lactobacillus acidophilus* [a], *L. alimentarius* [b], *L. brevis*, *L. casei* [a], *L. curvatus*, *L. fermentum*, *L. plantarum*, *L. pentosus*, *L. sakei* *Lactococcus lactis* *Pediococcus acidilactici*, *P. pentosaceus*
Actinobacteria	*Kocuria varians* [c] *Streptomyces griséus* *Bifidobacterium sp.* [a]
Staphylococcus	*S. xylosus, S. carnosus subsp. carnosus, S. carnosus subsp. utilis, S. equorum* [b]
Halomanadaceae	*Halomonas elongata* [b] (tested in dry cured ham)
Enterobacter	*Aeromonas sp.*
Mold	*Penicillium nalgiovense, P. chrysogeum, P. camemberti*
Yeast	*Debaryomyces hansenii, Candida famata*

Table 1. Microorganism species most commonly used as starter cultures in fermented meat products SOURCE: [15-17].
[a] Used as probiotic cultures.
[b] Used in commercial tests in industrial scale (Laboratorium Wiesby, Niebüll and Rudolf Müller and Co)
[c] formerly known as *Micrococcus varians.*

The selection of starter cultures for use in fermented meat products must be carried out according to the product formulation and the technological processing employed, since environmental factors can select a limited number of strains with the ability to compete and overcome on product. Typically, the species used as the starter culture are selected from strains naturally predominant in meat products and hence, well adapted to this environment. Therefore, these species present a tendency to have greater metabolic capacity which is reflected on the development of the proper sensory and physical-chemical characteristics on the product [6].

Given the adverse conditions of the meat matrix for a number of microorganisms, including those considered probiotics, several studies suggest the selection of probiotic properties in lactic bacteria from commercial starter culture traditionally used in fermented meat products and therefore, already adapted to grow in these conditions. These cultures will provide to the product the same sensory and technological characteristics than the traditional starter cultures, and exert beneficial effects to health [8, 15, 18]. Among the starter lactic acid bacteria, *Lactobacillus brevis, L. plantarum, L. fermentum* and *Pedioccus pentosaceus* have been characterized as probiotics [19-21]. Strains of *L. sakei* and *P. acidilactici* have also been proposed as potential probiotic in meat products, due to its survival under acid conditions and high concentrations of bile [22]. Probiotic cultures can also be selected from the lactic acid bacteria (LAB) naturally presented in fermented meat products [7, 21, 23-25].

2.2. Probiotic fermented sausages

Although the concept of including probiotics in meat products is not entirely new, only a few manufacturers consider the use of fermented sausages as vehicles for probiotics [7, 17].

Several meat products containing probiotics with claims for health benefits have been commercialized. A salami containing three intestinal LAB (*Lactobacillus acidophilus*, *Lactobacillus casei* and *Bifidobacterium* spp.) was produced by a German company in 1998. In the same year, a meat spread containing an intestinal LAB (*Lactobacillus rhamnosus* FERM P-15120) was produced by a Japanese company [26-28].

Fermented sausages are suitable for the incorporation of probiotic bacteria since mild or no heat treatment is usually required by dry fermented meat products, thus providing the suitable conditions required for the survival of probiotics [3, 14, 26]. The sausage has to be designed in such a way as to keep the number and viability of probiotic strain in the optimum range. Thus, reduction in pH (e.g. < 5.0), extended ripening (e.g. >1 month), dry or excessive heating has to be avoided if the beneficial effects of probiotic are to be harvested [3, 7].

In meat sector, meat cultures are generally added to fermented meat products with the function of inhibiting pathogens and increasing shelf-life, rather than introducing functional or physiological qualities. Those cultures are called protective starter cultures and do not promote significant changes in physical and sensory characteristics of the product. On the other hand, probiotic cultures are, by definition, those that after ingestion in sufficient number employ health benefits in addition to their nutritional effects [6, 8, 15]. However, often, the probiotic cultures have also been used in meat products as protective cultures, since both of these cultures have the ability to survive in adverse environments and to produce organic acids and bacteriocins [18]. Likewise, probiotics added to meat products are also known as functional starter cultures since they contribute to safety, can provide sensory and nutritional benefits and promote health [6].

The success of probiotics in other types of foods, especially dairy products, is based on scientific evidence of beneficial effects provided by some microorganisms. In meat products, the beneficial effects must be proven with the consumption of these products. From the good results obtained with dairy products it is not possible to conclude that a probiotic species will have the same effect on another type of product. This is due to the fact that the performance and properties of microorganisms are environment-dependent. Furthermore, there are few studies about the proper number of probiotic bacteria that should be ingested in meat products to achieve the desired effect [1, 15].

The estimated number of viable cells of probiotic bacteria to be ingested to obtain beneficial effects and temporary colonization of the intestine is around 10^9 to 10^{10} CFU/ g of product, in accordance with the counts of 10^6 to 10^8 viable cells found in 1 g of feces. Therefore, in a fermented meat product containing 10^8 CFU/ g, the minimum daily consumption might be 10-100 g of product [1, 29]. Rivera-Espinoza and Gallardo-Navarro [17] recommended the concentration of probiotic viable cells of at least 10^8 to 10^9 CFU/ g of the product to obtain the physiological effects associated with the use of probiotic food.

Despite the known health benefits provided by the use of probiotics such as the improvement of intestinal transit and digestion, improvement of symptoms of lactose intolerance, increase in immune response, reduction of diarrhea episodes, prevention or suppression of colon cancer and reduction of blood cholesterol [30, 31], much attention has paid to the use of probiotics in meat products in order to increase product safety and few studies evaluated the health benefits associated with the consumption of these products [7, 8, 15].

2.3. Most used probiotic cultures in meat products

Probiotics are mainly the strains from species of *Bifidobacterium* and *Lactobacillus*. Other than these, some species of *Lactococcus, Enterococcus, Saccharomyces* and *Propionibacterium* are considered as probiotics due to their ability to promote health in the host [32].

In fermented meat products several studies have demonstrated the feasibility of using probiotic *Lactobacillus*.

Arihara et al. [33] studied the use of *Lactobacillus gasseri* to improve the microbiological safety of fermented meat product. The use of *Lactobacillus rhamnosus* and *L. paracasei* subsp. *paracasei* for the fermentation of meat products has been studied by Sameshima et al. [9], while Pennacchia et al. [20] report the use of *Lactobacillus plantarum* and *Lactobacillus paracasei* as probiotics in meat products.

Erkkilä et al. [22] conducted experiments using probiotic strains of *L. rhamnosus* GG and potentially probiotic strains of *L. rhamnosus* LC-705, *L. rhamnosus* VTT-97800 and *L. rhamnosus* VTT for the manufacture of dry sausage.

Andersen [10] demonstrated the ability of mix of a traditional starter culture, Bactoferm T-SPX (Chr Hansen), and the potential probiotic cultures of *L. casei* LC-01 and *Bifidobacterium lactis* Bb-12 to ferment meat product.

Also Erkkilä et al. [11] used strains of *Lactobacillus gasseri, L. rhamnosus, L. paracasei* subsp. *paracasei, L. casei* and *Bifidobacterium lactis* for the manufacture of salami.

Pediococcus acidilactici PA-2 and *Lactobacillus sakei* Lb3 showed good survival characteristics in fermented sausages, being considered as probiotic candidates for meat products [7], as well as *Lactobacillus casei* and *Lactobacillus paracasei* isolated from fermented sausages which showed *in vitro* functional abilities [25].

Macedo et al. [34] investigated the viability of the use of probiotic *Lactobacillus paracasei, L. casei* e *L. rhamnosus* in fermented dry sausage with the maintenance of the technological and sensory characteristics of the product.

Vuyst et al. [7] and Khan et al. [3] stated that *Lactobacillus* species currently used as meat starter cultures, as *L. plantarum* and *L. casei*, can have a significant scope for being utilized in probiotic sausage manufacture.

2.3.1. Criteria for the selection of probiotic cultures for meat products

The criteria for a microbial culture to be considered probiotic are the stomach acidity resistance, lysozyme and bile resistance and the ability to colonize the human intestinal tract using mechanisms of adhesion or binding to intestinal cells [7, 8, 23, 35]. Other authors have also included the ability to tolerate pancreatic enzymes as a required characteristic of probiotic cultures [16].

Additionally to the criteria described above, the probiotic bacteria need to have *GRAS* (*Generally Recognized as Safe*) status [36]. Currently, this concept also includes the antibiotic resistance evaluated by Qualified Prediction Security Program suggested by EFSA (*European Food Safety Authority*). The ability of probiotic bacteria used in meat products to resist to some antibiotics can be genetically transmitted to other bacteria. Scientific studies report genetic determinants for bacterial resistance to chloramphenicol, erythromycin and tetracycline [14]. Normally, the lactic acid bacteria are sensitive to penicillin G, ampicillin, tetracycline, erythromycin, chloramphenicol and aminoglycosides, quinolones and glycopeptides [18]. Thus, the selection of probiotic cultures for meat products implies confirmation of the absence of antibiotic resistance transferable gens in selected strains [14].

However, among the criteria for the selection of probiotic cultures, the main condition to be evaluated is the ability of strains to promote beneficial effects in the host through interactions probiotic/ host and to prevent diseases [37]. These effects on human health may occur in three different ways according to the specificity of the strain: the antagonist action against other microorganisms in the same environment (by nutrient competition, bacteriocin production or competitive exclusion), the barrier effect on the intestinal mucosa and the boosting of immune system [7, 36].

2.3.2. Technological characteristics of probiotic cultures for meat products

For addition in fermented meat products, the probiotic bacteria need to maintain their viability towards the adverse conditions generated during the fermented sausages manufacture: low pH (<5.0), high salt content (2-3%), high nitrite content (around 120 ppm) and low water activity (<0.85). The probiotic cultures should also be capable of growing fast during the fermentation, be easily cultivated on an industrial scale, resist to freezing and lyophilization processes, provide longer shelf life to the product as well as contribute to the sensory quality of the final product [7, 11].

Probiotic cultures can be added in fermented sausage as part of the starter culture or as an additional culture incorporated during the mass mixing (Figure 1).

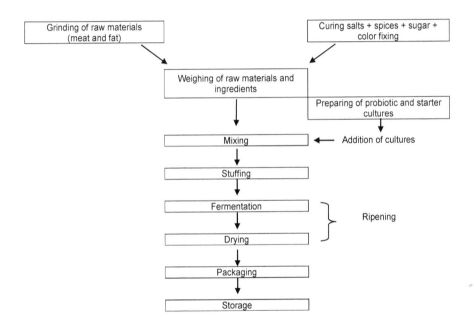

Figure 1. Basic flowchart of the processing of fermented dry sausage with the addition of probiotic cultures

Probiotic cultures may be added to the sausage batter as liquid inoculum, in high concentrations, or lyophilized. However, the addition of lyophilized culture can delay the fermentation time and reduce the culture viability in the final product. These effects can be reduced with the culture microencapsulation prior to lyophilization. This procedure is also indicated when probiotic strains are inhibited by ingredients of the sausage composition [6, 38].

Microencapsulation increases the viability of bacteria due to the protective effect of a polymeric membrane formed around the bacterial cells. The methods used for microencapsulation of lactic acid bacteria are extrusion and emulsification. Extrusion produces microcapsules with 2-3 mm in diameter which are 60 times greater than the microcapsule formed by emulsification. The materials most commonly used for the microencapsulation of probiotics include alginate, starch, k-carrageenan, guar gum, xanthan gum, gelatin and milk whey proteins. Muthukumarasamy and Holley [38] tested the microencapsulation of *Lactobacillus reuteri* ATCC 55730 in alginate for use in fermented meat product and found no adverse effect on the sensory quality of the product. Despite the microcapsules were visible to naked eye, they were detected as fat particles by the panelists due to their size and color similarity.

Rivera-Espinoza and Gallardo-Navarro [17] encapsulated *Bifidobacterium longum* and *Lactobacillus reuteri* in alginate to increase the survival of probiotics in fermented meat. Recently, Poulin, Caillard, and Subirade [39] created succinylated β-lactoglobulin tablet to protect *B. longum* strain and proved its protection effect *in-vivo* and *in-vitro*. Heidebach, Först and Kulozik [40] reported higher viability of *Lactobacillus* F19 encapsulated with casein during freeze storage compared to *Bifidobacterium* Bb12. Furthermore, the same authors [41] microencapsulated these two strains with rennet-induced gelation of milk, obtaining higher yields and improved survival rates.

2.3.2.1. Lactic acid production

One of the most important characteristics of *Lactobacillus* in fermented meat products is the production of lactic acid. The acidification has positive effects on safety and on the sensory characteristics of the product. The pH decrease in fermented sausages provides the coagulation of myofibrillar proteins, resulting in the increase of firmness and cohesiveness of the final product, and contributes to the flavor and red color. Inhibition of spoilage and pathogenic microorganisms is also provided by the fast decrease of pH and lactic acid production in appropriate quantities. The fast decrease in pH values during fermentation of sausages can also contribute to the prevention of the accumulation of biogenic amines, which are harmful to health [14].

However, it is important to confirm that the lactic acid bacteria used as probiotic produce the L(+) isomer lactic acid and do not produce the D(-) isomer lactic acid, due to the higher inhibitory effect on undesirable microorganisms of the L(+) lactic acid. Moreover, the D(-) lactic acid form is not metabolized by the human body and may cause health problems in consumers [7, 14, 42].

2.3.2.2. Resistance to salt (NaCl) and nitrite (NO₂)

According to Arihara and Itoh [43] and Sameshima et al. [9], the addition of 3% sodium chloride (NaCl) and 200 ppm sodium nitrite (NaNO₂) to fermented sausage is mandatory in Japan in order to maintain the microbiological safety of the product. Thus, the use of cultures resistant to curing salts is the first condition for the production of sausage with probiotic properties [23].

Sameshima et al. [9] tested the resistance of 202 Lactobacillus species of intestinal origin to sodium nitrite and sodium chloride in liquid medium and found that strains of L. paracasei ssp. paracasei, L. rhamnosus and L. acidophilus were tolerant to these salts. Similar results were obtained by Macedo et al. [44] who found resistance of Lactobacillus rhamnosus, Lactobacillus paracasei and Lactobacillus casei to the simultaneous use of sodium chloride and sodium nitrite at the concentrations of 3% and 200 ppm, respectively.

2.3.2.3. Bacteriocin production in meat products

Bacteriocins are peptides or proteins produced by microorganisms which destroy or inhibit the growth of gram positive bacteria, in particular Listeria monocytogenes. The use of bacteriocin-producing cultures in meat products may represent a considerable benefit to the consumers health and safety of the product, since bacteriocins do not pose toxicological hazards arising from their consumption and act as a natural form of preservation in the products. The production of bacteriocins has been detected in several lactic acid bacteria isolated from meat products such as L. sakei, L. curvatus, L. plantarum, L. brevis and L. casei [6].

2.3.3. Physiological characteristics of probiotic cultures for meat products

2.3.3.1. Resistance to low pH

The tolerance to acidity and bile salts are two fundamental properties that indicate the ability of a probiotic microorganism to survive through the gastrointestinal tract, resisting the acidic conditions of the stomach and the bile salts in the initial portion of the small intestine [22, 45].

The acidity is considered the most important deleterious factor that affects the viability and growth of lactic acid bacteria, since its growth is greatly inhibited at pH lower than 4.5. Such inhibition is related to a reduction in intracellular pH of the bacteria caused by non-dissociated lactic acid form, which due to its lipophilic nature, it diffuses through the cell membrane and causes collapse of the electrochemical gradient, promoting bacteriostatic or bactericidal effects [14, 36].

The survival of the probiotic to the gastric juice depends on its ability to tolerate low pH. At the time of hydrochloric acid excretion, the stomach pH is 0.9, however, during the digestive process the pH increases to around 3 due to the presence of food, remaining under this condition for a period of 2-4 hours [1, 22].

Due to the sensitivity of most bacteria to the low pH of the stomach, probiotic bacteria have to be ingested with food, because it acts as a buffer on the high acidity of the stomach, allowing the survival of the bacteria during gastric transit [46]. Meat, as well as milk, has buffers characteristics in acid environment and can thereby protect the probiotic from the adverse environment of the stomach [1].

Erkkilä and Petäjä [22] reported the resistance of species of *Lactobacillus pentosus*, *L. sakei*, *Pediococcus pentosaceus* e *P. acidilactici* to low pH and observed that at pH 4 and pH 5, the number of viable cells of these species remained unchanged compared to its initial value, indicating that the growth of the cultures was not affected by low pH.

Taking into account the pH conditions of stomach and the digestion time, probiotic bacteria ingested with food must be capable of resisting pH value 3 for a period of 2-4 hours to allow their survival during gastric transit. Macedo et al. [44] found that *Lactobacillus paracasei* used in probiotic salami was able to resist and grow in a medium at pH 3, showing a 20% increase in the initial number of cells during the 4 hours of exposure to this acidic condition.

Pennacchia et al. [20] tested the resistance of *Lactobacillus* isolated from 10 different types of salami to low pH. The authors found that from a total of 14 lactic acid bacteria that survived at pH 2.5 during 3 hours, 5 belonged to the *Lactobacillus casei* group. These authors also mention studies on the resistance of 20 strains of *Lactobacillus* isolated from infant faeces to acidic conditions and report the high viability rate of 3 strains of *L. paracasei* and one of *L. rhamnosus* at low pH.

2.3.3.2. Resistance to bile salts

Bile plays an important role in intestinal defense mechanism. The intensity of its inhibitory effect on microorganisms is determined by the concentration of salts in the bile composition [47]. Bile salts act by destroying the lipid layer and the fatty acids of the cell membrane of microorganisms. However, some *Lactobacillus* strains are able to hydrolyze bile salts by excreting bile salt hydrolase enzyme that weakens the detergent power of the bile [23]. *Lactobacillus* bile resistance has also been associated with other factors such as the stress response system as well as with the elements that involve the maintenance of cellular wall integrity, the energetic metabolism, the amino acid transport and the fatty acid biosynthesis [48].

According to Erkkilä and Petaja [22] and Pennacchia et al. [20], the average concentration of bile salts in the human intestinal tract is 0.3%, thus this is the critical concentration used for the selection of probiotic bacteria. Papamanoli et al. [23] consider as bile salts tolerance when a bacterial population reduces the number of viable cells from 10^6 - 10^7 CFU/ mL to 10^5 CFU/ mL in a 4 hour period.

Erkkilä and Petaja [22] observed a reduction of 1 log cycle in the initial number of viable cells of *Lactobacillus curvatus* and *Pediococcus acidilactici* when grown in a medium containing 0.3% bile salts and pH 6 after 4 hours of exposure.

From a total of 63 bacterial strains isolated from fermented sausages, canned fish, bakery dough and jellies, 9 strains of *Lactobacillus* sp. were able to survive at pH 2.5, while only strains of *Lactobacillus casei* e *Lactobacillus plantarum* showed survival at pH 2 and in the presence of bile salt [49].

Macedo et al. [44] found resistance of *Lactobacillus paracasei* to 0.3% bile salt.

Meat has also been reported to protect microbes against bile [50]. During meat sausage processing, *Lactobacillus* added to the batter are encapsulated by the matrix consisting of meat and fat. Due to the protection exerted by the food, the survival of *Lactobacillus in vivo* during transit through the stomach and intestine appears to be higher than that observed by the *in vitro* exposure of the microorganisms to low pH and bile salts [1, 22].

2.3.3.3. Detoxification capacity of biogenic amines produced in meat products

The biogenic amines, organic bases with aliphatic, aromatic or heterocyclic structures, are produced by the microbial decarboxylation of amino acids present in meat products, either by naturally occurring microorganisms or from the starter culture. The biogenic amines such as histamine, tryptamine, tyramine, cadaverine, putrescine and spermidine can cause toxic effects, especially in consumers with amino oxidase deficiency. In fermented meat products, biogenic amines producing microorganisms have a favorable environment due to the high protein content and the intense proteolytic activity that occurs during the long ripening time of these products. However, some strains of *Lactobacillus* are able to produce amino acid descarboxylase that prevents the accumulation of biogenic amines in the product. Thus, the selection of probiotic bacteria for use in fermented meat products must also be based on its ability to oxidate biogenic amines formed in the product and to prevent the formation of new amine by the rapid drop of pH that inhibits the growth of amine producing microorganisms. In fermented meat products, amine oxidase activity was detected in strains of *Lactobacillus casei* and *L. plantarum* [6, 14].

Ergönül and Kundakçi [51] found low biogenic amine contents in a Turkish fermented sausage manufactured by using three different probiotic starter culture combinations (*Lactobacillus casei*, *L. acidophilus* or their combination). Putrescine contents of the samples were ranging between 1.98 and 35.48 ppm during manufacturing and refrigerated storage (8 months), respectively, whereas the values were 0.96–18.50 ppm for cadaverine, 1.41– 10.84 ppm for histamine and 1.75–9.36 ppm for tyramine.

2.4. Beneficial effects associated with the consumption of probiotic meat products

As described earlier, most research involving probiotics in meat products focuses on the survival of probiotic species in the meat matrix and its influence on the technological and sensory characteristics of the final product. Few studies report the effects of consumption of these products on host health [7]. This condition is mainly due to the fact that *in vivo* tests are expensive, require more time for experimentation and the approval by ethics committees [36].

One of the few studies reporting the effects of the consumption of probiotic meat product on the human health was carried out by Jahreis et al. [52]. These authors evaluated the effect of daily consumption of 50g of probiotic salami containing *L. paracasei* LTH 2579 on the immunity system and blood triglycerides and cholesterol levels of healthy volunteers for a few week period, and obtained moderately satisfactory results. Although it has been observed effect on immunity of the host, small effect was observed on the plasmatic lipid levels.

In laboratory animals probiotic administration has shown to decrease the blood cholesterol level and increase the feed-conversion rate [53]. *L. plantarum* administration was reported to increase CD-8 and CD-4 lymphocytes in lab rats [54].

Other important physiological properties to be considered for the potential probiotics are the adhesive capacity toward Caco-2 cells and the antagonism toward pathogenic organisms [3].

Klingberg et al. [21] evaluated the ability of probiotic cultures to colonize the human intestinal tract by *in vitro* study using Caco-2 cells isolated from human colon adenocarcinoma. The starter strains *Pediococcus pentosaceus*, *Lactobacillus pentosus* and *L. plantarum* showed higher ability to adhere to cells in comparison to *Lactobacillus rhamnosus* used as control strain in the experiment.

Lactobacillus plantarum isolated from sausages exhibited superior adhesive properties toward Caco-2 cell lines as compared to *L. paracasei* and *L. brevis* [55].

The majority of studies on probiotic meat products focuses on the inhibition of pathogens by probiotics, increasing the safety of meat products. Mahoney and Henriksson [56] tested the inhibition of colonization and virulence of *Listeria monocytogenes* in the intestinal tract of rats by the consumption of fermented meat product with the addition of starter cultures, probiotic cultures and *Listeria monocytogenes*. The results showed that the starter culture consisting of *Pediococcus pentosaceus* and *Staphylococcus xylosus*, and the probiotic culture consisting of *Lactobacillus acidophilus*, *L. paracasei* and *Bifidobacterium* sp. were able to inhibit the growth of *Listeria monocytogenes* during its passage through the gastrointestinal tract. There was also a possible protective effect of the sausage on the intestinal mucosa by involving the pathogenic bacteria in its matrix and thus, not allowing it to adhere and colonize the intestine.

Autoaggregation of probiotic strains appears necessary for their adhesion to intestinal epithelial cells and coaggregation presents a barrier that prevents colonization by pathogenic microorganisms. Yuksekdag and Aslim [57] reported autoaggregation capacity of five *Pediococcus* strains isolated from a Turkish-type fermented sausages (sucuk) ranging from 35% to 84%. The high EPS (exopolysaccharide) producing *P. pentosaceus* Z12P and Z13P strains showed greater autoaggregation (79% and 84%, respectively) than the other strains. The coaggregation scores of those *Pediococcus* species with *L. monocytogenes* ATCC 7644 ranged from good (Z12P and Z13P) to partial (Z9P, Z10P, and Z11P).

Growth inhibition of *Escherichia coli* O157:H7 by the use of *Lactobacillus reuteri* ATCC 55730 and *Bifidobacterium longum* ATCC 15708 in the production of salami was confirmed by Muthukumarasamy and Holley [38]. Sameshima et al. [9] found that *Lactobacillus rhamnosus* FERM P-15120, *L. paracasei* subsp. *paracasei* FERM P-15121 and starter culture *L. sakei* were able to inhibit the growth and the toxin production of *Staphylococcus aureus* in fermented meat product.

Nedelcheva et al. [58] demonstrated the ability of *Lactobacillus plantarum* NBIMCC 2415 to inhibit the growth of pathogenic microorganisms such as *Escherichia coli* ATCC 25922, *Escherichia coli* ATCC 8739, *Proteus vulgaris* G, *Salmonella* sp., *Salmonella abony* NTCC 6017, *Staphylococcus aureus* ATCC 25093, *Staphylococcus aureus* ATCC 6538 P and *Listeria monocytogenes* at drying temperature (15-18 °C) for use in raw-dried meat products.

In addition to the studies related to the improvement of the safety of meat products with the use of probiotics, these bacteria have also been assessed for *in situ* production of nutraceutical compounds in meat products. Ammor and Mayo [14] describe studies related to high production of folate (vitamin B11) by a genetically modified *Lactobacillus plantarum*. Likewise, the production of conjugated linoleic acid (CLA), which has anticancer, antiobesity, antidiabetic, and antiatherogenic properties as well as stimulates the immune response, has been reported in some probiotic bacteria. Thus, the property of some probiotic bacteria to produce micronutrients and nutraceuticals compounds may allow *in situ* fortification of meat products, making them more nutritious and healthy.

The combined effect of the addition of probiotics and other active ingredients such as dietary fiber in meat products has also been studied. Sayas-Barberá et al. [59] reported that the addition of *Lactobacillus cas*ei CECT 475 to a traditional Spanish dry-cured sausage (*Longaniza de Pascua*) accelerates the curing process and that the incorporation of 1% orange fiber promotes the growth and survival of lactobacilli and micrococci, enhancing the microbial quality and safety of the sausages.

3. Conclusion

The fermented sausages fit perfectly in the current consumption trend due to their ease of preparation (ready to eat), ease of conservation, versatility of use (individually or as an garnish in cooking plates), nutritional appeal and variety of forms of presentation [60]. In this regard, probiotic fermented meat products might be the trend setters for development of innovative meat products.

Despite the selling of probiotic meat products occurs since 1998 in countries like Germany and Japan, further human-based studies are needed to establish documented proofs of the beneficial effect of these products, mainly with research on health promotion in humans [7]. Only after these studies will be possible to confirm the intrinsic value of fermented meat products and contribute to the recognition of such products as health foods.

Author details

Renata Ernlund Freitas de Macedo*
School of Agricultural Sciences and Veterinary Medicine, Pontifical Catholic University of Parana, Sao Jose dos Pinhais, Parana, Brazil

Sérgio Bertelli Pflanzer and Carolina Lugnani Gomes
Food Technology Department, Faculty of Food Engineer, State University of Campinas, Campinas, Sao Paulo, Brazil

4. References

[1] Työppönen S, Petäjä E, Mattila-Sandholm T. Bioprotectives and probiotics for dry sausages. International Journal of Food Microbiology 2003;83:233-244.

[2] Erkkilä S, Petäjä E, Eerola S, Lilleberg L, Mattila-Sandholm T, Suihko ML. Flavour profiles of dry sausages fermented by selected novel meat starter cultures. Meat Science 2001b;58:111-116.

[3] Khan MI, Arshad MS, Anjum FM, Sameen A, Aneeq-ur-Rehman, Gill WT. Meat as a functional food with special reference to probiotic sausages. Food Research International 2011;44(10):3125-3133.

[4] Santos FL, Ferreira CLLF, Costa NMB. Modulação da colesterolemia por meio de prebióticos e probióticos. In: Célia Lúcia de Luces Fortes Ferreira, editor. Prébióticos e Probióticos: Atualização e Prospecção. Viçosa, Rubio; 2003.

[5] Bejder HC. Probiotics: today dairy, tomorrow the world. Danish Dairy & Food Industry 2004;14:42-43.

[6] Leroy F, Verluyten J, Vuyst L. Functional meat starter cultures for improved sausage fermentation. International Journal of Food Microbiology 2006;106:270-285.

[7] Vuyst LD, Falony G, Leroy F. Probiotics in fermented sausages. Meat Science 2008;80:75-78.

[8] Lücke FK. Utilization of microbes to process and preserve meat. Meat Science 2000;56:105-115.

[9] Sameshima T, Magome C, Takeshita K, Arihara K, Itoh M, Kondo Y. Effect of intestinal *Lactobacillus* starter cultures on the behaviour of *Staphylococcus aureus* in fermented sausage. International Journal of Food Microbiology 1998;41:1-7.

[10] Andersen L. Fermented dry sausages produced with the admixture of probiotic cultures. In: Proceedings of the 44th International Commitment of Meat Science and Technology;1998; Barcelona, Spain. Barcelona: Institut de Recerca i Tecnologia Agroalimentaries, 1998. P. 826-827.

[11] Erkkilä S, Suihko ML, Eerola S, Petäjä E, Mattila-Sandholm T. Dry sausage fermented by *Lactobacillus rhamnosus* strains. International Journal of Food Microbiology 2001a;64:205-210.

*Corresponding Author

[12] Ferreira CLLF. Grupo de bactérias lácticas – Caracterização e aplicação tecnológica de bactérias probióticas. In: Célia Lúcia de Luces Fortes Ferreira, editor. Prébióticos e Probióticos: Atualização e Prospecção. Viçosa, Rubio; 2003.

[13] Campbell-Platt G. Fermented meats - a world perspective. In: Campbell-Platt G, Cook PE, editor. Fermented Meats. Glasgow: Chapman & Hall, 1995.

[14] Ammor M, Mayo B. Selection criteria for lactic acid bacteria to be used as functional starter cultures in dry sausage production: An update. Meat Science 2007;76(1):138-146.

[15] Hammes WP, Hertel C. New developments in meat starter cultures. Meat Science 1998;49:125-138.

[16] Ruiz-Moyano S, Martín A, Benito MJ, Nevado FP, Córdoba MG. Screening of lactic acid bacteria and bifidobacteria for potential probiotic use in iberian dry fermented sausage. Meat Science 2008;80:715-721.

[17] Rivera-Espinoza Y, Gallardo-Navarro Y. Non-dairy probiotic products. Food Microbiology, doi: 101016/ j.fm.2008.06.008, 2008.

[18] Maragkoudakis PA, Mountzouris KC, Psyrras D, Cremonese S, Fischer J, Cantor MD, Tsakalidou E. Functional properties of novel protective lactic acid bacteria and application in raw chicken meat against *Listeria monocytogenes* and *Salmonella enteritidis*. International Journal of Food Microbiology 2009;130:219-226.

[19] Silvi S, Oripianesi MC, Cresci A. Functional foods, gut microflora and healthy ageing. Isolation and identification of *Lactobacillus* and *Bifidobacterium* strains from faecal samples of elderly subjects for possible probiotic use in functional foods. Journal of Food Engineering 2003;56:195-200.

[20] Pennacchia C, Ercolini D, Blaiotta G, Pepe O, Mauriello G, Villani F. Selection of *Lactobacillus* strains from fermented sausages for their potential use as probiotics. Meat Science 2004;67:309-317.

[21] Klingberg TD, Axelsson L, Naterstad K, Elsser D, Budde BB. Identification of potential probiotic starter cultures for Scandinavian-type fermented sausage. International Journal of Food Microbiology 2005;105:419-431.

[22] Erkkilä S, Petäjä E. Screening of commercial meat starter cultures at low pH and in the presence of bile salts for potential probiotic use. Meat Science 2000;55:297-300.

[23] Papamanoli E, Tzanetakis N, Litopoulou-Tzanetaki E, Kotzekidou P. Characterization of lactic acid bacteria isolated from a Greek dry-fermented sausage in respect of their technological and probiotic properties. Meat Science 2003;65:859-867.

[24] Villani F, Mauriello G, Pepe O, Blaiotta G, Ercolini D, Casaburi A. Technological and probiotic characteristics of *Lactobacillus* and coagulase negative *Staphylococcus* strains as starter for fermented sausage manufacture. Italian Journal of Animal Science 2005;4:498.

[25] Rebucci R, Sangalli L, Fava M, Bersani C, Cantoni C, Baldi A. Evaluation of functional aspects in *Lactobacillus* strains isolated from dry fermented sausages. Journal of Food Quality 2007;30:187-201.

[26] Arihara K. Strategies for designing novel functional meat products. Meat Science 2006;74: 219–229.

[27] Arihara K, Ohata M. Functional meat products. In F. Toldra, editor. Handbook of meat processing (pp. Ames, Iowa: Wiley-Blackwell, 2010. P. 423-439.

[28] Toldrá F, Reig M. Innovations for healthier processed meats. Trends in Food Science & Technology 2011;22(9):517-522.

[29] Penna ALB. Probióticos & Saúde. In: Proceedings of the XVIII Congresso Brasileiro de Ciência e Tecnologia de Alimentos; 2002; Porto Alegre, Brazil. Porto Alegre: SBCTA, 2002. P. 4045-4046.

[30] Heenan CN, Adams MC, Hosken RW. Growth medium for culturing Probiotics bacteria for applications in vegetarian food products. Lebensmittel-Wissenschaft und-Technologie 2002;35:171-176.

[31] Tharmaraj N, Shah NP. Selective enumeration of *Lactobacillus delbrueckii ssp. Bulgaricus, Streptococcus thermophilus, Lactobacillus acidophilus, Bifidobacteria, Lactobacillus casei, Lactobacillus rhamnosus, and Propionibacteria*. Journal of Dairy Science 2003;86:2288-2296.

[32] Zhang W, Xiao S, Samaraweera H, Lee EJ, Ahn DU. Improving functional value of meat products. Meat Science 2010; 86(1):15-31.

[33] Arihara K, Ota H, Itoh M, Kondo Y, Sameshim T, Yamanaka H. *Lactobacillus acidophilus* group lactic acid bacteria applied to meat fermentation. Journal of Food Science1998;63:544-547.

[34] Macedo REF, Pflanzer SB, Terra NN, Freitas RJS. Desenvolvimento de embutido fermentado por *Lactobacillus* probióticos: características de qualidade. Ciência e Tecnologia de Alimentos 2008;28:509-519.

[35] Pidcock K, Heard GM, Henriksson A. Application of nontraditional meat starter cultures in production of Hungarian salami. International Journal of Food Microbiology 2002;76:75-81.

[36] Pan X, Chen F, Wu T, Tang H, Zhao Z. The acid, bile tolerance and antimicrobial property of *Lactobacillus acidophilus* NIT. Food Control 2009;20:598-602.

[37] FAO/WHO [Internet]. 2009 [updated 2001; cited 2009 May 25] Evaluation of health and nutritional properties of probiotics in food including powder milk with live lactic acid bacteria. Report of a joint FAO/WHO expert consultation, Córdoba, Argentina. 2001. Available from:
http://www.who.int/foodsafety/publications/fs_management/probiotics/en/index.html

[38] Muthukumarasamy P, Holley RA. Microbiological and sensory quality of dry fermented sausages containing alginate-microencapsulated *Lactobacillus reuteri*. International Journal of Food Microbiology 2006;111:164-169.

[39] Poulin JF, Caillard R, Subirade M. -Lactoglobulin tablets as a suitable vehicle for protection and intestinal delivery of probiotic bacteria. International Journal of Pharmaceutics 2011;405(1-2):47-54.

[40] Heidebach T, Först P, Kulozik U. Microencapsulation of probiotic cells by means of rennet-gelation of milk proteins. Food Hydrocolloids 2009;23(7):1670-1677.

[41] Heidebach T, Först P, Kulozik U. Influence of casein-based microencapsulation on freeze-drying and storage of probiotic cells. Journal of Food Engineering 2010;98(3):309-316.

[42] Caplice E, Fitzgerald GF. Food fermentations: role of microorganisms in food production and preservation. International Journal of Food Microbiology 1999;50:131-149.

[43] Arihara K, Itoh M. UV-induced *Lactobacillus gasseri* mutants resisting sodium choride and sodium nitrite for meat fermentation. International Journal of Food Microbiology 2000;56:227-230.

[44] Macedo REF, Pflanzer SB, Terra NN, Freitas RJS. Características de culturas lácticas probióticas para uso em produtos cárneos fermentados: sensibilidade aos sais de cura e uso de antibióticos para contagem seletiva. Boletim do CEPPA 2005;23(1):123-134.

[45] Annuk H, Shchepetova J, Kullisaar T, Songisepp E, Zilmer M, Mikelsaar M. Characterization of intestinal lactobacilli as putative probiotic candidates. Journal of Applied Microbiology 2003;94:403-412.

[46] Collado MC, Sanz Y. Method for direct selection of potencially probiotic *Bifidobacterium* strains from human feces based on their acid-adaptation ability. Journal of Microbiological Methods 2006;66:560-563.

[47] Charteris WP, Kelly PM, Morelli L, Collins JK. Effect of conjugated bile salts on antibiotic susceptibility of bile salt-tolerant *Lactobacillus* and *Bifidobacterium* isolates. Journal of Food Protection 2000;63(10):1369-1376.

[48] Taranto MP, Perez-Martinez G, Valdez GF. Effect of bile acid on the cell membrane functionality of lactic acid bacteria for oral administration. Research in Microbiology 2006;157:720-725.

[49] Haller D, Scherenbacher P, Bode C, Hammes WP. Selection of potentially probiotic bacteria. Zeitschrift fuer Ernaehrungswissenschaft 1997;36(1):87.

[50] Gänzle MG, Hertel C, van der Vossen JMBM, Hammes WP. Effect of bacteriocin-producing lactobacilli on the survival of *Escherichia coli* and *Listeria* in a dynamic model of the stomach and the small intestine. International Journal of Food Microbiology 1999;48:21-35.

[51] Ergönül B, Kundakçı A. Microbiological attributes and biogenic amine content of probiotic Turkish fermented sausage. Journal für Verbraucherschutz und Lebensmittelsicherheit 2011;6(1):49-56.

[52] Jahreis G, Vogelsang H, Kiessling G, Schubert R, Bunte C, Hammes WP. Influence of probiotic sausage (*Lactobacillus paracasei*) on blood lipids and immunological parameters of health volunteers. Food Research International 2002;35:133-138.

[53] Alkhalf A, Alhaj M, Al-Homidan I. Influence of probiotic supplementation on immune response of broiler chicks. Egypt Poultry Science 2010;30(1):271-280.

[54] Mao Y, Nobaek S, Kasravi B, Adawi D, Stenram U, Molin G, Jeppsson B. The effects of *Lactobacillus* strains and oat fiber on methotrexate-induced enterocolitis in rats. Gastroenterology 1996;111(2):334-44.

[55] Pennacchia C, Vaughan EE, Villani F. Potential probiotic *Lactobacillus* strains from fermented sausages: Further investigations on their probiotic properties. Meat Science 2006;73(1):90-101.

[56] Mahoney M, Henriksson A. The effect of processed meat and meat starter cultures on gastrointestinal colonization and virulence of *Listeria monocytogenes* in mice. International Journal of Food Microbiology 2003;84:255-261.

[57] Yuksekdag ZN, Aslim B. Assessment of potential probiotic- and starter properties of *Pediococcus* spp. Isolated from Turkish-type fermented sausages (sucuk). Journal of Microbiology and Biotechnology 2010;20(1):161-168.

[58] Nedelcheva P, Denkova Z, Denev P, Slavchev A, Krastanov A. Probiotic strain *Lactobacillus plantarum* NBIMCC 2415 with antioxidant activity as a starter culture in the production of dried fermented meat products. Biotechnology and Biotechnological Equipment 2012;24(1):1624-1630.

[59] Sayas-Barberá E, Viuda-Martos M, Fernández-López F, Pérez-Alvarez JA, Sendra-Nadal E. Combined use of a probiotic culture and citrus fiber in a traditional sausage *'Longaniza de pascua'*. Food Control 2012; doi 10.1016/j.foodcont.2012.04.009.

[60] Monfort JM. Los productos carnicos crudos curados. In: Proceedings of the XVIII Congresso Brasileiro de Ciência e Tecnologia de Alimentos; 2002; Porto Alegre, Brazil. Porto Alegre: SBCTA, 2002. P. 3984-3992.

Chapter 2

Use of Probiotics in Aquaculture

Rafael Vieira de Azevedo and Luís Gustavo Tavares Braga

Additional information is available at the end of the chapter

1. Introduction

The term probiotics was first used by Lilly & Stillwell in 1965. Probiotic was defined as the microbiological origin factor that stimulates the growth of other organisms. In 1989 Roy Fuller introduced the idea that probiotics generate a beneficial effect to the host. He defined probiotics as live microorganisms which, when administered in adequate amounts, confer benefit to the host's health, improving the balance of the microbiota in the intestine.

Probiotics are defined by Food and Agriculture Organization/World Health Organization as "live microorganisms which when administered in adequate amounts confer a health benefit on the host" [1].

The purpose of its use is to install, improve or compensate for the functions of the indigenous microbiota that inhabit the digestive tract or the surface of the body.

The idea of using fermented foods for some health benefits is not new, being mentioned in the Persian version of the Old Testament (Genesis 18:8) that "Abraham attributed his longevity to the consumption of sour milk". Later, in 76 BC, a Roman historian, Pline, recommended the use of fermented milk products for the treatment of gastroenteritis cases [2].

However, a scientific approach, recognizing the beneficial role of certain microorganisms was applied only in the first decades of the 20th century, with the suggestion of using *Lactobacillus* (in 1907 Elie Metchnikoff attributed the longevity of Bulgarian populations to yoghurt consumption); *Bifidobacterium* (in 1906 Henri Tissier observed a greater presence of *Bifidobacteria* in the feces of breastfed healthy children); and *Saccharomyces boulardii* (Henri Boulard emphasized the use of a tropical fruit colonized by this yeast to treat diarrhea of local populations in the East during an episode of cholera in 1920) [3].

Several clinical studies have shown the benefits of probiotics to human health. For example, diarrhea treatment [4]; lactose intolerance [5]; irritable bowel syndrome [6]; allergies [7]; cancer [8]; among others.

The use of growth promoters allows improving the zootechnical performance of animals. Initially a large variety of substances with antibiotic function was used to improve performance of poultry, pigs and cattle, especially penicillin and tetracycline.

The use of antibiotics as additives to feeds showed great benefits to animal husbandry, expressed primarily in improved weight gain and feed conversion.

Antibiotics were used for decades, but are being banished from the zootechnical activity, mainly due to the risks posed by antibiotic-resistant bacteria, which can result in problems for animal and human health.

Accordingly, probiotics have deserved attention from researchers seeking alternatives to the use of traditional growth promoters in the field of animal nutrition.

Probiotics have also received special attention from researchers seeking animal nutrition alternatives to the use of traditional growth promoters (antibiotics). Therefore, the use of probiotics is being increasingly seen as an alternative to the use of antibiotics in animal production.

Many scientific papers show the beneficial effects of supplementation with probiotic strains in diets for poultry, pigs, cattle, fish, crustaceans, mollusks and amphibians [9-13].

Probiotics have been incorporated through diet in order to maintain the balance of the intestinal flora of animals, preventing digestive tract diseases, improving the digestibility of feed, leading to increased use of nutrients and causing better zootechnical performance of animals [14, 15].

2. Probiotic organisms

The requirements that a probiotic organism must meet are [16]:

i.   Resistance to the acid stomach environment, bile and pancreatic enzymes;
ii.   Accession to the cells of the intestinal mucosa;
iii. Capacity for colonization;
iv.   Staying alive for a long period of time, during the transport, storage, so that they can colonize the host efficiently;
v.   Production of antimicrobial substances against the pathogenic bacteria; and
vi.   Absence of translocation.

The species normally used as probiotics in animal nutrition are usually non-pathogenic normal microflora, such as lactic-acid bacteria (*Bifidobacterium, Lactobacillus, Lactococcus, Streptococcus* and *Enterococcus*) and yeasts as *Saccharomyces* spp. (Table 1).

3. Mechanisms of action

The mechanisms of action of bacteria used as probiotics, although not yet fully elucidated, are described as [14, 15, 18]:

a. Competition for binding sites: also known as "competitive exclusion", where probiotics bacteria bind with the binding sites in the intestinal mucosa, forming a physical barrier, preventing the connection by pathogenic bacteria;
b. Production of antibacterial substances: probiotic bacteria synthesize compounds like hydrogen peroxide and bacteriocins, which have antibacterial action, mainly in relation to pathogenic bacteria. They also produce organic acids that lower the environment's pH of the gastrointestinal tract, preventing the growth of various pathogens and development of certain species of *Lactobacillus*;
c. Competition for nutrients: the lack of nutrients available that may be used by pathogenic bacteria is a limiting factor for their maintenance;
d. Stimulation of immune system: some probiotics bacteria are directly linked to the stimulation of the immune response, by increasing the production of antibodies, activation of macrophages, T-cell proliferation and production of interferon.

Aspergillus	*A. niger, A. orizae*
Bacillus	*B. coagulans, B. lentus, B. licheniformis, B. subtilis*
Bifidobacterium	*B. animalis, B. bifidum, B. longun, B. thermophylum*
Lactobacillus	*L. acidophillus, L. brevis, L. bulgaricus, L. casei, L. cellobiosis, L. fermentarum, L. curvatus, L. lactis, L. plantarum, L. reuterii, L. delbruekii,*
Pediococcus	*P. acidilacticii, P. cerevisae, P. pentosaceus, P. damnosus*
Saccharomyces	*S. cerevisiae, S. boulardii*
Streptococcus	*S. cremoris, S. faecium, S. lactis, S. intermedius, S. thermophyllus, S. diacetylatis*

Table 1. Microorganisms recognized as safe and used as probiotics in animals. Source: [17]

The mechanism of action of yeasts still needs substantiation by means of research. A likely mechanism of action of yeasts is related to total inhibition (*in vitro*) or partial inhibition of pathogens. Inactive yeasts contain large quantities of protein and polysaccharides in its walls, which can act positively in the immune system and in the absorption of nutrients. In addition, yeasts produce nutritious metabolites in digestive tract that boost animal performance, besides possessing minerals (Mn, Co, Zn) and vitamins (A, B_{12}, D_3) that enhance the action of beneficial microorganisms [19].

Although some mechanisms had been suggested on the action of probiotics, they are not completely clarified, but it is known that they inhibit growth of pathogenic microorganism by producing antimicrobial compounds; they compete with pathogens for adhesion sites and nutrients; and they model immune system of the host [20].

4. Selection of probiotics

Briefly, for the use of a given microorganism as probiotic, it is necessary its isolation, characterization and testing certifying its probiotic efficiency (Figure 1).

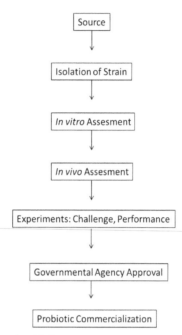

Figure 1. Diagram for selection of probiotics

First a source of microorganisms (e.g. digestive tract of healthy animals) must be selected.

After, the microorganisms with which the work is to be carried out are isolated and identified by means of selective culture.

Then a new culture with only the colonies of interest for conducting *in vitro* evaluations (inhibition of pathogens; pathogenicity to target species; resistance conditions of host; among others) is performed.

In case of the absence of restrictions on the use of the target species, experiments with *in vivo* supplementation, and small and large scale, are carried out to check if there are real benefits to the host.

Finally, the probiotic that presented significantly satisfactory result can be produced commercially and utilized.

5. Use of probiotic in aquaculture

Probiotics in aquaculture may act in a manner similar to that observed for terrestrial animals.

However, the relationship of aquatic organisms with the farming environment is much more complex than the one involving terrestrial animals.

Because of this intimate relationship between animal and farming environment, the traditional definition of probiotics is insufficient for aquaculture.

In this sense, Verschuere and colleagues [21] suggest a broader definition:

"It is a microbial supplement with living microorganism with beneficial effects to the host, by modifying its microbial community associated with the host or its farming environment, ensuring better use of artificial food and its nutritional value by improving the host's response to diseases and improving the quality of the farming environment."

The microorganisms present in the aquatic environment are in direct contact with the animals, with the gills and with the food supplied, having easy access to the digestive tract of the animal.

Among the microorganisms present in the aquatic environment are potentially pathogenic microorganisms, which are opportunists, i.e., they take advantage of some animal's stress situation (high density, poor nutrition) to cause infections, worsening in zootechnical performance and even death.

For this reason, the use of probiotics for aquatic organisms aims not only the direct benefit to the animal, but also their effect on the farming environment.

Bergh and colleagues [22] observed that, when starting its first feeding, the intestinal flora of the Atlantic halibut (*Hippoglossus hippoglossus*) changed from a prevalence of *Flavobacterium* spp. to *Aeromonas* spp./*Vibrio* spp. showing the influence of the external environment and food on the microbial community of this fish.

Vibrio spp., *Plesiomonas shigelloides*, and *Aeromonas* spp. are the main causative agents of diseases in aquaculture, and may even cause food infections in humans.

The interaction between the environment and the host in an aquatic environment is complex. The microorganisms present in the water influence the microbiota of the host's intestine and vice versa.

Makridis and colleagues [23] demonstrated that the provision of two strains of bacteria via food directly into the farming water of the incubators of turbot larvae (*Scophthalmus maximus*) promoted the maintenance of the bacteria in the environment, as well as the colonization of the digestive tract of the larvae.

Changes in salinity, temperature and dissolved oxygen variations, change the conditions that are favorable to different organisms, with consequent changes in dominant species, which could lead to the loss of effectiveness of the product.

Accordingly, the addition of a given probiotic in the farming water of aquatic organisms must be constant, because the conditions of environment suffer periodic changes.

Thus, the variety of microorganisms present must therefore be considered in the choice of probiotic to be used in aquaculture.

Intensive farming systems utilize high stocking densities, among other stressors (e.g. management), which often end up resulting in low growth and feed efficiency rates, besides of weakness in the immune system, making these animals susceptible to the presence of opportunistic pathogens present in the environment.

In this sense, the effect of probiotics on the immune system has led to a large number of researches with beneficial results on the health of aquatic organisms, although it has not yet been clarified how they act.

In addition, probiotics can also be used to promote the growth of aquatic organisms, whether by direct aid in the absorption of nutrients, or by their supply.

Probiotics most used in aquaculture are those belonging to the genus *Bacillus* spp. (*B. subtilis*, *B. licheniformis* and *B. circulans*), *Bifidobacterium* spp. (*B. bifidum*, *B. lactis, and B. thermophilum*), lactic-acid bacteria (*Lactobacillus* spp. e *Carnobacterium* spp.) and yeast *Saccharomyces cerevisiae* [24,25].

The benefits observed in the supplementation of probiotics in aquaculture include [21, 26-28]:

1.   Improvement of the nutritional value of food;
2.   Enzymatic contribution to digestion;
3.   Inhibition of pathogens;
4.   Growth promoting factors;
5.   Improvement in immune response; and
6.   Farming water quality.

Among the most recent studies that point to the effect of the use of probiotics for various aquatic organisms stand those for fish [21], shrimps [26], mollusks [30] and frogs [29].

5.1. Results of probiotics in fish farming

5.1.1. Immune system

Gatesoupe [31] observed that turbot larvae (*Scophthalmus maximus*) fed rotifera enriched with lactic-acid bacteria increased resistance against infection by *Vibrio* spp.

The joint administration of *Lactobacillus fructivorans* and *Lactobacillus plantarum* through dry or live feed promoted the colonization of the intestine of sea bream larvae (*Sparus aurata*) and the decrease in mortality of animals during larviculture and nursery [32].

Gram and colleagues [33] showed that the use of *Pseudomonas fluorescens* AH2 as probiotics decreased the mortality of juveniles of rainbow trout (*Oncorhynchus mykiss*) exposed to *Vibrio anguillarum*.

Kumar and colleagues [34] observed higher survival rate of carp *Labeo rohita* fed *Bacillus subtilis*, submitted to intraperitoneal injection with *Aeromonas hydrophila*.

Oral administration of *Clostridium butyricum* increased phagocytic activity of leucocytes of rainbow trout [35].

Nikoskelainen and colleagues [36] observed that the administration of *Lactobacillus rhamnosus* at 105 UFC g^{-1}, stimulated the respiratory burst in rainbow trout.

Other studies showed an increase in immune response with the use of probiotics for different species, such *Carnobacterium maltaromaticum* B26 and *Carnobacterium divergens* B33 for rainbow trout [38], *Lactobacillus belbrüeckii*, *Bacillus subtilis* and *Debaryomyces hansenii* for gilthead seabream [39-41], *B. subtilis* and *Pseudomonas aeruginosa* for *Labeo rohita* [42,43], *Lactococcus lactis* for Nile tilapia (*Oreochromis niloticus*) [44] and *B. simplex* DR-834 to carp (*Cyprinus carpio*) [45].

5.1.2. Performance

Tovar and colleagues [37] incorporated the yeast *Debaryomyces hansenii* to the feed of sea bass larvae and observed improvement in the maturation of the digestive tract of this species. According to the authors this satisfactory effect was due to the high secretion rate of spermine and spermidine by yeasts.

Increase of weight gain and survival was observed for turbot larvae fed rotifera enriched with acid-lactic bacteria [31].

Queiroz and Boyd [46] observed enhancement of the zootechnical performance and survival of channel catfish (*Ictalurus punctatus*) when a mixture of *Bacillus* spp. was added to the farming water.

Using yeast *Saccharomyces cerevisiae* as probiotic for Israeli carp, Noh and colleagues [47] observed an increase in the food efficiency of this species.

Lara-Flores and colleagues [48] concluded that the use of *Saccharomyces cerevisiae* as probiotic for fry of Nile tilapia resulted in better growth and food efficiency, suggesting that this yeast promotes adequate growth in tilapia farming. In this study it was observed that fish fed control diet showed reduced survival and digestibility of feed with increased storage density, considered a stressful factor for growing fish. This result highlighted the efficiency of the use of this probiotic in stressful situations.

Other positive results of the probiotic on the performance of fish are found for *Labeo rohita* fingerlings [49], Nile tilapia [50] and common carp [51].

5.2. Results of the use of probiotics in shrimp farming

5.2.1. Immune system

In relation to farmed shrimp, bacterial diseases are considered as the largest cause of mortality in larvae.

The administration of a mixture of bacteria (*Bacillus* spp. and *Vibrio* spp.) positively influenced on survival and had protective effect against *Vibrio harveyi* and the white spot syndrome virus (WSSV) [15]. This result was due to stimulation of the immune system, by increasing phagocytosis and antibacterial activity.

The administration of a commercial probiotic for the larvae of *Marsupenaeus japonicus* resulted in increased survival (97%) being significantly higher than the control treatment [52].

Thus, the use of *Bacillus coagulans* SC8168 as probiotic for postlarvae of *Litopenaeus vannamei* resulted in higher survival of animals [53].

In a study with tiger shrimp (*Penaeus monodon*), the inoculation of *Bacillus* S11, a saprophyte strain, resulted in higher survival of postlarvae challenged by a luminescent pathogenic bacterial culture [54].

Bacillus subtilis and *Lactobacillus plantarum* for *Litopenaeus vannamei* [55-58], *Pediococcus acidilactici* to *Litopenaeus stylirostris* [59] and *Bacillus* NL110 and *Vibrio* NE17 for *Macrobrachium rosenberguii* [60] also proved effective in improving the immune system of these animals.

5.2.2. Performance

Lin and colleagues [61] used *Bacillus* spp. in the diet of *Litopenaeus vannamei* enhancing digestibility rates of the feed.

Ziaei-Nejad and colleagues [26] added the probiotic *Bacillus* spp. in the farming of *Fenneropenaeus indicus* larvae and observed survival increase, and also an increase in the activities of lipase, protease and amylase enzymes in the digestive tract of shrimps.

Several studies have shown that the bacteria of the genus *Bacillus* spp. secrete exoenzymes (proteases, lipases and carbohydrases) that can help improve digestion and nutrient absorption increase, resulting in better use of food and animal growth [62].

5.3. Results from the use of probiotics in the farming of others aquatic organisms

5.3.1. Mollusks

The culture of oysters and scallops has been introduced in many countries, however, mass mortalities of larvae have frequently occurred and to prevent these mortalities, most farmers use antibiotics [63]. Thus, the use of probiotic bacteria has been fueled, especially during the hatchery [64].

Riquelme and colleagues [65] identified a bacteria (*Alteromonas haloplanktis*) capable of reducing the mortality of Chilean scallop larvae (*Argopecten purpuratus*) when exposed to 10^3 colony forming units per milliliter (UFC ml^{-1}) of *Vibrio anguillarum*.

Cultures of *Alteromonas media* control *Vibrio tubiashii* infections in larvae of Pacific oysters (*Crassostrea gigas*) [66].

Other bacteria with probiotic potential for mollusks such as Pacific oysters (*Alteromonas* spp.) [67, 68], Scallop larvae (*Roseobacter* spp., *Vibrio* spp., *Pseudomonas* spp., *Arthrobacter* spp.) [69-71], promoted growth, survival and immune response of animals.

5.3.2. Frogs

For Bull Frog (*Lithobates catesbeianus*) with an average weight of 3.13 g, the addition of probiotic *Bacillus subtilis* in different doses (2.5, 5.0 and 10 g kg^{-1} feed) resulted in improved weight gain, feed conversion and apparent survival, when compared to control treatment (without added probiotic); however, the immunostimulant effect was demonstrated through the increased phagocytic capacity of animals [72].

Likewise, Dias and colleagues [29] observed the beneficial effect of two commercial probiotics on the immune system of *L. catesbeianus*.

5.4. Probiotics and quality of water in aquaculture

Another aspect of the use of probiotics in aquaculture is the improvement of the quality of the water in the farming nurseries. Increases in organic load, levels of phosphorous and nitrogen compounds are growing concerns in aquaculture.

Boyd [73] noted the beneficial effect of probiotics on organic matter decomposition and reduction of the levels of phosphate and nitrogen compounds.

Aerobic denitrifying bacteria are considered good candidates to reduce nitrate or nitrite to N_2 in aquaculture waters.

To this end some bacteria were isolated in shrimp farming tanks. *Acinetobacter*, *Arthrobacter*, *Bacillus*, *Cellulosimicrobium*, *Halomonas*, *Microbacterium*, *Paracoccus*, *Pseudomonas*, *Sphingobacterium* and *Stenotrophomas* are some of the denitrifying bacteria already identified [28].

Reduction in levels of phosphorous and nitrogen compounds in the farming water of shrimp *Litopenaeus vannamei* was also observed when commercial probiotics were added to the water [27].

Similarly, for the shrimp *Penaeus monodon*, an improvement in the quality of farming water was observed with the addition of *Bacillus* spp. as probiotic [74].

Gram-positive bacteria are better converting organic matter into CO_2 than gram-negative bacteria. Thus, during a production cycle, higher levels of these bacteria can reduce the accumulation of particulate organic carbon. Thus, maintaining higher levels of these gram-positive bacteria in production pond, farmers can minimize the buildup of dissolved and particulate organic carbon during the culture cycle while promoting more stable phytoplankton blooms through the increased production of CO_2 [21].

6. Conclusion

The results reported so far with the use of probiotics for aquatic organisms are promising. However, many works have not achieved satisfactory results.

Sometimes in experiments in which aquatic organisms are challenged by some pathogenic agent, the probiotic organism does not exhibit inhibiting action against the pathogen, resulting in mortality.

Similarly, the conditions to which the animals are subjected during farming may directly influence the effectiveness of probiotics. Thus, when not subjected to stressful situations, the results often do not show a significant effect of probiotics on the performance of animals.

In general, the effects of adding probiotics tend to be most striking in unsuitable operating conditions or in conditions of stress, when the microflora is unbalanced, primarily in young animals.

Among these factors, the most commonly featured are: temperature above or below the thermal comfort zone; presence of pathogens; poor sanitary conditions; stressful management; change in nutrition; transport; high storage density; after treatment with antibiotics; sudden change of environment.

Also, the results obtained in experiments with probiotics may be affected by factors such as: type of probiotic microorganism; method and quantity administered; condition of the host; condition of intestinal microbiota; age of the animal.

Author details

Rafael Vieira de Azevedo
State University of Norte Fluminense Darcy Ribeiro,
Center for Agricultural Science and Technology, Campos dos Goytacazes, Rio de Janeiro, Brazil

Luís Gustavo Tavares Braga*
State University of Santa Cruz, Department of Agricultural and Environmental Sciences, Ilhéus, Bahia, Brazil

7. References

[1] WHO/FAO. Joint World Health Organization/Food and Agricultural Organization Working Group. Guidelines for the Evaluation of Probiotics in Food 2002. Ontario, Canada.

---

* Corresponding Author

[2] Schrezenmeir J, de Vrese M. Probiotics, prebiotics, and symbiotic – approaching a definition. The American Journal of Clinical Nutrition 2001; 73(2) 361S-364S.

[3] Shortt C. The probiotic century: historical and current perspectives. Trends in Food Science & Technology 1999; 10(12) 411-417.

[4] DeVrese M, Marteau PR. Probiotics and Prebiotics: Effects on diarrhea. The Journal of Nutrition 2007; 137(3) 803S-811S.

[5] He T, Priebe MG, Zhong Y, Huang C, Harmsen HJ, Raangs GC, Antoine JM, Wellingand GW, Vonk RJ. Effects of yogurt and bifidobacteria supplementation on the colonic microbiota in lactose-intolerant subjects. Journal of Applied Microbiology 2008; 104(2) 595-604.

[6] Nagala R, Routray C. Clinical case study multispecies probiotic supplement minimizes symptoms of irritable Bowel Syndrome. US Gastroenterology & Hepatology Review 2011; 7(1) 36-37.

[7] Jain S, Yadav H, Sinha PR, Kapila S, Naito Y, Marotta F. Anti-allergic effects of probiotic Dahi through modulation of the gut immune system. Turkish Journal of Gastroenterology 2010; 21(3) 244-250.

[8] Chen X, Fruehauf J, Goldsmith J, Xu H, Katchar K, Koon H, Zhao D, Kokkotou E, Pothoulakis C, Kelly C. *Saccharomyces boulardii* inhibits EGF receptor signaling and intestinal tumor growth in Apc(min) mice. Gastroenterology 2009; 137(3) 914-923.

[9] Aly SM, Abd-El-Rahman AM, John G, Mohamed MF. Characterization of some bacteria isolated from *Oreochromis niloticus* and their potential use as probiotics. Aquaculture 2008; 277(1-2) 1-6.

[10] Ignatova M, Sredkova V, Marasheva V. Effect of dietary inclusion of probiotic on chickens performance and some blood. Biotechnology in Animal Husbandry 2009; 25(5-6) 1079-1085.

[11] Soleimani NA, Kermanshahi RK, Yakhchali B, Sattari TN. Antagonistic activity of probiotic lactobacilli against *Staphylococcus aureus* isolated from bovine mastitis. African Journal of Microbiology Research 2010; 4(20) 2169-2173.

[12] Veizaj-Delia E, Piub T, Lekajc P, Tafaj M. Using combined probiotic to improve growth performance of weaned piglets on extensive farm conditions. Livestock Science 2010; 134(1) 249-251.

[13] Gatesoupe FJ. The use of probiotics in aquaculture. Aquaculture 1999; 180(1) 147-165.

[14] Fuller R. Problems and prospects. In: Fuller R. (ed.) Probiotics – The scientific basis. London: Chapman & Hall; 1992. p377-386.

[15] Balcázar JL, Blas I, Zarzuela-Ruiz I, Cunningham D, Vendrell D, Músquiz JL. The role of probiotics in aquaculture. Veterinary Microbiology 2006; 114(1) 173-186.

[16] Capriles VD, Silva KEA, Fisberg M. Prebióticos, probióticos e simbióticos: Nova tendência no mercado de alimentos funcionais. Revista Nutrição Brasil 2005; 4(6) 327-335.

[17] Lyons P. Yeast: out of the black box. Feed Manangement 1986; 37(10) 8-14.

[18] Jin LZ, Ho YW, Abdullah N, Jalaludin S. Probiotics in poultry: modes of action. World's Poultry Science Journal 1997; 53(4) 351-368.

[19] Hill J, Tracey SV, Willis M, Jones L, Ellis AD. Yeast culture in equine nutrition and physiology. In: Proceedings of Alltech's Annual Symposium 2006. Available from: http://eNo.engormix.com/MA-equines/nutrition/articles/yeast-culture-equine-nutrition-t279/p0.htm (acessed 31 April 2012).

[20] Oelschlaeget T. Mechanisms of probiotic actions – A review. International Journal of Medical Microbiology 2010; 300(1) 57-62.

[21] Verschuere L, Rombaut G, Sorgeloos P, Verstraete W. Probiotic bacteria as biological control agents in aquaculture. Microbiology and Molecular Biology Review 2000; 64(4) 655-671.

[22] Bergh Ø, Hansen GH, Taxt RE. Experimental infection of eggs and yolk sac larvae of halibut, *Hippoglossus hippoglossus* L. Journal of Fish Diseases 1992; 15(5) 379-391.

[23] Makridis P, Fjellheim AJ, Skjermo J, Vadstein O. Colonization of the gut in first feeding turbot by bacterial strains added to the water or biencapusated in rotifers. Aquaculture International 2000; 8(5) 367-380.

[24] Lee YK, Nomoto K, Salminen S, Gorbash SL. Handbook of probiotics. New York: Wiley; 1999.

[25] Sanders ME, Klaenhammer TR. Invited review: the scientific basis of *Lactobacillus acidophilus* NCFM functionality as a probiotic. Journal of Dairy Science 2001; 84(2) 319-331.

[26] Ziaei-Nejad S, Rezaei M, Takami G, Lovett D, Mirvaghefi A, Shakouri M. The effect of *Bacillus* spp. bacteria used as probiotics on digestive enzyme activity, survival and growth in the Indian white shrimp *Fenneropenaeus indicus*. Aquaculture 2006; 252(2-4) 516-524.

[27] Wang Y, Xu Z, Xia M. The effectiveness of commercial probiotics in Northern White Shrimp *Penaeus vannamei* ponds. Fisheries Science 2005; 71(5) 1034-1039.

[28] Wang A, Zheng G, Liao S, Huang H, Sun R. Diversity analysis of bacteria capable of removing nitrate/nitrite in a shrimp pond. Acta Ecologica Sinica 2007; 27(5) 1937-1943.

[29] Dias DC, De Stéfani, MV, Ferreira CM, França FM, Ranzani-Paiva MJT, Santos AA. Hematologic and immunologic parameters of bullfrogs, *Lithobates catesbeianus*, fed probiotics. Aquaculture Research 2010; 41(7) 1064-1071.

[30] Macey BM, Coyne VE. Improved growth rate and disease resistance in farmed *Haliotis midae* through probiotic treatment. Aquaculture 2005; 245(1-4) 249-261.

[31] Gatesoupe FJ. Lactic acid bacteria increase the resistance of turbot larvae, *Scophthalmus maximus*, against pathogenic Vibrio. Aquatic Living Resource 1994; 7(1) 277-282.

[32] Carnevali O, Zamponi MC, Sulpizio R, Rollo A, Nardi M, Orpianesi C, Silvi S, Caggiano M, Polzonetti AM, Cresci A. Administration of probiotic strain to improve

sea bream wellness during development. Aquaculture International 2004; 12(4-5) 377-386.

[33] Gram L, Melchiorsen J, Spanggard B, Huber I, Nielsen T. Inhibition of *Vibrio anguillarum* by *Pseudomonas fluorescens* AH2, a possible probiotic treatment of fish. Applied and Environmental Microbiology 1999; 65(3) 969-973.

[34] Kumar R, Mukherjee SC, Prasad KP, Pal AK. Evaluation of *Bacillus subtilis* as a probiotic to indian major carp *Labeo rohita* (Ham.). Aquaculture Research 2006; 37(12) 1215-1221.

[35] Sakai M, Yoshida T, Astuta S, Kobayashi M. Enhancement of resistance to vibriosis in rainbow trout, *Oncorhynchus mykiss* (Walbaum) by oral administration of *Clostridium butyricum* bacterin. Journal of Fish Disease 1995; 18(2) 187-190.

[36] Nikoskelainen S, Ouwehand AC, Bylund G, Salminen S, Lilius EM. Immune enhancement in rainbow trout (*Oncorhynchus mykiss*) by potential probiotic bacteria (*Lactobacillus rhamnosus*). Fish & Shellfish Immunology 2003; 15(5) 443–452.

[37] Tovar D, Zambonino J, Cahu C, Gatesoupe FJ, Vázquez-Juárez R, Lésel R. Effect of live yeast incorporation in compound diet on digestive enzyme activity in sea bass (*Dicentrarchus labrax*) larvae. Aquaculture 2002; 204(1-2) 113-123.

[38] Kim D, Austin B. Innate immune responses in rainbow trout (*Oncorhynchus mykiss*, Walbaum) induced by probiotics. Fish & Shellfish Immunology 2006; 21(5) 513-524.

[39] Salinas I, Cuesta A, Esteban MA, Meseguer J. Dietary administration of *Lactobacillus delbrüeckii* and *Bacillus subtilis*, single or combined, on gilthead seabream cellular innate immune responses. Fish & Shellfish Immunology 2005; 19(1) 67-77.

[40] Reyes-Becerril M, Salinas I, Cuesta A, Meseguer J, Tovar-Ramirez D, Ascencio-Valle F, Esteban MA. Oral delivery of live yeast *Debaryomyces hansenii* modulates the main innate immune parameters and expression of immune-relevant genes in the gilthead seabream (*Sparus aurata* L.). Fish & Shellfish Immunology 2008; 25(6) 731-739.

[41] Salinas I, Abelli L, Bertoni F, Picchietti S, Roque A, Furones D, Cuesta A, Meseguer J, Esteban MA. Monospecies and multispecies probiotic formulations produce different systemic and local immunostimulatory effects in the gilthead seabream (*Sparus aurata* L.). Fish & Shellfish Immunology 2008; 25(1-2) 114-123.

[42] Nayak SK, Swain P, Mukhrjee SC. Effect of dietary supplementation of probiotic and vitamin C on the immune response of Indian major carp, *Labeo rohita* (Ham.). Fish & Shellfish Immunology 2007; 23(4) 892-896.

[43] Giri SS, Sen SS, Sukumaran V. Effects of dietary supplementation of potential probiotic *Pseudomonas aeruginosa* VSG-2 on the innate immunity and disease resistance of tropical freshwater fish, *Labeo rohita*. Fish & Shellfish Immunology 2012; 32(6) 1135-1140.

[44] Zhou X, Wang Y, Yao J, Li W. Inhibition ability of probiotic *Lactococcus lactis*, against *A. hydrophila* and study of its immunostimulatory effect in tilapia (*Oreochromis*

niloticus). International Journal of Engineering, Science and Technology 2010; 2(7) 73-80.

[45] Wang G, Liu Y, Li F, Gao H, Lei Y, Liu X. Immunostimulatory activities of *Bacillus simplex* DR-834 to carp (*Cyprinus carpio*). Fish & Shellfish Immunology 2010; 29(3) 378-387.

[46] Queiroz F, Boyd C. Effects of a bacterial inoculum in channel catfish ponds. Journal of the World Aquaculture Society 1998; 29(1) 67-73.

[47] Noh SH, Han K, Won TH, Choi YJ. Effect of antibiotics, enzyme, yeast culture and probiotics on the growth performance of Israeli carp. Korean Journal of Animal Science 1994; 36(1) 480-486.

[48] Lara-Flores M, Olvea-Novoa MA, Guzman-Mendez BE, López-Madrid W. Use of the bacteria *Streptococcus faecium* and *Lactobacillus acidophilus*, and the yeast *Saccharomyces cerevisiae* as growth promoters in Nile tilapia (*Oreochromis niloticus*). Aquaculture 2003; 216(1-4) 193-201.

[49] Ghosh K, Sen SK, Ray AK. Supplementation of *Lactobacillus acidophilus* in compound diets for *Labeo rohita* fingerlings. Indian Journal of Fisheries 2004; 51(4) 521-526.

[50] El-Haroun ER, Goda AMAS, Chowdhury MAK. Effect of dietary Biogen® supplementation as a growth promoter on growth performance and feed utilization of Nile tilapia *Oreochromis niloticus* (L.). Aquaculture Research 2006; 37(14) 1473-1480.

[51] Faramarzi M, Kiaalvandi S, Iranshahi F. The effect of probiotics on growth performance and body composition of common carp (*Cyprinus carpio*). Journal of Animal and Veterinary Advances 2011; 10(18) 2408-2413.

[52] El-Sersy NA, Abdel-Razek FA, Taha SM. Evaluation of various probiotic bacteria for the survival of *Penaeus japonicus* larvae. Fresenius Environmental Bulletin 2006; 15(12A) 1506-1511.

[53] Zhou X, Wang Y, Li W. Effect of probiotic on larvae shrimp (*Penaeus vannamei*) based on water quality, survival rate and digestive enzyme activities. Aquaculture 2009; 287(3-4) 349-353.

[54] Rengpipat ST, Phianphak W, Piyatiratitivorakul S, Menasaveta P. Effects of a probiotic bacterium in black tiger shrimp *Penaeus monodon* survival and growth. Aquaculture 1998; 167(3-4) 301-313.

[55] Tseng D, Ho P, Huang S, Cheng S, Shiu Y, Chiu C, Liu C. Enhancement of immunity and disease resistance in the white shrimp, *Litopenaeus vannamei*, by the probiotic, *Bacillus subtilis* E20. Fish & Shellfish Immunology 2009; 26(2) 339-344.

[56] Liu K, Chiu C, Shiu Y, Cheng W, Liu C. Effects of the probiotic, *Bacillus subtilis* E20, on the survival, development, stress tolerance, and immune status of white shrimp *Litopenaeus vannamei* larvae. Fish & Shellfish Immunology 2010; 28(5-6) 837-844.

[57] Silva EF, Soares MA, Calazans NF, Vogeley JL, Valle BC, Soares R, Peixoto S. Effect of probiotic (*Bacillus* spp.) addition during larvae and postlarvae culture of the white shrimp *Litopenaeus vannamei*. Aquaculture Research 2011; 1-9.

[58] Kongnum K, Hongpattarakere T. Effect of *Lactobacillus plantarum* isolated from digestive tract of wild shrimp on growth and survival of white shrimp (*Litopenaeus vannamei*) challenged with *Vibrio harveyi*. Fish & Shellfish Immunology 2012; 32(1) 170-177.

[59] Castex M, Lemaire P, Wabete N, Chim L. Effect of *Pediococcus acidilactici* on antioxidant defences and oxidative stress of *Litopenaeus stylirostris* under *Vibrio nigripulchritudo* challenge. Fish & Shellfish Immunology 2010; 28(4) 622-631.

[60] Rahiman KMM, Jesmi Y, Thomas AP, Hatha AAM. Probiotic effect of Bacillus NL110 and Vibrio NE17 on the survival, growth performance and immune response of *Macrobrachium rosenbergii* (de Man). Aquaculture Research 2010; 41(9) 120-134.

[61] Lin HZ, Guo Z, Yang Y, Zheng W, LI ZJ. Effect of dietary probiotics on apparent digestibility coefficients of nutrients of white shrimp *Litopenaeus vannamei* Boone. Aquaculture Research 2004; 35(15) 1441-1447.

[62] Ninawe AS, Selvin J. Probiotics in shrimp aquaculture: Avenues and challenges. Critical Reviews in Microbiology 2009; 35(1) 43-66.

[63] Farzanfar A. The use of probiotics in shrimp aquaculture. FEMS Immunology and Medical Microbiology 2006; 48(2) 149-158.

[64] Vaseeharan B, Ramasamy P. Control of pathogenic *Vibrio* spp. by *Bacillus subtilis* BT23, a possible probiotic treatment for black tiger shrimp *Penaeus monodon*. Letters in Applied Microbiology 2003; 36(2) 83-87.

[65] Riquelme C, Hayashida G, Araya R, Uchida A, Satomi M, Ishida Y. Isolation of a native bacterial strain from the scallop *Argopecten purpuratus* with inhibitory effects against pathogenic vibrios. Journal of Shellfish Research 1996; 15(2) 369-374.

[66] Gibson LF, Woodworth J, George AM. Probiotic activity of *Aeromonas media* on the Pacific oyster, *Crassostrea gigas*, when challenged with *Vibrio tubiashii*. Aquaculture 1998; 169(1-2) 111-120.

[67] Douillet P, Langdon CJ. Effects of marine bacteria on the culture of axenic oyster *Crassostrea gigas* (Thunberg) larvae. Biological Bulletin 1993; 184(1) 36–51.

[68] Douillet AP, Langdon CJ. Use of a probiotic for the culture of larvae of the Pacific oyster (*Crassostrea gigas*, Thunberg). Aquaculture 1994; 119(1) 25-40.

[69] Ruiz-Ponte C, Samain JF, Sánchez JL, Nicolas JL. The benefit of a *Roseobacter* species on the survival of scallop larvae. Marine Biotechnology 1999; 1(1) 52-59.

[70] Riquelme C, Araya R, Escribano R. Selective incorporation of bacteria by *Argopecten purpuratus* larvae: implications for the use of probiotics in culturing systems of the Chilean scallop. Aquaculture 2000; 181(1-2) 25-36.

[71] Riquelme CE, Jorquera MA, Rojas AI, Avendaño RE, Reyes N. Addition of inhibitor-producing bacteria to mass cultures of *Argopecten purpuratus* larvae (Lamarck, 1819). Aquaculture 2001; 192(2-4) 111-119.

[72] França FM, Dias DC, Teixeira PC, Marcantônio AS, De Stéfani MV, Antonucci A, Rocha G, Ranzani-Paiva MJT, Ferreira CM. Efeito do probiótico *Bacillus subtilis* no crescimento,

sobrevivência e fisiologia de rãs-touro (*Rana catesbeiana*). Boletim do Instituto de Pesca 2008; 34(3) 403-412.

[73] Boyd CE. Aquaculture sustainability and environmental issues. World Aquaculture 1999; 30(2) 10-72.

[74] Dalmin G, Kathiresan K, Purushothaman A. Effect of probiotics on bacterial population and health status of shrimp in culture pond ecosystem. Indian Journal of Experimental Biology 2001; 39(9) 939-942.

The Use of Probiotic Strains as Silage Inoculants

Yunior Acosta Aragón

Additional information is available at the end of the chapter

1. Introduction

To secure the health and good performance of animal husbandry, animals need a constant supply of high quality nutrients the whole year round. The preservation of feed for use during periods of underproduction is a universal problem. All farmers worldwide face the challenge of guaranteeing feed for their animals throughout the year, and not only in terms of quantity but also quality [1, 2].

Thus, a major concern of any farm that seeks to operate economically is the need to preserve the quality of feedstuffs. On-farm feed preservation plays an important role in maintaining the nutritive value of feed while avoiding losses caused by micro-organisms and contamination with undesirable toxins, for instance, mycotoxins. Grain prices have risen steadily due to poor harvests in key producing countries, supply constraints in rice-growing economies and fast-growing demand for bio-fuel [3]. A price decrease is not expected in the coming years. This is one of the reasons why producers have to maximise animal performance by using locally produced feedstuffs that are found in abundance, such as pastures, silages and industrial by-products.

The preservation of feed value is an important topic for animal performance. The aim is to inhibit the growth of undesirable micro-organisms and the spoilage of the feedstuffs while minimizing nutrient and energy losses.

A common technique used to preserve feed involves manipulating the presence or lack of oxygen. Grains and hay are usually preserved aerobically with the addition of different preservatives. Ensiling is a classic example of an anaerobic preservation technique.

The practice of ensiling was originally a management tool used mainly in ruminant production to fulfill feed demand by storing and preserving any excess feed resources from periods of overproduction for later use during periods of lack. However, its importance has been increasing, especially in high input "zero-grazing" systems that enhance productivity per animal per area unit [4-6]. Today, silage is the world's largest fermentation process, with an estimated 287 million tons produced in the EU alone [2].

Ensiling is a process in which lactic acid bacteria (LAB) convert sugars into mainly lactic acid and other by-products, such as acetic or butyric acid [7], under anaerobic conditions. This decreases the pH value, keeps the feed value, inhibits the growth of undesirable micro-organisms, and preserves forages for long periods of time under normal conditions of up to one to two years and even more. Though ensiling is used mainly to preserve voluminous feed, many other substrates including grains, by-products like fish residues, wet distillery grains with solubles or WDGS and brewer's grains can also be ensiled.

The major advantages of silage are:

a.　that crops can be harvested almost independent of weather conditions,
b.　harvesting losses are reduced and more nutrients per area are harvested, and
c.　ensiling permits the use of a wide range of crops [8, 9].

The necessary pre-requisites for the ensiling of any material are:

a.　easily fermentable sugars (Water Soluble Carbohydrates, WSC),
b.　anaerobic conditions,
c.　lactic acid bacteria (LAB) and
d.　factors allowing their proliferation like dry matter (DM) content and buffer capacity.

The DM content plays a huge role in the fermentability of a substrate. This key point seems to be easy to guarantee but under practical conditions, is actually not. Due to different weather conditions, it is a real challenge to harvest crops with adequate DM content.

On the other hand, bacteria, and specifically lactic acid bacteria originating from the epiphytic microflora or silage inoculants, are able to survive only under specific conditions. One such condition is the DM content, as it determines the osmotic pressure and the aw-value of the substrates.

The ensiling process can be divided into four main phases:

1.　Aerobic phase: This refers to the respiration and proteolysis by the plant's own enzymes. This can be reduced by optimizing particle length and proper compacting of the material (Picture 1). This phase takes about three days under normal ensiling conditions.
2.　Fermentation: This refers to the acidification caused mainly by lactic acid produced by lactic acid bacteria (LAB). This phase takes two to three weeks. Under anaerobic conditions, lactic acid bacteria produce considerable amounts of lactic acid and the pH decreases, inhibiting the growth of undesirable micro-organisms (especially *Clostridia* and *Enterobacteria*). LAB ferments the substrate homofermentatively (only lactic acid) or heterofermentatively (lactic acid + acetic acid). However, LAB represent only between 0.1 to 1.0 % of the normal epiphytic microflora. Therefore the use of bacterial inoculants to secure the fermentation has increased in recent years.

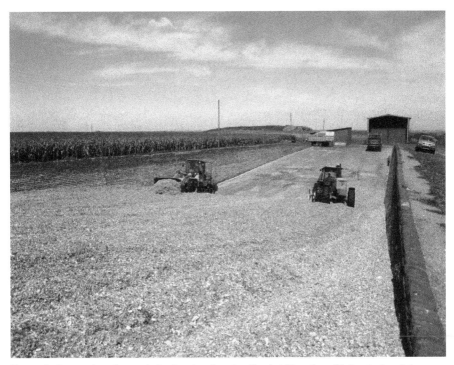

Picture 1. Compacting of corn whole plant for silage in a South African farm (Y. Acosta Aragón)

3. Stable phase: Fermentation ceases due to a lack of carbohydrate substrates, and the pH remains constant, depending on the anaerobic conditions created.

4. Feed out phase: Once the silo is opened and during feeding, portions of the silage are exposed to oxygen (Picture 2). Aerobic micro-organisms, primarily yeasts and molds, will grow, consume dry matter (sugar, lactic acid and other chemical substances), and cause heating and high losses (CO_2 and H_2O). This phase is decisive because the nutrient losses could be considerably high. Aliphatic short chain acids (acetic, propionic and butyric acid) [10] inhibit the growth of yeasts and molds and that is why biological inoculants containing heterofermentative bacteria are used. The response to additives depends not only on the forage to be treated, but also the dry matter (DM) content [11], sugar content, and buffering capacity of the original material [12]. The characteristics of inoculants include a rapid growth rate (to compete with other micro-organisms), tolerance of low pH, ability to reduce pH quickly, non-reactivity towards organic acids, tolerance towards a wide temperature range, ability to grow in high DM materials, absence of proteolytic activity and an ability to hydrolyze starch.

In recent years, producers have begun to pay more attention to silage additives, [13] which have been the focus of a tremendous amount of research over the last 20 years. Some of this research has focused on increasing the nutritional value of silage by improving fermentation so that storage losses are reduced, and increasing the aerobic stability of silage after the opening of silos [14].

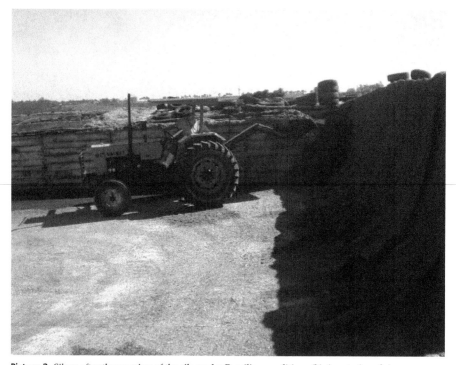

Picture 2. Silage after the opening of the silo under Brazilian conditions (Y. Acosta Aragón)

2. Silage microbiology

Silage making is based on microbiology. Silage inoculants are additives containing LAB that are used to manipulate and enhance fermentation in silages like grass, alfalfa, clover and other silages, as well as aerobic stability (mainly in corn silage). The most common LAB in commercial inoculants is *Lactobacillus plantarum* and other *Lactobacilli*, followed by *Enterococci* (for instance, *E. faecium*) and some *Pediococci* [15]. The main criteria for their selection are:

- high production of lactic and/ or acetic acid
- above all, quick growth in the first phase of the ensiling process in order to inhibit undesirable micro-organisms
- high osmotolerance
- fermentation under technical conditions
- no antibiotic resistances

One the most important classifications of the LAB is according to whether their influence on the ensiling process is homo- or heterofermentative. Homofermentative LAB produce mainly lactic acid (more than 90% of the whole fermentation products) with energy losses close to zero. On the other hand, heterofermentative LAB use WSC not only to produce lactic acid but also acetic or propionic acid, ethanol, mannitol, etc.

The philosophy behind the first silage inoculants at the end of the 80s was that, in order to achieve good results in the ensiling process, the substrate needs to acidify very deeply and quickly. Since the drop in pH value is highly correlated (r^2 from -0.8 to -0.9) with the lactic acid content, a major goal was to increase the amount of lactic acid through the use of homofermentative LAB. However producers and researchers very soon found that the best fermented silages often showed a worsened aerobic stability after the opening of the silo. Those aerobic instabilities, reflected in heating and energy losses, are caused mainly by yeasts. Yeasts are aerobic, mostly unicellular, eukaryotic micro-organisms classified as fungi, which convert carbohydrates to CO_2 and alcohols, mainly ethanol. It is a metabolic exothermic process with an energy loss of approx. 40 %. However, yeasts are sensitive to short-chain organic acids like acetic and propionic acids. This was the reason for the start of the use of heterofermentative LAB to prevent aerobic silage instability.

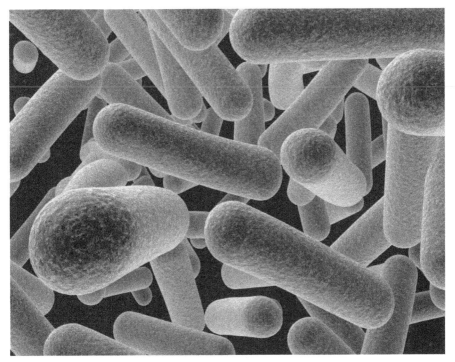

Picture 3. Listeria monocytogenes (iStock_000002507254Large©Sebastian Kaulitzki)

The main harmful micro-organisms present in silages are microbes with different characteristics (classification, physiology, pathogenesis, detection, epidemiology, routes of infection, infectious cycles, etc.) [16]. Good agricultural practices can help to prevent infections transmitted by the ingestion of contaminated silages.

Listeria monocytogenes: These are gram-positive bacterium that can move within eukaryotic cells (Picture 3). Clinical symptoms, such as meningoencephalitis, abortions and mastitis in ruminants, are frequently recognized by veterinarians. The bacterium lives in the soil and in poorly made silage, and is acquired by ingestion. It is not contagious; over the course of a 30-year observation period of sheep disease in Morocco, the disease only appeared in the late 2000s when ensiled feed-corn bags became common. In Iceland, the disease is called silage sickness [17]. *L. monocytogenes* usually cannot survive below pH 5.6, but in poorly consolidated silage with some oxygen, it may survive at pH levels as low as 3.8. As these conditions also favor the growth of certain molds, moldy silage generally presents a high risk of listeriosis [18].

Clostridia: These are gram-positive obligate anaerobic bacterium that can form spores (Picture 4).

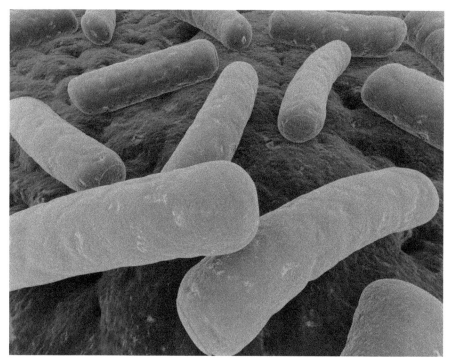

Picture 4. Clostridia (iStock_000008522722XLarge©Sebastian Kaulitzki)

Crops for ensiling are often harvested in relatively wet conditions and have a low dry matter content (<25 %). This presents a risk of contamination with Clostridia, which increases the nutrient (protein) losses in silages and causes fermentation to butyric acid. Another important consequence is that animals may reject silage due to its low palatability. Clostridia can be prevented by a rapid and sudden pH decrease (pH below 4.5) [19].

Entereobacteria (coli forms): These are gram-negative, non-spore forming, facultative anaerobes (Picture 5). They commonly enter silages from slurry, manure and soil in the early stages of fermentation and convert the water-soluble carbohydrates into acetic acid, ethanol, CO_2, and ammonia, resulting in high energy losses [20]. Their growth is reduced by anaerobiosis, low pH values and fermentation acids. The optimal pH value for growth is around 7; lower pH values markedly decrease the growth [20].

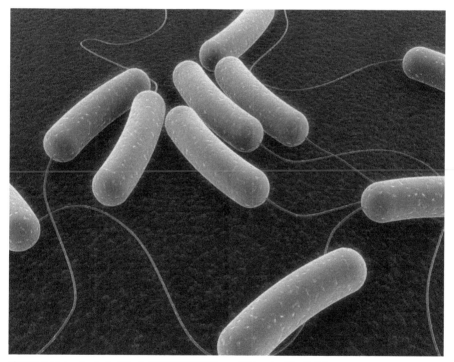

Picture 5. Enterobacteria (iStock_000003187348XLarge©Sebastian Kaulitzki)

Yeasts: These are eukaryotic unicellular aerobic micro-organisms (fungi) that use organic compounds as a source of energy, mostly from hexoses and disaccharides, and do not require sunlight to grow (Picture 6).

There are no known yeast species that only grow anaerobically (obligate anaerobes) [21]. Yeasts grow best in a neutral or slightly acidic pH environment. During the feed-out phase in the absence of inhibiting substances like acetic and propionic acid, yeasts can grow very rapidly and surpass 1 000 000 cfu/g silage, causing aerobic instability but also increasing the

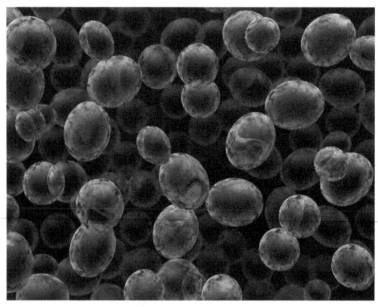

Picture 6. Yeasts (iStock_000012250997XLarge©Dmitry Knorre)

Micro-organisms	Author	Year	Statement
Saccharomyces rouxii and *Torulopsis versatilis*	Noda *et al.* [23]	1982	An increased toxic effect in brine fermentation of soy sauce from pH 5.5 to 3.5
Candida krusei and *Pichia subpelliculosa*	Danner *et al.* [24]	2003	Acetic acid has the greatest inhibitory effect on yeast growth. 20 g liter^{-1} of acetic acid in the test mixture was enough to completely inhibit the growth of the selected yeasts at pH 4.
Silage yeasts	Driehuis and van Wikselaar [25] Oude Elferink *et al.* [18]	1996 1999	High levels of formic or acetic acid reduce survival during storage (in silages)
Silage yeasts	Driehuis *et al.* [26] Oude Elferink *et al.* [18]	1999 1999	Lactic acid is degraded anaerobically to acetic acid and 1,2-propanediol, which in turn causes a significant reduction in yeast numbers

Table 1. Effect of acetic acid on different yeasts

risk of diarrhea in domestic animals. They compete with lactic acid bacteria for sugars, which they ferment to create mainly ethanol. Ethanol has little (if any) preservative effect in the silage but causes extremely dry matter and high energy losses of 48.9 and 0.2 %

respectively [20]. A level of acetic acid of 1.5 to 3.0 % in the dry matter could prohibit yeast growth in silages exposed to air in the feed out phase [22]. However, higher levels diminish the silage palatability. An overview of results in the scientific literature about inhibition of yeast by acetic acid is presented in Table 1.

Molds: These grow in multicellular filaments and derive energy from the organic matter in which they live, for example silages (Picture 7).

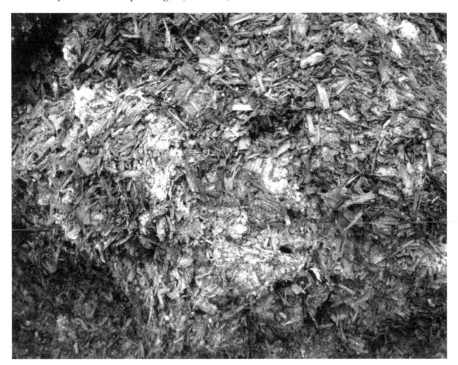

Picture 7. Molds in silages (Y. Acosta Aragón)

Mold spores can remain airborne indefinitely, live for a long time, cling to clothing or fur, and survive extremes of temperature and pressure. Many molds also secrete mycotoxins which, together with hydrolytic enzymes, inhibit the growth of competing micro-organisms. The mycotoxins secreted can negatively affect the performance of domestic animals. Milk contamination, decreased milk production, mastitis, laminitis, poor reproductive performance and several gastrointestinal disorders are some of the effects on dairy cattle which have been extensively described. The main mycotoxins found in silages were ZON, DON and fumonisins [27] as well as roquefortine. The majority of fungi are strict aerobes (require oxygen to grow) [28]; and only a few of them are micro aerobic (*Mucor spp.)* [29]. The main parameters for controlling the growth of the micro-organisms as described above are summarized in *Table 2*.

Parameter	Micro-organisms				
	Listeria monocytogenes	Clostridia	Enterobacteriae	Yeasts	Molds
Nutrients (Water-soluble carbohydrates)	+++	+++	+++	+++	-
Anaerobiosis	+++	-	+++	+++	+++
pH*	+++	+++	+++	-	-
Lactic acid* (fermentation)	+++	+++	+++	-	-
Acetic acid* (feed out phase)	+	+	++	+++	+++

Table 2. The control of harmful micro-organisms present in silages
*- Low inhibition, + High inhibition. * Factors influenced by the use of silage inoculants*

3. Use of probiotic strains in silages

Fermentation characteristics are generally improved with inoculation [30]. [31] reported that inoculation improved fermentation characteristics in over 90% of 300 silages, including alfalfa, wheat, corn, and forage sorghum silages. With any forage preservation technique, the quantity and quality of material available at the end of storage is always below that of the original. Thus, the primary goal of forage preservation is to minimize the spoilage and losses of dry matter (DM) which will be reflected in the energy content of the silage, a limiting factor for milk production.

Silage inoculants can be classified according to their effect on the ensiled matter or their mode of action. The main effects of inoculants are:

a.   to prevent undesirable fermentations and
b.   to prevent silage spoilage during the feed out phase.

To achieve these effects, producers can utilize three different products or a combination of:

a.   acids,
b.   their salts and solutions respectively, and
c.   biological silage inoculants.

Other silage additives with more limited uses than the above are molasses [32] and enzymes. Salts and acids are used to cause an abrupt decrease in the pH value when the dry matter content of the raw material is out of the optimal range. In cases of low dry matter content, these products inhibit, above all, the growth of *Clostridia*. High dry matter content very often means bad conditions for the compaction of raw materials; air stays inside the ensiled matter, thereby hindering the anaerobic conditions required for good silage. The advantage of the use of salts is that they are non-corrosive and easier and safer in application compared with their corresponding acids.

Biological silage inoculants have been used and are established on the market because of:

a.   their proven effectiveness in accelerating fermentation and improving aerobic stability,
b.   higher recovery of dry matter and energy content compared with non-treated silages,
c.   safety during usage and
d.   relatively lower cost per treated ton compared with acids.

The quality of good biological silage inoculants must be selected, first, on the basis of the included strains and their proportions in the product. Multi-strain inoculants have the advantage of possibly using different sources of energy, with each strain having a different desirable effect (rapid pH decrease, higher production of lactic acid, or acetic acid production for a better aerobic stability). It is, therefore, possible to change the mode of action of a product containing the same strains but with different proportions of the bacterial strains. On the other hand, different strains of the same micro-organism will grow faster on different substrates, temperature conditions or moisture content (osmotolerance).

Another aspect to take into account is the number of bacteria in the product and per gram of silage. A review of the products existing on the silage additive market shows a variation of 100 000 to 1 000 000 cfu/ g of silage [33].

The effectiveness of a biological silage additive can be measured using different methods. It is very difficult, under practical conditions, to measure success in terms of higher performance (milk and/ or meat production) because the whole process is conditional upon many factors. The first aspect to be taken into account is silage quality, worded in simple parameters such as pH value, fermentation acids and energy content, compared with the normal values for the ensiled crop or against a negative (no additive) or a positive (with other additive) control.

In selecting the right biological silage additive, some pre-requisites, such as the crop to be ensiled, should be taken into account. According to [33] there are three types of crops from the point of view of "ensilability", which are classified according to their fermentability coefficient (FC):

FC = DM + 8 x (sugar content / puffer capacity)

The following criteria are used to interpret the FC values:

-   poor ensilability (FC < 35)
-   average ensilability(35 < FC < 45) and
-   good ensilability (FC > 35)

For substrates of poor ensilability, the recommended biological silage additive should contain (principally) homofermentative bacteria which produce mostly lactic acid. This dramatically reduces the pH value (high negative correlation coefficient of more than 0.80 between lactic acid content and pH values). For substrates of good ensilability such as in whole maize crop, the aim should be to increase the aerobic stability, because such substrates are very rich in nutrients and spoil very quickly when in contact with air, and therefore yeasts and molds [26, 34]. In the last case (improvement of aerobic stability), biological silage additives with a higher ratio of heterofermentative bacteria are preferred due to a higher production of acetic or propionic acid and the corresponding inhibition of undesirable spoilage micro-organisms [35, 36]. Nevertheless the use of propionate-producing propionic bacteria appears to be less suitable for the improvement of silage aerobic stability, due to the fact that these bacteria are only able to proliferate and produce propionate if the silage pH remains relatively high [37].

A real challenge for probiotic strains is the inoculation of haylage because of the high DM content and the concomitant higher osmotic pressure. Very often, the term haylage is used indistinctly and there are definitions which claim that "a round bale silage (a baleage) is also sometimes called haylage". [38] considered baleage, big bale haylage and round bale silage as different names given to the same preserved feedstuff. Both processes are anaerobic but the first one (haylage) is related to the DM content at ensiling; and the second one (baleage) is the procedure used to protect the material against spoiling (baling, wrapping). That is the reason why we fully agree with [8] when he writes "wrapped haylage bales". Haylage may be preserved wrapped but also in other type of silos (bunker, trench, etc.). Another controversial topic is the right DM content range for haylage. A review on this topic is shown in Figure 1.

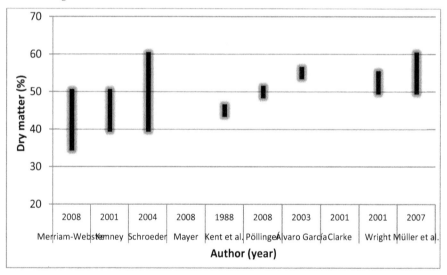

Figure 1. Dry matter content of haylage according to different sources

The range varies from 35 to 60 % DM. Moreover, many companies produce haylage for horses and consider it a special feed made of wilted grass silage with 65 % DM. In our context, where we refer to the use of silage inoculants in haylage for cattle, we will consider a range of 40 to 50 % DM, since anything below 40 % DM would be normal wilted silage. Anything over this range (55 % DM) and the feed would be more suited to horses due to the higher fiber content *(see Figure 1)*. Two very important aspects should be taken into account: a) the high DM content is out of the optimal values for LAB and b) the material, due to the high DM content, is difficult to compact.

The process of making haylage is the same as that for silage making, except that it takes longer for wilting to reach the desired DM content. The advantages of the use of haylage are:

- Free from spores and dust (very important for horses!)
- Lower storage losses than in silage making
- Weather independent compared with hay making
- Higher density of nutrients per volumetric unit compared with silages

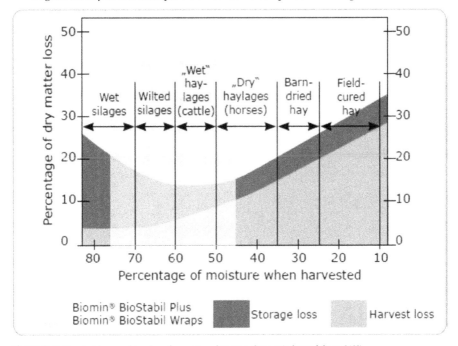

Figure 2. Estimated hay and haylage harvest and storage losses (adapted from [43])

The storage and harvest losses with different moisture contents are given in *Figure 2*. Note that total losses are minimized at a moisture level of between 50 and 60 % (40 to 50 % DM), which represents a great advantage of the use of haylage. According to [39], the quality parameters for haylage are not determined strictly enough. A major aim in haylage making should be to reduce pH values to below 5, ideally below 4.5 to diminish the risk of botulism [40] and listeriosis [41]. Since the DM is higher compared with that in silages, the production of fermentation products will be lower. Common values for haylage containing lactic and acetic acid would be from 15 to 50, and less than 20 g/ kg DM respectively. In haylage as in silage, butyric acid and ethanol are equally undesirable. Due to the often slower acidification process, some amounts of one or both of these acidic substances may appear.

The effects silage inoculants in haylages should be the same as the effects in silages, namely. a quicker and deeper acidification and/ or enlarged aerobic stability, in addition to improved animal performance. [42] found a tendency towards higher DM intake (20.4 vs. 18.1 kg/ day) among cows in early lactation fed treated haylage (alfalfa haylage of 45 % DM; P < 0.32). The use of inoculants decreased the pH value from 5.29 vs. 5.11 for the control and the treated haylage groups respectively.

4. The control of harmful micro-organisms present in deficient silages

The examples are based on the results obtained in field trials with silages inoculated with blends of homo- and heterofermentative bacteria (Biomin® BioStabil Plus - 20 grass silages and Biomin® BioStabil Mays - 24 corn silages). Different substrates were used to refer to the silage quality parameters. In this study [44], only the parameters that can be directly influenced by the use of silage inoculants were selected (pH value, lactic and acetic acid and aerobic stability).

The results of the trials conducted with silages that have and have not been treated with silage inoculants are presented in Figure 3.

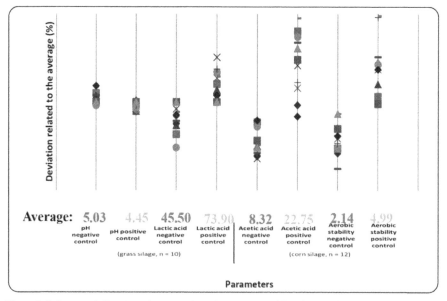

Figure 3. Influence of silage inoculants on selected parameters of the silage quality

As shown in Figure 3, the use of a silage inoculant improves the fermentation and lactic acid production (on average, 0.58 and in 28.4g/kg of dry matter respectively) in grass silages. The use of a silage inoculant that contains heterofermentative lactic acid bacteria (*L. brevis*) improves the acetic acid production and the aerobic stability in corn silages in 14.43g/kg of dry matter (+173 %) and 2.85 days (+133 %) respectively.

5. Results using probiotic strains in silages

The trial results were obtained with blends of homo- (*L. plantarum* and *E. faecium*) and heterofermentative bacteria (*L. brevis*) in different concentrations, as specified in each paragraph.

5.1. The use of silage inoculants in milk production

The use of silage inoculants can improve silage quality. Better silage means better hygiene and therefore improvements in animal performance can be expected. The results of a trial discussed below give an example of how milk production can be improved [45]. In the trial, mixed grass-legume sward wilted for 6 – 8 hours to 320 g DM/ kg (174 g of crude protein/ kg DM; 6.68 MJ NEL/ kg DM) was ensiled. The calculated fermentation coefficient was 49. The sward was cut and picked with a precision chop forage harvester (theoretical particle length of 30 mm). The grass-legume sward was treated with BSP (Biomin® BioStabil Plus, blend of *L. plantarum, E. faecium* and *L. brevis*; 2 x 10^5 cfu/ g of forage, 4 g of product applied in 4 liters of water/ ton), to be compared with a control treatment similarly collected from field but without inoculation after wilting. Representative samples of harvested and wilted grass mixtures were taken throughout harvesting. Silages were sampled every other week during the feeding experiment, which began 90 days after ensiling.

Aerobic stability was measured using data loggers which recorded the temperature once every six hours. The boxes were kept at a constant room temperature (21°C). Aerobic deterioration was denoted by the number of hours in which the temperature of the silage did not surpass the ambient temperature by more than 2°C.

Twenty-four Lithuanian black-and-white dairy cows were selected for the experiment from a larger group (from a herd of 120 dairy cows) according to parity, lactation, date of calving, present milk yield, last year's milk yield, and live weight using a multi-criteria method. The dairy cows were group-fed twice a day, bedded on straw and had access to water *ad libitum*. The cows were individually fed common commercial compound feed and their intake recorded.

Cows were milked twice a day and their milk yield was registered weekly. Milk samples were taken once a week from the morning and evening milking and the fat, protein, lactose contents and somatic cell count were analyzed. Data were analyzed using variance analysis to test for the effect of silage treatments with the software Genstat/ 1987. The Fisher's least significant difference (LSD) procedure at the 5% significance level was used to determine differences in treatment means.

There were no significant differences in the dry matter and crude fiber content (Table 3) between the untreated and treated silages. However, treatment with BSP resulted in significantly lower DM losses (+17.9 g/ kg of DM, P<0.01), significantly higher crude protein (149.4 vs. 159 g/ kg of DM; P<0.05) and digestible protein concentrations (108.9 vs. 117.8 g/ kg of DM; P<0.01). Kramer (2002) found higher dry matter losses due to fermentations that differed from the homofermentative and respirative processes in the ensiled material. Higher protein content was also found in silages treated with an inoculant by, for instance, [47] (legume grass mixture) and [48] (red clover). A quick reduction in the silage pH limits the breakdown of protein due to inactive plant proteases [49]. The net energy lactation (NEL) content was also significantly higher in the treatment with BSP (+0.08 MJ/ kg DM respectively).

Parameters	Unit	Treatments		P
		Control	BSP	
		X ± SD	X ± SD	
Dry matter (DM)	g/ kg	315.4 ±3.12	319.2 ±5.96	0.079
DM losses	g/ kg DM	106.2 ±6.30	88.3 ±6.75	**
Crude protein		149.4 ±6.37	159.0 ±6.91	*
Digestible protein		108.9 ±5.92	117.8 ±6.42	**
Crude ash		70.7 ±5.04	71.2 ±4.51	0.826
Net Energy Lactation (NEL)	MJ/ kg DM	6.42 ±0.09	6.50 ±0.07	*

Table 3. Effect of Biomin® BioStabil Plus treatment on the chemical composition of ensiled grass-legume
* and ** denote statistical significance at level 0.05 and 0.01 respectively

The treatment with BSP increased fermentation rates, resulting in a significant pH decrease (P<0.05) and a significant increase in the concentration of total fermentation acids (P<0.05) compared with the control silage (Table 4). The inoculant produced more lactic acid (P<0.01), which reflects the results obtained by [50, 51, 52]; and numerically higher acetic acid content compared with that of the control silage. [6] gave a reference value of 1% for acetic acid in fresh matter to denote proper aerobic stability and good silage intake, whereas [53] gave a value of 2 – 3% in DM.

Both the butyric acid and ammonia nitrogen contents were significantly 10 times lower when BSP was used (P<0.01 in both cases). Butyric acid is the main product of the *Clostridia* metabolism, which can be controlled by a quick and deep acidification [46, 49]. [54] found no butyric acid in well fermented inoculated silages (pH of 4.1-4.2), while silages which were not inoculated contained certain amounts of that acid. In more than 60% of reviewed literature, [52] reported lower ammonia nitrogen contents in silages treated with inoculants.

Parameters	Unit	Treatments		P
		Control X ± SD	BSP X ± SD	
pH	-	4.38 ±0.09	4.25 ±0.08	*
Total organic acids		67.16 ±7.49	76.62 ±8.60	*
Lactic acid		36.74 ±5.26	44.15 ±5.93	**
Acetic acid	g/ kg DM	28.23 ±3.18	32.17 ±5.43	0.051
Butyric acid		2.15 ±1.98	0.23 ±0.36	**
Ethanol		7.87 ±1.16	7.06 ±0.69	0.059
Ammonia N	g/ kg total N	57.5 ±7.24	46.0 ±4.03	**

Table 4. Effect of Biomin® BioStabil Plus treatment on the fermentation characteristics of ensiled grass-legume
* and ** denote statistical significance at level 0.05 and 0.01 respectively.

The non-inoculated control silage was already heated after 54 hours and after 108 hours, had reached a temperature exceeding the ambient temperature by 2°C (Figure 4). The temperature rise in inoculated silage was small and first heated after 102 hours; however, no temperature rise of 2°C over the ambient temperature was observed during the 10-day exposure to air. This is due to a higher acetic acid content, which stops yeast growth. Increased concentrations of acetic acid in silage treated with BSP had a positive effect on the aerobic stability of the silage [24, 55].

Classical microbial inoculants, containing only homolactic bacteria, were shown to have no effect on and could even cause the aerobic stability of the silage to deteriorate [52, 56]. [57] found no positive effect on aerobic stability when a blend of homolactic lactic acid bacteria was used. Several authors have discovered that heterolactic lactic acid bacteria positively improve aerobic stability [24, 58].

Silages and dry matter intake are presented in Table 5. Based on the data recorded during the experimental period (92 days) the feed intake of silage DM was higher by 6.5% for treated silage than that of the untreated silage, corresponding to the results from [59]. The intake of compound feed did not differ as it was restricted to a certain amount for both treatments. The energy intake (digestible energy and net energy lactation) was also higher for the silage treated with BSP (+6.1 and 5.3 % respectively) compared with the untreated control treatment. The Energy Corrected Milk (ECM) production was also higher in the BSP treatment (+1.4 liter of ECM/ cow/ day). [55] reported a milk production increase of 3 – 5%. [52] reported increased milk production in approx. 50% of the reviewed studies, with a statistically significant average improvement of +1.41 l/ day.

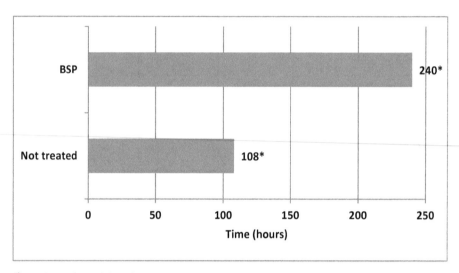

Figure 4. Aerobic stability of grass-legume silages treated or not with a silage inoculant
(* and ** denote statistical significance of means at 0.05 and 0.01 levels respectively)

Parameters	Unit	Treatments		P
		Control $\mathbf{X} \pm$ SD	BSP $\mathbf{X} \pm$ SD	
Silage intake		10.7 ±1.51	11.4 ±1.26	0.225
Compound feed	kg DM/ cow/ day	4.0 ±0.61	4.0 ±0.49	0.988
Total Dry matter intake		14.7 ±2.12	15.4 ±1.74	0.382
Total Net energy lactation intake	MJ	103.0 ±14.94	108.5 ±12.33	0.341
Daily energy corrected milk (ECM) production	kg/ cow/ day	17.4 ±2.69	18.8 ±2.40	0.183
Feed Conversion (FC)	NEL MJ/ 1 kg ECM	5.93 ±0.08	5.77 ±0.09	**

Table 5. The effect of inoculant Biomin® BioStabil Plus on silage intake, milk yield and feed conversion
* and ** denote statistical significance at level 0.05 and 0.01 respectively.

The feed conversion, calculated as the quotient between the NEL intake and the ECM production, denoted better efficiency in the conversion of energy into milk in the treatment with the BSP inoculant: cows fed the treated silage needed less energy (5.77 MJ NEL/ 1 liter of ECM) than others fed an untreated silage (5.93 MJ NEL/ 1 liter of ECM). This difference of 0.16 MJ was of high statistical significance ($P<0.01$), in spite of the fact that the differences in the parameters silage intake and milk production were not statistically significant. According to [55], feed efficiency can be increased by up to 9%.

The milk composition and somatic cell count are shown in Table 6. The protein, fat and lactose contents were higher in the BSP treatment, but not statistically significant ($P>0.05$). The somatic cell count of the milk from cows fed the treated silage was of statistically lower significance ($P<0.05$) than that of the control treatment (125,000 $vs.$ 222,000). This correlates with improved hygiene in the treated silage. This parameter of milk quality should be considered as a consequential effect of better silage hygiene. It is well known that the somatic cell count is a polyfactorial parameter [60, 61].

Parameters	Unit	Treatments		P
		Control $X \pm SD$	BSP $X \pm SD$	
Fat		4.30 ±0.40	4.43 ±0.28	0.376
Protein	%	3.36 ±0.15	3.42 ±0.22	0.451
Lactose		4.80 ±0.15	4.87 ±0.19	0.317
Somatic cell count	1000	222.3 ±152.13	125.1 ±30.98	*

Table 6. The effect of inoculant Biomin® BioStabil Plus on milk constituents and the somatic cell count * and ** denote statistical significance at level 0.05 and 0.01 respectively.

The biological silage inoculant had a significant effect on the quality characteristics of legume-grass silage, in terms of lower pH, due to a higher lactic acid fermentation caused by the homofermentative lactic acid bacteria. Similarly, inoculated silage showed higher ($P<0.05$) net energy lactation concentrations by 1.25%, compared with untreated silage. Inoculant treatment significantly decreased butyric acid content, N-NH$_3$ fraction and dry matter losses.

Improved silage fermentation with BSP increased silage intake and milk production. Better utilization of feed energy was reflected in the significantly higher efficiency of the conversion of feed-NEL into milk. Significantly lower somatic cell counts in milk from cows fed with the treated silage, indicate a higher hygiene quality in the milk compared with that of the control treatment.

5.2. The use of silage inoculants in meat production

The use of silage inoculants in the production of meat has been widely investigated [62, 63]. In spite of the sometimes controversial results, several trials have shown advantages from their use, reflected in better silage quality, aerobic stability and animal performance. The results of a trial conducted by [64] will be discussed in detail in the following paragraphs.

The aim of this trial was to study the effect of a silage inoculant on the nutrient content, silage quality, aerobic stability and nutritive value of ensiled whole plant corn, as well as on the feed intake and growth performance of fattening young cattle.

The effect of inoculation for whole plant corn silage treated with a commercial product (Biomin® BioStabil Mays, BSM, blend *Enterococcus faecium, Lactobacillus plantarum* and *Lactobacillus brevis,* DSM numbers 3530, 19457 and 23231 respectively; 4 g of product/ton of silage diluted in 4 l of water, 1×10^5 cfu/g of material), was compared with a control treatment with no silage additives (CT). The material had a DM of 323 g/kg, crude protein and water soluble carbohydrate concentrations of 87.9 and 110.5 g/kg DM respectively.

The inoculant was applied uniformly using an applicator. The silos were filled within 48 hours, covered with polythene sheet and weighted down with tires. The raw material as well as each silage was sampled. Volatile fatty acid and lactic acid, as well as alcohol concentrations, were determined by gas-liquid chromatography.

Aerobic stability was measured using data loggers which recorded temperature readings once every six hours. The boxes were kept at a constant room temperature of 21°C. Aerobic deterioration was denoted by days (or hours) until the start of a sustained increase in temperature by more than 2°C above the ambient temperature.

For the animal feeding trial 40 young beef cattle (eight to nine months old) with similar mean live weights were used and divided into two analogous groups (20 animals each). The experimental period lasted 100 days.

The animals were bedded on straw and had free access to water. Fresh silages were offered *ad libitum* twice daily, allowing for at least 10% orts (as-fed basis). Silage DM intake was calculated per group as the difference between the amount of silage supplied and the amount of silage remaining. Barley straw was included in the diet (1 kg/ animal/ day; 88 % of DM, energy value of 3.9 MJ ME/ kg DM). The animals were individually weighed on the first day of the experimental period, subsequently once per month, and on the final day of the experiment. The average weight gain and growth rates were calculated for each animal and for each group. Feed conversion ratio was calculated as the ratio between feed intake and body weight gain. Data were analyzed using variance analysis to test for the effect of silage treatments by Genstat/ 1987. A probability of $0.05<P<0.10$ was considered a near-significant trend.

The use of BSM significantly improved the silage quality compared with the CT (Table 7). The silage treated with BSM showed statistically significant higher DM recovery and digestible protein, coinciding with [65]; lower DM losses (P<0.01 for all) and higher crude protein content (P<0.05). The digestible energy content was highly significant in the treated silage compared with the untreated silage. There were no significant differences between the untreated and treated silages in terms of crude fiber NDF content.

Parameters	Unit	Treatments		P
		Control	BSM	
		X ±SD	X ±SD	
Dry matter (DM)	g/ kg	305.8 ±4.30	312.2 ±4.66	**
DM losses		70.2 ±15.87	40.9 ±2.60	**
Crude protein		80.2 ±4.94	84.7 ±3.24	*
Digestible protein	g/ kg DM	48.2 ±2.96	52.5 ±2.01	**
Crude fiber		214.8 ±4.59	210.2 ±7.30	0.074
Crude ash		45.2 ±3.26	44.4 ±4.10	0.622
Digestible Energy (DE)	MJ/ kg DM	12.8 ±0.06	13.1 ±0.07	**
Metabolizable Energy (ME)		10.8 ±0.08	10.9 ±0.13	*

Table 7. Effect of the treatment with a commercial product BSM on the chemical composition and fermentation characteristics of ensiled whole plant corn
* and ** denote significance at level 0.05 and 0.01 respectively

BSM treatment increased fermentation rates in whole crop corn silages, resulting in a significant pH decrease (P<0.01) and a significant increase in total organic acids concentration (P<0.05) compared with the CT (Table 8). The lactic acid content in the BSM treatment was also significantly higher (P<0.01) since homofermentative LAB were used [66]. The acetic acid content of the BSM treatment was numerically higher than that of the CT. Silage inoculation with BSM significantly decreased concentrations of butyric acid, ethanol and ammonia-N (P<0.01) of corn silage compared with the CT. Homofermentative silage inoculants by improving silage fermentation can reduce wasteful end-products such as ammonia-N and volatile fatty acids, which result in poorer feed conversion efficiency and higher in-silo dry matter losses [67-70].

The use of silage inoculants containing homofermentative lactic acid bacteria to increase lactic acid production and enhance the rate and extent of pH decline [12, 37, 70] can also lead to a reduction in protein breakdown [65]. As shown in Table 2, the BSM silage treatment decreased DM losses by 3.0 % (P<0.01) and had higher digestible energy (DE) and metabolic energy (ME) concentrations by 2.3 and 1.00 % (P<0.01 and P<0.05) respectively compared with the untreated CT silage.

Parameters	Unit	Treatments		P
		Control X ±SD	BSM X ±SD	
pH	-	3.89 ±0.09	3.71 ±0.03	**
Total organic acids		80.0 ±4.33	93.3 ±10.52	**
Lactic acid		50.3 ±2.60	61.4 ±5.88	**
Acetic acid	g/ kg DM	29.0 ±2.16	31.5 ±4.87	0.116
Butyric acid		0.4 ±0.30	0.1 ±0.11	**
Ethanol		13.2 ±2.10	9.3 ±2.41	**
Ammonia N	g/ kg total N	51.0 ±10.29	38.0 ±7.77	**

Table 8. Effect of the treatment with a commercial product BSM on the fermentation characteristics of ensiled corn
* and ** denote significance at level 0.05 and 0.01 respectively

During aerobic exposure after opening the silos, the CT (Figure 5) had a temperature increase of more than 2°C above the ambient temperature after 84 hours. In the BSM treatment, the increase of more than 2°C above the ambient temperature occurred only after 156 hours.

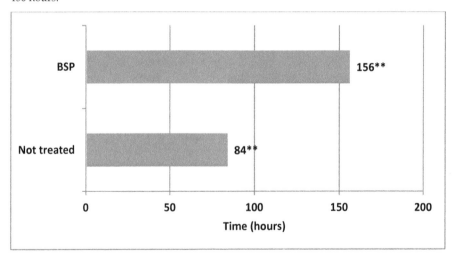

Figure 5. Aerobic stability of corn silages treated or not with a silage inoculant
(* and ** denote statistical significance of means at 0.05 and 0.01 levels respectively)

The stability of BSM silage was improved by 72 hours (3 days) compared with the CT. Recently, silage studies with whole crop corn silages using obligatory heterofermentative LAB *L. buchneri* as an inoculant, showed a 20-fold increase in the aerobic stability of the silage, which increased from approximately 40 hours for untreated silages to more than 790 hours for the inoculated silages [26]. Other studies [58, 71] have provided more definitive evidence of the existence of certain LAB strains with the power to inhibit yeast and mold growth, and to improve aerobic stability. Some authors have described the positive aspect of the formation of acetic acid by heterofermentative lactic acid bacteria, which inhibits spoilage organisms [7, 72].

Average daily weight gains (ADWG) for BSM and CT are shown in Table 9.

Treatment/ statistical parameter	n	Trial period in days (kg, X ±SD)			
		0 - 31	32 - 63	64 - 100	0 - 100
Control	20	0.931 ±0.124	0.981 ±0.129	1.068 ±0.074	0.998 ±0.087
Commercial product BSM	20	0.940 ±0.081	1.062 ±0.129	1.206 ±0.089	1.078 ±0.078
Standard error	-	0.016	0.021	0.017	0.014
P level	-	0.778	0.055	**	**

Table 9. Average daily body weight gain of the beef cattle in different trial periods
** *denotes significance at level 0.01*

From 0 to 31 trial days, neither statistically nor numerically marked differences in ADWG were found between the treatments. However in the trial period between 32 to 63 days, the differences in ADWG show a near-significant trend ($0.05 < P < 0.10$) with a P value of 0.055. The ADWG in the last third of the feeding trial period (from 64 to 100 days), and throughout the whole trial period (0 to 100 days), showed a statistically significant difference ($P < 0.01$) of 138 and 80g respectively.

In order to avoid differences due to different moisture contents, the intake is shown in Table 10 on the DM basis. The silage DM intake for BSM was higher by 6.14% compared with the CT (3.97 *vs.* 3.74 kg DM/ animal/ day), and showed a near-significant trend (P=0.065). As expected, because of the restricted feeding, no differences were found in compound feed DM intake. These results were similar to those reported by [52]; however, some researchers found that feeding microbial inoculated silage to cattle does not affect dry matter intake compared with non-inoculated silage [73]. A combination of increased DM intake and higher energy in the silage treated with BSM, led to a significant increase (P<0.05) in metabolizable energy intake compared with those animals fed with the CT. The animals receiving BSM had a better conversion of energy into body weight compared with that of the CT because they needed 2.37 MJ of ME (3.4 %) less for a 1 kg increase in body weight. However, this difference was not statistically proven.

Parameter	Unit	Treatment		p
		Control X ±SD	BSM X ±SD	
Silage DM intake	kg DM/ animal/ day	3.74 ±0.12	3.97 ±0.17	0.065
Compound feed DM intake		1.74 ±0.0	1.74 ±0.0	0.000
Total DM intake[1]		6.36 ±0.12	6.59 ±0.17	0.065
Total Metabolizable Energy (ME) intake	MJ/ animal/ day	69.27 ±1.33	72.34 ±1.97	*
Feed Conversion Rate	MJ of ME / kg gain	69.52 ±3.49	67.15 ±2.26	0.298

Table 10. The effect of the treatment with the commercial product BSM on silage DM, energy intake, and feed conversion rate
* denotes statistical significance at level 0.05
[1] 1 kg/ animal/ day of barley straw (88% of DM, 3.9 MJ ME/ kg DM) was included in the diet for both treatments

The inoculation with the microbial silage inoculant had a significant positive effect on whole crop corn silage quality in terms of:

- lowering pH and shifting fermentation towards lactic acid,
- suppressing butyric acid, ethanol and ammonia-N formation,
- significantly reducing DM losses,
- statistically increasing digestible and metabolizable energy,
- statistically significant improvements in aerobic stability, and
- improvements in the silage intake and performance of beef cattle, and a positive effect on the utilization of feed energy.

6. Limiting factors in the use of probiotic strains for silages on the farm

Many factors have been associated with failures in the use of probiotic strains as silage inoculants. They could be related to ambient factors, to the strains themselves and to the application.

6.1. Limiting factors related to the ambient

- **Water soluble carbohydrates (WSC)**: These are main sources of energy for lactic acid bacteria. There is a lack of WSC in crops wilted for long periods [74]. Low concentrations of WSC in herbage, even in inoculated ones, can lead to a decrease in silage quality [75, 76].
- **Water content and water activity in the crop**: The lack of water in the material to be ensiled can seriously affect the growth of LAB. Harvesting at low moisture levels worsens the compacting and therefore the exclusion of oxygen in the ensiled material.

- **Ambient temperatures at ensiling**: Extreme low or high temperatures can affect the performance of probiotic strains used as silage inoculants. Regions in Northern Europe and Canada could be affected by low temperatures in September/ October, in some cases below 0°C during the night. However it is important to note that daytime temperatures which coincide with the time of silage making are more important. Ambient temperatures of around 10°C during silage making could be considered the lowest limit for the activity of probiotic strains [77]. On the other hand, a combination of high temperatures (>35°C) and high humidity could negatively influence the ensiling process. It is well known that *Pediococci* are more resistant to higher temperatures than *Lactobacilli* [78], which could lead to the possibility of developing silage inoculants for tropical regions.

6.2. Limiting factors related to probiotic strains

- **Viability of the probiotic strains**: This is closely related to storage conditions. High temperatures and/ or high humidity have been associated with lower survival rates in available commercial products (DLG, 2011). The shelf life varies between six months (granulates) and 18 to 24 months (powders for liquid application).
- **Competitiveness vs. epiphytic microflora**: Bacteria contained in the silage inoculants have to compete successfully against the wild microflora living on plants. Many probiotic strains fail in the selection process for silage additives due to their low capacity to grow more rapidly or suppress other undesirable micro-organisms. A classic example is *Propionibacterium* where the production of propionic acid could be of great importance in extending the duration of silage aerobic stability. Unfortunately *Propionibacterium* grows more slowly than other bacteria and is affected by low pH values [79, 80].
- **Concentration of the probiotic strains in commercial products**: The scientific community [78] and manufacturers [33] agree that the minimal concentration of lactic acid bacteria is 1×10^5 cfu/ g of silage. The concentration in the silage can be easily calculated by multiplying the concentration in the product by the dosage per ton, and dividing by 1×10^6. As simple as this seems, big differences between declared concentrations and real concentrations have been found in our own research. However, the concentration of in cfu/ g of silage cannot be the only criterion for selecting a silage inoculant. Selection must also include the ability to decrease the pH value (high lactic acid production) and/ or improve the aerobic stability (for example acetic acid production).

6.3. Limiting factors related to the application

- **Quality of diluted water**: It is a well-researched fact that chlorinated water can decrease the effectiveness of probiotic strains. One important aspect is also the microbiological quality of water. Often, water is contaminated with *E. coli*, the bacterium responsible for nutrient losses and fecal odor in the silage.

-   **Tank shelf life**: Storage conditions in the applicator tank differ in terms of temperature, chlorine content, toxic residues and sunlight. It is therefore strongly recommended that products are used within 24 to 48 hours after dilution. The user should be aware that he is working with live micro-organisms which can survive and be effective only if favorable conditions are created for them. An important selling point, for example, was in Australia where the tank shelf life was extended by over one week. Special attention should be paid to that: it is not about what is easier, but what is more effective.
-   **Dry application vs. powder application**: Addition of bacteria to water was more effective than a dry application of the same bacteria in lowering the pH of wilted grass silage and wilted alfalfa silage (450 and 550 g DM/ kg) [81, 82, cited by 74].

Abbreviations

BSM	Biomin® BioStabil Mays
BSP	Biomin® BioStabil Plus
cfu	Colony forming units
CT	Control treatment
DE	Digestible energy
DM	Dry matter
ECM	Energy corrected milk
LAB	Lactic acid bacteria
ME	Metabolizable energy
NEL	Net energy lactation
WSC	Water soluble carbohydrates

Author details

Yunior Acosta Aragón
Biomin Holding GmbH, Herzogenburg, Austria

7. References

[1] Caneva G, Nugari MP and O. Salvadori Plant Biology for Cultural Heritage: Biodeterioration and Conservation. ISBN 978-0-89236-939-3, 70. (2009)

[2] Wilkins RJ, Syrjala-Qvist L and Bolsen KK. The future role of silage in sustainable animal production. Proceedings of the XIIth International Silage Conference. Uppsala, Sweden. 1999, 23-40. (1999)

[3] UN News Centre. World cereal prices surge to 10-year highs due to poor harvests, biofuel demand– UN. Available from: http://www.un.org/apps/news/story.asp?NewsID=20878&Cr=food&Cr1   (accessed 30.06.2008). (2006)

[4] Klein CAM and Ledgard SF. An analysis of environmental and economic implications of nil and restricted grazing systems designed to reduce nitrate leaching from New

Zealand dairy farms. I. Nitrogen losses. New Zealand Journal of Agricultural Research, 2001. Vol. 22. 201-215. (2001):

[5] Muller CJC and Botha JA. Production responses of lactating Jersey cows on two intensive grazing systems versus a zero-grazing system. 32nd Congress of the Grassland Society of Southern Africa. 20 - 23 Jan., 1997. 90. (1997)

[6] Ogle B. Suggestions for intensive livestock-based smallholder systems in semi-arid areas of Tanzania. Livestock research for Rural Development. Vol. 2, 1. Available from: www.cipav.org.co/lrrd/lrrd2/1/ogle.htm (accessed 14.07.2009). (1990)

[7] Rooke JA. Acetate silages: microbiology and chemistry. Landbauforschung Voelkenrode Sonderheft 123, 309-312. Schroeder, J. W. (2004): Silage fermentation and preservation. NDSU Extension Service, North Dakota State University. Available from: www.ext.nodak.edu/extpubs/ansci/dairy/as1254w.htm (accessed 22.05.2011). (1991)

[9] Macaulay A. Silage Production – Introduction. Available from: http://www1.agric.gov.ab.ca/$department/deptdocs.nsf/all/for4912 (accessed 12.01.2011). (2003)

[10] Moon NJ. Inhibition of the growth of acid tolerant yeasts by acetate-lactate and propionic and their synergistic mixture. J. Appl. Bacteriol., 55: 435-460. (1983)

[11] Burns H, Piltz J, Kaiser A, Blackwood I and Grifiths N. Making high quality silage. Research Update for Growers- Southern Region (High Rainfall)- August 2005. Available from: www.grdc.com.au/growers/res_upd/hirain/h05/burns.htm (accessed 04.02.2012). (2005)

[12] McDonald P, Henderson AR and Heron SJE (eds). The Biochemistry of Silage. Second Edition. Chalcombe Publications. Bucks, England. (1991)

[13] Knický M. Possibilities to improve silage conservation. Effects of crop, ensiling technology and additives. Doctoral thesis at the Swedish University of Agricultural Science Uppsala, 2005, 9. (2005)

[14] Jones CM, Heinrichs AJ, Roth GW and Ishler VA. From harvest to feed: Understanding silage management. Available from: www.das.psu.edu/dairynutrition/documents/silage2004.pdf (Accessed 17.03.2011). (2004)

[15] Weddell JR, Agnew R and Cottrill B. The UK Forage Additives Approval Scheme - Developments and Products Approvals. Proceedings of the XIIIth International Silage Conference. Auchincruive, Scotland. 2002, 230-231. (2002)

[16] Ziggers D. Good or bad guys determine silage quality. Dairy and beef. Vol. 2, 27-29. (2003)

[17] Fiedoruk K and Zaremba ML. Performance Estimation of Nested PCR-Based Assays for Direct Detection of *Listeria monocytogenes* in Artificially Contaminated Materials. Polish J. of Environ. Stud. Vol. 19, No. 2 (2010), 293-299. (2009)

[18] Oude Elferink SJWH, Driehuis F, Gottschal JC and Spoelstra SF. Silage fermentation processes and their manipulation (Paper 2.0). Silage Making in the Tropics with Particular Emphasis on Smallholders. ISSN 0259-2517. Proceedings of the FAO Electronic Conference on Tropical Silage, 01.09. to 15.12.1999. (1999)

[19] Wilkinson JM. Silage. Chalcombe publications. ISBN 0 94861750 0. p: 1-20, 107. (2005)

[20] McDonald P. The biochemistry of silages. ISBN: 0 0471 X. pp: 91- 93, 174. (1981)

[21] Tucker G and Featherstone S. Essentials of Thermal processing. Wiley Blackwel. ISBN: 978-1-4051-9058-9, 288. (2011)

[22] Pahlow G. Praxishandbuch Futterkonservierung. 7th ed. DLG Verlag 2006. ISBN 3 7690 0677 1, 18-19. (2006)

[23] Noda F, Hayashi K, Mizunuma T. Influence of pH on inhibitory activity of acetic acid on osmophilic yeasts used in brine fermentation of soy sauce. Appl. Environ. Microbiol. 43: 245-246, 1982. 599. (1982)

[24] Danner H, Holzer M, Mayrhuber E and Braun R. Acetic acid increases stability of silage under aerobic conditions. Applied and Environmental Microbiology 69: 1, 562-567. (2003)

[25] Driehuis F and van Wikselaar PG. Effects of addition of formic, acetic or propionic acid to maize silage and low dry matter grass silage on the microbial flora and aerobic stability. p. 256-257. In: D.I.H. Jones, R. Jones, R. Dewhurst, R. Merry, and P.M. Haigh (ed.) Proc. 11th Int. Silage Conference, Aberystwyth, UK. 8-11 September 1996. IGER, Aberystwyth, UK. (1996)

[26] Driehuis F, Oude Elferink S JWH. and Spoelstra SF. Anaerobic lactic acid degradation during ensilage of whole crop corn inoculated with *Lactobacillus buchneri* inhibits yeast growth and improves aerobic stability. J. Appl. Microbiol. 87, 583-594. (1999)

[27] Acosta Aragón Y and Rodrigues I. Contaminación de ensilados con micotoxinas. Proceedings of the XIVth Latin American Congress of Buiatrics 2009. Lima, Peru. (2009)

[28] Sumarah MW, Miller JD and Blackwell BA. Isolation and metabolite production by *Penicillium roqueforti, P. paneum* and *P. crustosum* isolated in Canada. Mycopathologia. Volume 159, Number 4 (2005), 571-577. (2005)

[29] Walker C. Relationship between dimorphology and respiration in *Mucor genevensis* studied with chloramphenicol. J. Bacteriol. 1973 Nov; 116(2): 972-80. (1973)

[30] Saarisalo E, Skyttä E, Haikara A, Jalava T and Jaakkola S. Screening and selection of lactic acid bacteria strains suitable for ensiling grass. Journal of Applied Microbiology, 102, 327-336. (2007)

[31] Bolsen KK, Ashbell G and Wilkinson JM. Silage additives. In: Biotechnology in Animal Feeds and Animal Feeding. Edited by R. J. Wallace and A. Chesson. Weinheim: 33-54. (1995)

[32] Hinds MA, Bolsen KK, Brethour I, Milliken G and Hoover J. Effects of molasses, urea and bacterial inoculant additives on silage quality, dry matter recovery and feeding value for cattle. Anim. Feed Sci. Technol., 12: 205-205. (1985)

[33] DLG (Deutsche LandwirtschaftsGesellschaft). Praxishandbuch Futter- and Substratkonser-vierung. 8. Vollständig überarbeitete Auflage. DLG Verlag, ISBN 978-3-7690-0791-6, 284-327. (2011)

[34] Kung LJr and Ranjit NK. The effect of Lactobacillus buchneri and other additives on the fermentation and aerobic stability of barley silage. Journal of Dairy Science, v.84, n.5, p.1149-1155, 2001. (2001)

[35] Filya I, Karabulut A and Sucu E. The effect of *Lactobacillus plantarum* and *Lactobacillus buchneri* on the fermentation, aerobic stability and ruminal degradability of corn silage in warm climate. Proceedings of the XIII International Silage Conference. (2002)

[36] Dawson E, Rust RS and Yokoyama MT. Improved fermentation and aerobic stability of ensiled, high moisture corn with the use of Propionibacterium acidipropionici. J. Dairy Sci. 81:1015-1021. (1998)

[37] Weinberg ZG and Muck RE. New trends and opportunities in the development and use of inoculants for silage. FEMS Microbiol. Rev. 19, 53-68. (1996)

[38] Mayer R. Balage: A method of increasing usable forage value per acre. Available from: http://www.extension.iastate.edu/agdm/articles/mayer/MayAug99.htm (accessed 23.10.2010). (1999)

[39] Pöllinger A. Gärheu als alternative Konservierungsform für Grünlandfutter. 15. Alpenländisches Expertenforum. Grundfutterqualität – aktuelle Ergebnisse und zukünftige Entwicklungen 26. März 2009 LFZ Raumberg-Gumpenstein. (2009)

[40] Kenney D. Botulism in horses and haylage. Available from: http://www.omafra.gov.on.ca/english/livestock/horses/facts/info_botulism.htm (accessed 19.11.2008). (2001)

[41] Ryser TE and Marth EH. *Listeria*, listerosis and food safety, 3rd edition. Marcell. Dekker, N.Y. (2007)

[42] Kent BA, Arambel MJ and Walters JL. Effect of bacterial inoculant on alfalfa haylage: ensiling characteristics and milk production response when fed to dairy cows in early lactation. J. Dairy Sci. 71: 2457-2461. (1988)

[43] Omafra Staff. Forages: Harvest and Storage. Available from: http://www.omafra.gov.on.ca/english/crops/pub811/3harvest.htm (accessed 20.03.2012). (2011)

[44] Acosta Aragón Y. The contribution of silage inoculants in the disease prevention. Proceedings of the 14th International Conference on Production Diseases in Farm Animals, Gent, Belgium. (2010)

[45] Acosta Aragón Y, Jatkauskas J and Vrotniakiene V. The Effect of a Silage Inoculant on Silage Quality, Aerobic Stability and Milk Production. Iranian Journal of Animal Science. Accepted Dec. 2011. (2011)

[46] Kramer W. Neue Entwicklungen und Strategien im Bereich der Silierzusätze. 8. Alpenländisches Expertenforum, 9. – 10. April 2002, Bundsanstalt für alpenländische Landwirtschaft, Österreich. (2002)

[47] Jatkauskas J and Vrotniakiene V. Effect of *Lactobacillus rhamnosus* and *Propionibacterium freudenreichii* inoculated silage on nutrient utilization by dairy cows. ISSN 1392-2130. Veterinarija ir Zootechnika. T. 36 (58). 2006. (2006)

[48] Winters AL, Lloyd J, Leemans, D. Lowes K and Merry R. Effect of inoculation with *Lactobacillus plantarum* on protein degradation during ensilage of red clover. Proceedings of the XIIIth International Silage Conference, Auchincruive, Scotland, 108 - 109. (2002)

[49] Kung LJr. Use of forage additives in silage fermentation. 2000-01 Direct-fed Microbial, Enzyme and Forage Additive Compendium. The Miller Publishing Company, Minnesota, USA, 39-44. (2000)

[50] Filya I, Ashbell G, Hen Y and Weinberg ZG. The effect of bacterial inoculants on the fermentation and aerobic stability of whole crop wheat silage. Anim. Feed Sci. Technol., 2000; 88: 39-46. (2000)

[51] Muck RE, Filya I and Contreras-Govea FE. Inoculant effects on alfalfa silage: *In vitro* gas and volatile fatty acid production. J. Dairy Sci. vol. 90, 5115–5125. (2007)

[52] Muck RE and Kung LJr. Effects of silage additives on ensiling. Silage: Field to Feedbunk. NRAES-99. Northeast Reg. Agric. Eng. Serv., Ithaca, NY, 187-199. (1997)

[53] Spiekers H. Praxishandbuch Futterkonservierung. Grundlagen. Einleitung und Zielgrößen. 7. Auflage 2006. ISBN 3-7690-0677-1. 10. (2006)

[54] Ohmomo S, Tanaka O, Kitamoto HK and Cai Y. Silage and microbial performance, old story but new problems. Japanese Agricultural Research. 36 (2), 59-71. (2002)

[55] Weinberg ZG, Muck RE, Weimer PJ, Chen Y and Gamburg M. Lactic acid bacteria used in inoculants for silage as probiotics for ruminants. App. Biochem. and Biotechnol. Vol. 118, 2004. (2004)

[56] Weinberg ZG, Ashbell G, Hen Y, Azrieli A, Szakacs G and Filya I. Ensiling whole-crop wheat and corn in large containers with *Lactobacillus plantarum* and *Lactobacillus buchneri*. J. Ind. Microbiol. Biotechnol. Vol. 28, 7-11. (2002)

[57] Inglis GD, Yanke LJ, Kawchuk LM and McAllister TA. The influence of bacterial inoculants on the microbial ecology of aerobic spoilage of barley silage. Canadian J. of Microbiol./ Rev. Canadian Microbiol., 45 (1), 77-87. (1999)

[58] Ranjit NK and Kung LJr. The effect of *Lactobacillus buchneri, Lactobacillus plantarum,* or chemical preservative on the fermentation and aerobic stability of corn silage. J. Dairy Sci. vol. 83, 526-535. (2000)

[59] Winters AL, Fychan R and Jones R. Effect of formic acid and a bacterial inoculant on the amino acid composition of grass silage and on animal performance. Grass and Forage Science 2001. Vol. 56, 181-192. (2001)

[60] Pennington J. Reducing somatic cell count in dairy cattle. Cooperative Extension Service, Division of Agriculture, University of Arkansas, FSA 4002. http://www.uaex.edu/Other_Areas/publications/PDF/FSA-4002.pdf (Accessed 01.11.11) (2011)

[61] Schukken YH, Wilson DJ, Welcome F, Garrison-Tikofsky L and Gonzalez RN. Monitoring udder health and milk quality using somatic cell counts. Vet. Res. 34 (2003), 579-596. (2003)

[62] Fellner V, Phillip LE, Sebastian S. and Idziak EE. Effects of a bacterial inoculant and propionic acid on preservation of high moisture ear corn, and on rumen fermentation, digestion and growth performance of beef cattle. Can. J. Anim. Sci. 81, 273-280. (2001)

[63] Kamarloiy M and Yansari AT. Effect of microbial inoculants on the nutritive value of corn silage for beef cattle. Pakistan Journal of Biological Science. 11 (8): 1137-41. (2008)

[64] Acosta Aragón Y, Jatkauskas J and Vrotniakiene V. The Effect of a Silage Inoculant on Silage Quality, Aerobic Stability, and Meat Production on Farm Scale. ISRN Veterinary Science, vol. 2012, 6 pages, 2012. (2012)

[65] Merry RJ, Jones R. and Theodorou MK. The conservation of grass. In: Hopkins A. (ed.), Grass. Its Production and Utilisation, 3rd Ed. Oxford: UK, Blackwell Science Ltd. (2000)

[66] Marciňáková M, Lauková A, Simonová M, Strompfová V, Koreneková B and Naď P. Probiotic properties of *Enterococcus faecium* EF9296 strain isolated from silage. Czech Journal of Animal Science, 53, 336-345. (2008)

[67] Davies DR. Silage inoculants – Where Next? In: V. Jambor, S. Jamborova, B. Vosynkova, P. Prochacka, D. Vosynkova and D. Kumprechtova (eds). Proceedings of the 14th International Symposium Forage Conservation, Brno. Mendel University, Czech Republic, 32-39. (2010)

[68] Jatkauskas J and Vrotniakiene V. Fermentation characteristics and nutritive value of inoculated corn silage. Proceedings of the 20th general meeting of EGF, Luzern, Switzerland, 21-24 June, 1077-1079. (2004)

[69] Pahlow G and Honig H. The role of microbial additives in the aerobic stability of silage. Proceedings of the 15th general meeting of EGF, The Netherlands, 149-152. (1994)

[70] Kung L, Stokes MR and Lin CJ. Silage additives. In: D.R. Buxton, R.E. Muck and J.H. Harison (eds) Agronomy Series No. 42. Silage Science and Technology. Madison, Wisconsin, USA, 305-360. (2003)

[71] Reis RA, Almeida GR, Siqueira GR, Bernardes ER and Janusckiewicz E. Microbial changes and aerobic stability in high moisture corn silages inoculated with *Lactobacillus buchneri*. In Park R.S and Stronge M.D. (ed.). Proceedings of the XIVth International Silage Conference, July 2005, Belfast, Northern Ireland. 223. (2005)

[72] Cooke L. New strains slow silage spoilage. Agric. Res., 40: 17. (1995)

[73] Luther RM. Effect of microbial inoculation of whole-plant corn silage on chemical characteristics, preservation and utilization by steers. J. Anim. Sci., 63, 13-29. (1986)

[74] Kung LJr. Potential factors that may limit the effectiveness of silage additives. Proceedings of the XVth International Silage Conference. July 27-29 2009, Madison, Wisconsin, USA, 37-45. (2009)

[75] Davies DR, Merry RJ, Williams AP, Bakewell EL, Leemans DK and Tweed JKJ. Proteolysis during ensilage of forages varying in soluble sugar content. J Dairy Sci. Feb; 81 (2): 444-53. (1998)

[76] Tyrolová Y and Výborná A. Effect of the stage of maturity on the leaf percentage of lucerne and the effect of additives on silage characteristics. Czech Journal of Animal Science, 53, 330-335. (2008)

[77] Resch R. Personal communication. LFZ, Research Institute, Raumberg- Gumpenstein, Austria. (2010)

[78] Cai Y, Kumai S, Ogawa M, Benno Y and Nakase T. Characterization and Identification of *Pediococcus* Species Isolated from Forage Crops and Their Application for Silage Preparation. Appl. Environ Microbiol. 65(7): 2901–2906. (1999)

[79] Filya I, Sucu E and Karabulut A. The effects of *Propionibacterium acidipropionici* and *Lactobacillus plantarum*, applied at ensiling, on the fermentation and aerobic stability of

low dry matter corn and sorghum silages. Journal of Industrial Microbiology & Biotechnology. Volume 33, Number 5 (2006), 353-358. (2006)

[80] Weinberg ZG, Ashbell G, Bolsen KK, Pahlow G, Hen Y and Azrieli A. The effect of a propionic acid bacterial inoculant applied at ensiling, with or without lactic acid bacteria, on the aerobic stability of pearl-millet and maize silages, J. Appl, Bacteriol. 78 (1995), 430-436. (1995)

[81] Whiter AG and Kung LJr. The effect of a dry or liquid application of *Lactobacillus plantarum* MTD1 on the fermentation of alfalfa silage. J. Dairy Sci. 84:2195-2202. 2001.

[82] Pahlow G and Weissbach F. New aspects of evaluation and application of silage additives. Landbauforschung, Volkenrode 206 (special issue): 141-158. (1999)

Chapter 4

Protective Effect of Probiotics Strains in Ruminants

Everlon Cid Rigobelo and Fernando Antonio de Ávila

Additional information is available at the end of the chapter

1. Introduction

In last 15 years the use of probiotics strains in animal production has been increased. These probiotics strains can modulate the balance and activities of the gastrointestinal microbiota in which are responsible to gut homeostasis. The intake of probiotics supplemented in ration and provided to the animals, can strongly affect the structure and activities of the gut microbial communities leading to promoting health and improving the performance in livestock, when it is impaired by numerous factors, such as dietary and management constraints. The understanding of the digestive ecosystems in terms of microbial composition and functional diversity is fundamental to modulate the gastrointestinal tract (GIT) of domestic animals providing to them the possibility to maintain the homeostasis of these complex microbial communities, which can be composed of bacteria, protozoa, fungi, archaea, and viruses, thus promoting a reduction of the incidence of diseases. Therefore considerable researchs during 30 years are characterizing the domestic animals 'GIT. The welfare, health and feed efficiency of the animals can be affected by different factors, many of them, environmental factors. Among these factors, feeding practices, composition of animal diets, farms management and productivity constraints can influence the microbial balance in GIT, whose role is fundamental to gut homeostasis and its reduction consequently can affect efficiency digestive When occurs the reduction of microbial in GIT, some reactions as digestion and fermentation of plant polymers are impaired, since the action of the microbiota on gut is strongly related with the realization these reactions, and the animals also are impaired by the fact these polymers to be of particular importance to the herbivorous (Chaucheyras-Durand and Durand, 2010).

2. Use of antibiotics

The problem caused by indiscriminate use of antibiotic as growth promoter in feed to livestock is that this practice has been associated with emergence of resistance to antibiotics in zoonotic bacteria. The use of growth promoter in feed to livestock has been done since 1940 because this practice is correlated with higher health status and improves at performance of animals in terms of feed conversion. The use of antibiotics at animal has had a profound impact on animal health and welfare.

The problems found by this practice require the development of alternative intervention strategies for zoonotic livestock pathogens. Some these strategies could be vaccines in diarrhea in neonates and post weaning animals, limited access to livestock, control of vermin, modifying air flow, high level disinfection regimes, acidification of feed and the supply of probiotic into animals supplemented in ration by example are efficient management to reduce the occurrence of pathogen at the animal production.

3. Use of probiotics strains

All additives used in animal feed, including yeasts and bacteria, are strictly regulated within the EU legislative framework. Until May 2003, the risk assessment of animal feed additives for use in European was the responsibility of the Scientific Commitee of Animal Nutrition (SCAN) (Anadon et al., 2006). After this date, the European Food Safety Authority (EFSA) took over the functions of SCAN. While EFSA provide expert scientific advice to the European Commission the approval and risk management of a probiotic product is responsibility of the EC and its constituent member's states. For use of microorganism in United States as a feed additive is necessary before the product to be outgoing to approval by the Food and Drug Administration (FDA).

The requirements for a novel probiotic product required by EU regulations on animal feed additives are the identification and characterization to species level, and the efficacy data must be provided in support of any claims made for the product. Some characteristics are requested to product such as no adverse effects on the health of performance, the product must be safe for the operator, have no adverse effects upon exposure and also the product must not pose a risk to the safety of the end-consumer (SCAN, 2001).

4. Use of probiotics to control gastrointestinal diseases in livestock

The intensive production farmed livestock together with the veto of the use of antimicrobial feed supplements in the EU, this situation has increased the risk of contracting gastrointestinal diseases if prophylactic antimicrobial feed supplements are not utilized. The removal of growth promoters has led to a significant increase in the incidence of diseases and also with significant increases in feed costs, the reduced feed weight conversion.

5. Use of probiotics in animals

Although the mechanisms involved have not been fully elucidated a reduction in pathogen carriage and subsequent clinical disease is one possible mechanisms responsible by reduction of occurrence of disease when the growth promoter is utilized in livestock. After this prohibition many problems arisen and also the need of use of alternatives to resolve this situation. One of these alternatives is the use of probiotics as feed supplement or functional food which may be used for prophylaxis in animals and humans. There are numerous probiotics products commercially available for livestock. Currently commercial livestock probiotic can be separated into two categories, being these, competitive exclusion that are defined and those that are undefined.

6. Use of probiotic in ruminants

In ruminants that have four stomachs being them rumen, omasum, reticle and abomasums when these animals born they have the abomasums extremely big. This situation occurs because the type of food is liquids as milk. Usually the animal becomes ruminants when he from the third or fourth month of age. This development is due the installation of microbiota ruminal in gut and also by distention of organ due the fiber intake. The bacteria from rumen and bowel are acquired through the contact of cattle with the cow or other animal and also by grass intake.

The rumen is as fermentation chamber and it has approximately for 50-85% by use of dry matter from food. The saliva is mixed with food and has a control upon pH of rumen and the papillae existing in inner wall of the rumen increasing the absorption area.

The amount of bacteria from rumen is the approximately 10^{11} CFU/g of counts rumen, the fungi is the 10^3 CFU/g and the protozoa is 10^5 cell /g. There are most of 60 species of bacteria that grow into rumen microbita and this environment has CO_2, CH_4 and N_2 stomach gas maintaining the pH value among $6 - 6.5$. The temperature within the rumen is 39°C and the bacteria type living can be characterized according to theirs functions such as cellulolytic, proteolytic, amylolytic.

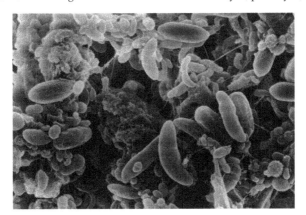

Picture 1. Picture took from Antibiotics and chemotherapeutic and probiotics
Avila et al Funep Publisher Brazil 83p.

The proteins and fibrous foods in rumen are converted at ammonia, organic acids and amino acids by microorganism's action. As the majority of amino acids are synthesized of rumen the animals need to be supplied with essential amino acids from ration or injectable. The main factors of stress feed that leaving to a decreasing of ruminal microbiota are dry grasslands, pastures in budding and seasonal changes. The decreasing of ruminal microbiota can be caused by antibiotics use and also environment changes as occur at auctions, expositions and pre-slaughter. The use of rumen bacteria into ruminants promotes the growth into gut before the establishment of pathogen in these animals causing the prevention of diarrhea occurrence. This situation decreases the weaning time and maintains the balance of rumen microbiota increasing the production of enzymes as cellulase, amylase, urease, protease consequently increasing improving the use fibrous foods. Others benefits to use of probiotics in ruminants are promotes the increasing of weight gain, increasing the milk production and decreasing of diarrhea period.

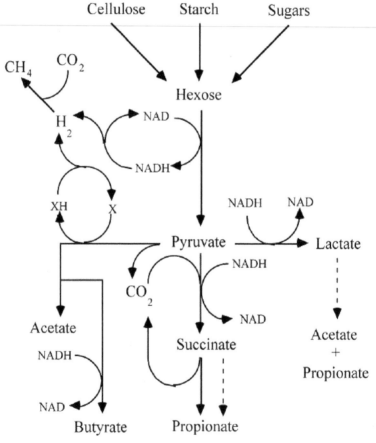

Picture 2. Picture took from Antibiotics and chemotherapeutic and probiotics Avila et al Funep Publisher Brazil 83p.

The advantages of the use of probiotics in livestock are the period of adaptation of animal is not necessary, doesn't hinder the management on the farm because it can be supplement to ration or mineral salt, and as probiotic is the natural product does not necessary the disposal of milk and also this product can be used during the slaughter of animals as cattle, sheep and buffaloes. According with FERREIRA, (2003) the probiotics microorganisms most used belong to the group of lactic bacteria as *Aerococcus, Atopobium, Bifidobacteirum, Brochothrix, Carnobacterium, Enterococcus, Lactobacillus, Weissella*. The lactic bacteria are positive Gram, anaerobic, negative catalase, presenting of cocos and bacillus way. The probiotics can counts ruminal bacterias as Ruminobacter and Succinovibrio with specifics characteristics that are used in supplementation of ruminants.

Some authors have been showed that some probiotics strains have seen resistant to the antibiotics effects and therefore these strains could be used together the administration of antibiotics in animals. The yeasts are unicellular microorganisms with capacity of survive in several mediums have a great spectrum of pH and many mediums can be saline or without oxygen. The *Saccharomyces boulardii* has been largely tested in human's trials (PENNA et al., 2000). And the *Saccharomyces cerevisiae* in animals showed promising results.

The *Lactobacillus* is constituted by cells that vary long and thin to short and curves with 1.5-6.0μm length and 0.6-0.9 width. The ideal temperature to growth is 45ºC and grows in pH 5.5-6.0. The Lactobacillus species known at moment is 56 and the most used as additive are *L. acidophilus, L. rhamnnosis and L. casei*.

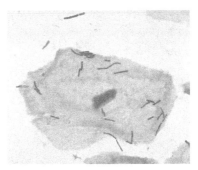

Picture 3. Picture took from Antibiotics and chemotherapeutic and probiotics Avila et al Funep Publisher Brazil 83p.

The genus *Bifidobacterium* includes 30 species. Many of these 10 are form humans dental caries, vagina and feces, 17 are from animal origin 2 are from wastewater and 1 of fermented milk. These bacteria present optimal growth among 37ºC and 41ºC and minimal growth among 25º C and 28ºC at pH 6-7. The *Bifidobacterium Bifidobacterium animallis, Bifidobacterium lactis, Bifidobacterium longum* species have probiotics characteristics also have capabilities to ferment complex carbon.

Some species of *Bacillus subtilis, Bacillus licheniformis* and *Bacillus cereus* are bacteria positive Gram in rods form. The Bacillus are the only that form spores allowing that these strains to be used in adverse conditions mainly in high temperature.

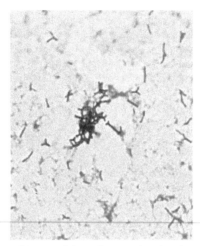

Picture 4. Picture took from Antibiotics and chemotherapeutic and probiotics Avila et al Funep Publisher Brazil 83p.

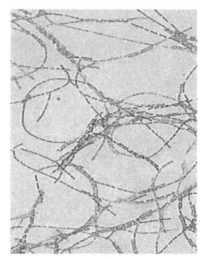

Picture 5. Picture took from Antibiotics and chemotherapeutic and probiotics Avila et al Funep Publisher Brazil 83p.

Enterococcus faecium is the microorganism belonged to the *Enterococcus* genus belonged to the Lancifield D group. This morphology identification requests the use of coloration by Gram and also catalase test in blade. These bacteria are positive Gram and present the characteristic form of streptococcus (chain cocos), negative catalase and no spore and faculty anaerobic. Through the chemical analysis the strain ferment the lactose, arabinose, mannitol, no ferment the sorbitol. This strain growth into MacConkey medium containing 6.5% of NaCl.

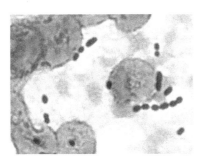

Picture 6. Picture took from Antibiotics and chemotherapeutic and probiotics Avila et al Funep Publisher Brazil 83p.

Ruminobacter amylophilum is the microorganism belonged to the Ruminobacter genus to its morphology identification is necessary to use Gram coloration this genus present as rods negative Gram. They have motility and no spores. This ferments the cornflour, maltose and liquefy gelatin. They synthesize lactic acid and CO_2 from formic acid.

7. Others benefits and action mode of probiotics strains

7.1. Immune modulation

The maturation of the humoral immune mechanisms can be conducted by microbial colonization, this events can promote the c circulation of the IgA and IgM secreting cells. The other important factor that can be affected by microbial colonization on the gut of different animals particularly the ruminants are the balance of the different T helper subsets. The memory B and T cells migrate to effectors sites in consequence these events.

Other mechanisms to immune modulation are followed by active proliferation local induction of certain cytokines and production of secretion antibodies as IgA. When the host is exposure to the antigen, immune cells respond releasing cytokines from host direct the subsequent immune responses. The low-dose tolerance immunity TGF-B associated in via local cytokine is the man mechanisms which the gut associated lymphoid tissue maintains homeostasis. Some lactic acid bacteria can induces the production of proinflammatory cytokines, tumor necrosis factors alpha and interleukin-6 from human peripheral blood mononuclear cells. A strain of *Lactobacillus casei* can inhibit the growth of pathogenic strains as *Pseudomonas aeruginosa* and *Listeria monocytogenes* leading to an increase in the level of macrophages. Others strains as *Lactobacillus acidophilus* and *Bifidobacterium bifidum* could inhance non-specific immunity and concluded that specific lactic acid bacteria could play a role in specific age groups, specific neonates or the elderly. The results can be observed when two groups of animals are compared itself in relation with their age. Usually the positive effect against the colonization by pathogenic bacteria upon the gut occurs most efficiently in neonates than oldest.

Some studies showed a significant increase in IgA immune response. In others, on children with mild to moderate stable Crohn´s Diseases, administration with strain GG improved the gut barrier function and clinical status after six months of therapy.

8. Antitumor activity

Some probiotic strains could decrease some enzymes synthesized by many microorganisms may convert procarcinogens into carcinogens and cause colon cancer, some of them azoreductase, β- glucuronidase and nitroreductase. *Lactobacillus acidophilus* could decrease nitroreductase, azoreductase and β glucuronidase activities in carnivorous animals. Another strain as *Lactobacillus rhamnosus* could bacterial β-glucuronidase activity in the large intestine.

Lactobacillus and Lactobacillus bulgaricus suppressed Ehrlich ascitis tumor or Sarcoma 180 in mice. Tumor suppression in associated with intact viable cells, intact dead cells and cell wall fragments or Lactobacilli and Bifidobacteria. When *Lactobaacillus casei* was provided into rats it had effective prevention against the recurrence of superficial bladder cancer.

Nitites used in food processing are converted to carcinogenic nitrosamines in the gastrointestinal tract in several people. Cellular uptake of nitites by *Lactobacillus* and *Bifidobacteria* has been shown in vivo. Also, Lactobacillus has been shown as a great reducer of bile salts. They are implicated in the initiation of colon carcinogens. These strains have been biotransformed of primary to secondary bile salts, this way, there are reduction the possible initiation of cancer. Other authors have been suggested that the decrease of intestinal pH, through metabolic activities of Lactobacillus acid bacteria, could inhibit the growth of putrefactive bacteria, can prevent large bowel cancer.

Many probiotics strains have a positive effect against mould growth and aflatoxin production. These aflatoxins are associated to cause cancer. Thus the reduction of these moulds decrease the occurrence of cancer caused by this mould.

9. Reduction of cholesterol

Some studies have showed the effect of fermented milk or milk containing probiotic strains producing lactic acid on serum cholesterol levels. These studies reported that a strain of *Streptococcus thermophilus* and *Lactobacillus acidophilus* reduced cholesterol levels in rats. Milk fermented with lactic acid bacteria and *Streptococcus cerevisae* led to lower serum cholesterol than control group, also phospholipids and bile acids in the fecal samples from mice were lower. When a trial was using rats inoculated with *E. faecium* , they presented a lower cholesterol levels. The same findings were observed in pigs that have been fed a high cholesterol diet.

Another results also, showed that the serum lipoprotein levels of 334 individuals remained unchanged when they were treated with *Lactobacillus acidophilus* and *L. delbrueckii* subsp *bulgaricus* and *E. faecium* administered over six weeks to adults and it resulted in a initial increase in total cholesterol and LDL followed by a sharp decrease two weeks after termination of treatment. The decrease corresponded with an increase in the reduction of iodonitrotetrazolium and superoxide production by peripheral neutrophils and an elevated production of IgG. Several studies don´t explain because there was the reduction in cholesterol levels and suggest that the reduction of cholesterol is not due to assimilation or to a direct interaction between the bacteria and cholesterol. This effect is due to the co-precipitation of cholesterol with deconjugated bile salts at pH value below 6.0. This would not explain the reduction of cholesterol in vivo as the pH of the bower gastrointestinal is neutral to alkaline. Probably there is a physical association between cholesterol and the cell surface.

10. Decreasing of lactose intolerance

Some descents from Asia and Africa usually are stricken by lack the intestinal mucosal enzyme β-galactosidase and therefore suffer from reduction in lactase activity. This situation can occur many times after an infection caused rotavirus gastroenteritis. There are much lactic bacteria which are capable to synthesize the enzyme β-galactosidase. Many of them as the bacteria *Streptococcus salivarius* subps *thermophilus* and *Lactobacillus delbrueckii* subps *bulgaricus*. The levels of enzyme produced by these bacteria are high and many products treated with this enzyme presented a low concentration of lactose. These species are sensitive to bile salts. These substances can lead to release of high levels of β-galactosidase in the gastrointestinal tract. Lactose from fermented milk containing the probiotic *Lactobacillus acidophilus* were better absorbed by many people with lower β-galactosidase activity. All symptoms from lactose intolerance were decreased.

11. Stool transit

The diarrhea occurrences in neonate are the main cause of death. This disorder affects animals of many species and also the human among them the children. *Lactobacillus* GG had a high decreasing in severity of acute watery diarrhea in young children. Patients treated on erythromycin reacted decreasing the period of diarrhea when they received *Lactobacillus* GG.

The symptoms caused by slow stool transit are diarrhea, stomach pain, abdominal pain and nausea. All symptoms were recovery quickly when the patients received *Lactobacillus* GG. Indeed one of the most severe diarrhea is that caused by *Clostridum difficile*. Usually people stricken by this disease recently passed by treatment with antibiotics. The supply of *Lactobacillus rhamnosus* improved the symptoms of intestinal disorders.

Patients who consumed milk fermented by the strain experienced less diarrhea than those that don't received. Many of them were patients that were being treated with pelvic radiotherapy. The effect of different LAB n different types of diarrhea has been showed in many studies. Yet are needed others studies to determine which mechanisms the LAB use to relieve diarrhea.

From now on this chapter will present some findings from some trials that were performed with the aim of verifying the protective effect of a probiotic mix that was kindly donated by IMEVE Biotecnology located in Jaboticabal São Paulo State against the colonization caused by STEC in sheep.

Abstract: Shiga toxin-producing *Escherichia coli* (STEC) strains are food-borne pathogens that cause human diseases, and ruminants are usually important reservoirs of STEC. The first step of enteric infection is colonization of the host's gut mucosal surface by pathogenic strains of bacteria. Probiotic bacteria can decrease the severity of infection by competing for receptors and nutrients and by synthesizing an acid that creates an unfavorable environment for the growth of several bacterial species. The aim of this study was to determine whether the inoculation of sheep with a mixture containing 5×10^8 (CFU) of *Lactobacillus acidophilus, Lactobacillus helveticus, Lactobacillus bulgaricus, Lactobacillus lactis, Streptococcus thermophilus* and *Enterococcus faecium* per animal decreases the shedding at animals previously inoculated with STEC nonO157. Sheep that received oral inoculums containing 2×10^9 viable bacteria of STEC carriers of *stx1, stx2* and *eae* genes were compared with others groups that did not receive inoculums. When probiotic was inoculated together with the STEC non-O157, the numbers of these same bacteria in a fecal sample were lower than the group did not receive. It occurred during the 3th, 5th, 6th and 7th weeks post-inoculation. Thus, we conclude that this mixture likely presented a potential protective effect in reducing colonization by STEC non-O157 and can be used as an alternative method to decreases STEC non-157 infection in sheep, thereby reducing transmission to humans.

12. STEC diseases

Healthy cattle, sheep and other ruminants can be reservoirs of Shiga-toxin-producing *Escherichia coli* (STEC) strains. STEC have been associated with human diseases such as hemorrhagic colitis and hemolytic uremic syndrome (Hussein 2007; Ramamurthy 2008). These bacteria can be transmitted from person to person (Belongia et al., 1993), but most outbreaks have been associated with the consumption contaminated beef products or a variety of other foods. Before colonization by STEC, it may be possible to determine whether to use the colonization of ruminal mucosa by oral administration of probiotic bacteria as a strategy (Ávila et al., 2000).

Probiotics are live microorganisms that, when administered in the appropriate amount, will benefit the health of the host (Food and Agriculture Organization of the United Nations, 2003; Sanders, 2003). Microbial interference is common to all genera and decreases the severity of infection by mechanisms involving nutrient competition, generation of an unfavorable environment, and competition for attachment or adhesion sites (Chaucheyras-Durand and Durand, 2010). Probiotics bacteria can stimulate the immune system through innate cell surface pattern recognition receptors or via direct lymphoid cell activation. Practical applications for this action of probiotics based on this characteristic include their use in anti-tumor, anti-allergy and immunotherapy treatments, but there is also increasing evidence that some probiotics can sufficiently stimulate a protective immune response to enhance resistance to microbial pathogens (Cross, 2002).

The benefits caused for use of probiotics strains in ruminants are known, however there are few information about the use of probiotics strains to reduction of shedding of STEC non-O157 in sheep.

This study verified the protective effect of probiotic treatment against the colonization of STEC non-O157 in sheep measured the number of STEC recovered from fecal simple.

13. Materials and methods

13.1. Animals and experimental locations

The study was performed with 20 sheep of Santa Ines race in the fattening stage, female previously screened by not be carrying of STEC non-O157 strains distributed in four groups with five animals each that were confined at a property located in São Paulo State. The experiment was made January to March 2012. The sheep were selected based on closeness of body weight (41 ± 2) kg and age (9-12) months. Then, all animals were ear-tagged and drenched with Ivomec (MSD- Agvet Merck) for internal parasite control at the rate of 2cc/46kg body weight. During three weeks pre-experimental adaptation period, were offered for all groups of sheep a diet of identical composition *ad libitum* consumption. Group I did not receive the probiotics strains or STEC non-O157 being the control group. Group II received an only oral dose of inoculums containing 2×10^9 viable cell of STEC non-O157 per animal. Group III received an only oral dose of inoculums containing 2×10^9 viable cell of STEC non-O157 per animal together with daily oral doses at concentration of 5×10^8 CFU of *Lactobacillus acidophilus, Lactobacillus helveticus, Lactobacillus bulgaricus, Lactobacillus lactis, Streptococcus thermophilus* and *Enterococcus faecium* per animal lyophilized provided directly in the mouth of animals with help of a cannula of application throughout the experiment. The inoculums were provided with help of a cannula of application and were diluted at 40mL of 0.9% saline solution. Group IV received the probiotics alone at the same number of cells viable and of the same way. During three weeks before of start of experiment always in same hour in the morning were collected feces samples directly of rectum of these animals. The samples were cultured in plate on MacConkey agar then the colonies that grew had their DNA extracted as described by Wani et al. (2003) to verify the absence of STEC non-O157 and *Salmonella*. After the third week the groups of animals were inoculated and monitored by seven weeks with weekly collections of their feces. All animals of present study were not carrying STEC non-O157 before inoculation and were kept in bays separated to avoid cross contamination throughout the experiment in an environmentally controlled building. Each pen had a concrete floor with individual drain, a feeding box and water through and was cleaned once a day and the fecal material deposited was transported to other place where it was composted.

This study was conducted in accordance with the ethical guidelines for investigations involving laboratory animals and was approved by the Ethics in Animal Research Committee (EARC) of UNESP-Univi Estadual Paulista and no adverse effects were observed in the animals receiving the *E. coli* (STEC) and probiotics during the experiment.

14. Probiotic

The probiotics bacteria used were *Bacillus cereus, Lactobacillus acidophilus* and *Enterococcus faecium* all strains in amount of 3×10^8 (CFU). These strains were isolated from sheep rumina and intestinal tracts following the recommendations of Hungate (1975) and Wolf et al.

(1975). These bacteria have the following features: they are nonpathogenic, enzyme-producing and resistant to lactic acid and low pH. These strains were kindly donated by Imeve Medications Veterinary Industry responsible by all tests realized concerning the quality and conditions of use.

15. STEC non-O157

To verify the protective effect of probiotics strains reducing the shedding of STEC was used a STEC non-O157 strain isolated from healthy sheep and characterized as described by Possé et al., (2007). It was kindly donated by Laboratory of bacteriological from UNESP Jaboticabal.

16. Samples

For seven weeks, post-inoculation feces samples in same hour in the morning were collected from the sheep and transported to the laboratory, where DNA was extracted. Bacterial strains grown overnight in nutrient broth (Sigma) at 37° C were pelleted by centrifugation at 12,000g for 1 min, resuspended in 200m L of sterile distilled water, and lysed by boiling for 10min. Lysates were centrifuged as described above, and 150m L of the supernatants was used as DNA template for the PCR (Wani et al. , 2003). All isolates were subjected to PCR; *stx1*, *stx2*, and *eae* genes were detected using the primers and PCR conditions described by China et al. (1996). Control reference strains were *E. coli* EDL 933 (O157:H7, *stx1*, *stx 2*, *eae*) and *E. coli* K12 (negative control).

17. STECs recuperated

The values of STEC in each sample were determined of two different methods of counting. In both 1 g of each fecal sample was collected, cultured on MacConkey agar, then it was incubated at 37°C for 24 h. In the first counting, all colonies grown displaying similar genome to STEC non-O157 strain previously inoculated orally were counted. In second counting were selected at least five colonies per sample grown and then separated in STEC non-O157 displaying pattern genome the others isolates from *E. coli* that did not display this specific DNA patterns.

18. *E. coli* STEC fingerprint by pulsed-field gel electrophoresis (PFGE) of chromosomal DNA

Genomic DNAs from STEC non-O157 isolates cultured from sheep were prepared as previously described by Barret et al., 1994. The agarose-embedded DNA was digested with 10U of *XbaI*/plug (Gibco BRL) at 37°C overnight. PFGE was performed in a CHEF-DR II unit (Bio-Rad Laboratories, Hercules, Calif.) using 1% PFGE grade Tris Borate EDTA buffer gels. The DNA was electrophoresed for 20 hours at a constant voltage of 200V (6V/cm) pulse time of 5 to 50 s, an electric field angle of 120° and a temperature of 15°C before being stained with ethidium bromide. Resulting patterns were analyzed on a DNA Pro Scan, ProRFLP program (DNA Proscan, Inc. Nashville, Tenn), and the size of the DNA fragments was used as the criteria for categorizing distinct patterns.

19. Results

The animals received inoculums containing only one isolate of STEC non-O157 carriers of *stx1, stx2* and *eae* genes. After three day post inoculations fecal samples were collected from these animals to make the re-isolating of the strains STEC non-O157 that had been previously inoculated into animals. All strains isolated from fecal samples had their DNA patterns compared with DNA pattern from STEC non-O-157 strain previously inoculated into animals and all those strains had the DNA similar to the strain previously inoculated were counted.

From strains isolated from fecal simples collected during the three weeks prior to inoculation of animals no STEC strain had the similar DNA to the DNA pattern from strains of STEC non-O157 previously inoculated into animals. The results showed that the STEC non-O157 strain previously inoculated into animals was the only strain recovered displaying this specific pattern of DNA. All strains isolated from fecal sample from animals from group I and IV also had no similar DNA patterns to the strain previously inoculated into animals these strains were classified as non-STEC (Table1).

	Group III	Group IV
Weeks without inoculation		
1	0.0	0.0
2	0.0	0.0
3	0.0	0.0
Weeks post-inoculation		
1	34/134	0.0
2	122/152	0.0
3	133/143	0.0
4	288/119	0.0
5	323/123	0.0
6	129/143	0.0
7	84/138	0.0

Table 1. Proportion of means of STEC with the means of ordinary *E. coli* grown on plate re-isolated from feces samples from sheep from Groups I to IV during three weeks without inoculation and then during seven weeks post-inoculation.

Ordinary strain of *E. coli* were all strains that not displayed similar DNA to the strains previously inoculated into animals

The relations among the means values of STEC non-O157 strains displaying the specific pattern of DNA previously inoculated with *E. coli* strains non-STEC from group II and III were respectively as follows: 21/123, 130/142, 146/135, 304/122, 352/132, 190/145 and 90/148;

34/134, 122/152, 133/143, 288/119, 323/123, 129/143 and 84/138 bacteria isolated per gram of feces. (Table1). The means values of STEC non-O157 strains displaying specific pattern of DNA previously inoculated in the animals from groups II and III were compared among itself within the same week to verify the possible reduction of isolates occurred in the animals from group III by administration of probiotics strains (Figure1).

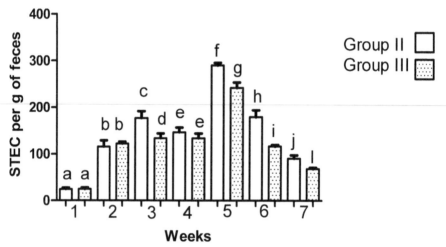

Figure 1. Comparison among the means of STEC from samples feces from Groups II and III. In each week the same letters show that the means not differs among them.

Comparing the means values of isolates of STEC non-157 strains from group II with the means values of isolates of STEC non-O157 strains from Group III within the same weeks verified that the difference was statistically significant among them only the third, fifth, sixth and seventh week post animals´ inoculation (Figure1). There was lowest shedding of STEC non-O157 displaying similar DNA to the pattern of STEC non-O157 previously inoculated into animals belonged to the Group III than Group II, except in the first, second, and fourth week. The Group III had been received probiotic together with the STEC non-O157.

When the quantification was made through the selection at least five colonies from fecal sample during seven weeks of 1 to 5 sheep the results were 24, 26, 29, 30 and 29 in the group II and 20, 15, 19, 18, 16 in the group III (Table.2 and Table.3). The results show that there was no isolating of STEC non-O157 from sheep before the inoculation of bacteria inoculated. The total number of isolates from animals from group III were lowest than from group II. However these values not differ statistically. The aim this second counting was to verify if the reduction of shedding of STEC non-O157 from group III compared with group II would be shown by other way. However, this last counting way did not show statistical difference among the isolates.

	Sheep1	Sheep2	Sheep3	Sheep4	Sheep5
Weeks post-inoculation					
1	2	2	3	3	2
2	2	3	5	5	4
3	5	4	5	4	5
4	5	5	5	5	5
5	4	5	4	5	5
6	3	4	3	4	4
7	3	3	4	4	4
Total	24	26	29	30	29

Table 2. Total values of STEC re-isolated from feces sample selecting at least five colonies grown per samples from Group II.

	Sheep1	Sheep2	Sheep3	Sheep4	Sheep5
Weeks post-inoculation					
1	3	2	3	3	2
2	3	2	3	2	2
3	4	1	3	2	2
4	3	3	2	3	3
5	1	4	3	3	3
6	4	2	3	2	3
7	2	1	2	3	1
Total	20	15	19	18	16

Table 3. Total values of STEC re-isolated from feces sample selecting at least five colonies grown per samples from Group III.

20. Discussion

Shiga-toxin-producing E. coli (STEC) strains are associated as a foodborne pathogen since 1982 and it has been identified as the cause of several outbreaks (Beutin et al., 2002; Karmali et al., 1989; Willshaw et al., 2001).

Probiotics are live microorganisms taken as food supplements that beneficially affect the host, maintaining a balance in their intestinal microbiota (Fuller, 1989). The ruminants including cattle, sheep and deer are reservoirs of STEC and the fecal shedding of these bacteria forms the vehicle of entry into the human food chain (Lema et al., 2001). The probiotics could be used as strategies to reduction of shedding these pathogens by animals (Chaucheyras-Durand et al. 2010).

In the present study we evaluated the protective effect of a mixture of probiotics strains to decrease the shedding of STEC non-O157 in sheep. The group III that received probiotic had fewer STEC non-O157 recovered from their feces when compared with the group II that did not receive the probiotics being that these differences were significant in 3th, 5th, 6th to 7th weeks. The probiotics strains failed to decrease the shedding of STEC non-O157 by feces during the first, second and fourth week post inoculation. In last three weeks of experiment there was a reduction in the shedding of the STEC non-O157 from feces from group III that received probiotic together with STEC non-O157 compared with the shedding of the STEC non-O157 from feces from group II which received STEC non-O157 only. For unknown reason the shedding of STEC non-O157 from group III was lower than group II during the third week post inoculation. However in the fourth week post inoculation there was no difference among the number of isolates of STEC non-O157 from both group III and II. As the probiotics beneficially affect the host, maintaining a balance in their intestinal microbiota (Fuller, 1989) probably the presence of probiotics strains hindered colonization and consequently the shedding these bacteria by feces.

Several mechanisms have been proposed to explain the beneficial effects of probiotics among them are the production of organic acids by bacterial probiotics can help decrease the gut pH, create more favorable ecological conditions for the resident microbiota and decrease the risk of pathogen colonization (Servin, 2004). The growth of pathogenic bacteria also can be hindered by synthesis of antimicrobial peptides, such as bacteriocins or production of enzymes able to hydrolyze bacterial toxins (Buts, 2004), stimulating the immune system, increasing the absorption of minerals and increasing the syntheses of vitamins (Thuory et al., 2003). Bactericins are produced by many lactic acid bacteria (LAB), including species normally found in the gastrointestinal tract as *L. acidophilus*-group as *L. acidophilus, Lactobacillus amylovorus, L. crispatus, L. crispatus, Lactobacillus gallinarum, L. gasseri and L. plantarum*, (De Vuyst et al., 1996 and Dicks & Botes, 2010).

Chaucheyras-Durand et al. (2010) indicated that some strategies may be used in the rumen to decrease the number of viable STEC cells as the use of *Lactobacillus acidophilus* supplemented in the ration, thereby preventing the contamination of food. These strategies are the administration of probiotics in the ruminants. The impact of probiotics and the physicochemical conditions of the rumen digesta on the survival of pathogenic strains could have significant implications for farm management practices and food safety and decrease the risk of food-borne illness.

In our study all sheep belonging to the group that received STEC non-O157 together with daily intake from probiotics strains had lower shedding this STEC non-O157. Some authors as Lema et al., (2001) verified that in lambs, the use of feed supplemented with lactic bacteria such as *Lactobacillus acidophilus* and *Enterococcus faecium* improved meat production. The mixture of probiotic strains used in this study contained strains of lactic bacteria, which probably allowed for the effect cited. Kritas et al., (2006) used *Bacillus licheniformis* and *Bacillus subtilis* supplemented in ration on sheep and verified although the mortality of sheep had not decreased there were beneficial effect on milk yields, fat and protein in milk.

As many bacterial species are present in the intestine, and under normal conditions the majority of these bacteria are strictly anaerobic. This composition makes the gut capable of responding to the possible anatomic and physicochemical variations that occur (Lee et al., 1999). The intestinal microbiota exercises a large influence on many biochemical reactions of the host. The balance maintained by probiotics hinders the growth of pathogenic microorganisms that are present. In contrast, an imbalance in the gut microbiota may cause the proliferation of pathogens and subsequent bacterial infection (Gibson, 1998).

The increased resistance against pathogens is the most important characteristic in developing effective probiotics. The use of probiotics strains excludes potentially pathogenic microorganisms and increases the natural defense mechanisms of the host (Puupponen-Pimiä et al., 2002). The modulation of intestinal microbiota by probiotic microorganisms occurs through a mechanism of competitive exclusion (Guarner and Malagelada, 2003). Also, the probiotics help to reset the intestinal microbiota through adhesion and colonization of the intestinal mucosa. This action hinders the adhesion or invasion of epithelial cells by pathogenic bacteria and decreases the synthesis of toxin. An imbalanced microbiota causes changes, such as the diarrhea associated with infections or treatment with antibiotics, allergic reactions to foods, and intestinal inflammatory diseases. Therefore, correcting an imbalance in the intestinal microbiota constitutes the basis for probiotic therapy (Isolauri et al., 2004). According Zhao et al. (1998), probiotics administered prior to exposure to pathogenic *E. coli* may reduce the levels of pathogenic *E. coli* carried in most animals. In this study we observed that concurrent inoculation of probiotics strains with STEC strains probably hindered the colonization of the pathogenic bacteria in the sheep, as compared with the groups that did not receive the probiotics treatment as well as by consequence decreasing thus the shedding by STEC non-O157. According to Batista et al. (2008), the administration *of Lactobacillus acidophilus,* decreased the number of days the animals displayed symptoms of diarrhea in the group of ruminants that received the probiotic compared with the group that did not receive any probiotic. Roos et al., (2010) verify that the use of *Bacillus cereus* and *Sacharomyces boulardii* enhanced the humoral immune response of lambs to the vaccines.

Some characteristics in probiotics strains are unwanted and much worrisome as well as antimicrobial resistance. Some lactic bacteria could present antibiotic resistance and these bacteria used for food is considered a major danger since this resistance could be transferred to pathogenic bacteria. The probiotics strains used in our study were tested to susceptibility to 27 antibiotics and verified that generally the *Lactobacillus* strains were inhibited to all antibiotics tested (Karapetkov et al., 2011).

In a study with cattle performed in Brazil, the authors used a probiotic contained strains of *Ruminobacter amylophilus, Ruminobacter succinogenes, Succinovibrio dextrinosolvens, Bacillus cereus, Lactobacillus acidophilus* and *Streptococcus faecium,* and these strains were administered at a dose of 3 x 10^8 live cells (CFU) of each strain resuspended in 250 mL of milk and administered orally. This study had many groups of animals. Some animals were vaccinated, others received probiotic and others both were vaccinated and received probiotic. These results showed that the combination of vaccine with the probiotic administered for 15 or 30 days were the most effective treatments for the control of diarrhea and weight gain (Ávila et al., 2000).

Some studies have indicated a higher prevalence of STEC in sheep than in cattle (Beutin et al., 1997; Sidjalat and Bensink, 1997; Urdahl et al., 2003), confirming that sheep are a significant reservoir of STEC. The findings of this study suggest that this probiotic likely presented a potential protective effect in reducing colonization by STEC non-O157 and can be used as an alternative method to decrease STEC non-157 infection in sheep, thereby reducing transmission to humans. Probiotic microorganisms, which benefit from a "natural image", can expect a promising future in animal nutrition (Chaucheyras-Durand and Durand, 2010).

Author details

Everlon Cid Rigobelo and Fernando Antonio de Ávila

UNESP Animal Science Faculty of Dracena, UNESP Department of Veterinary Pathology, Brazil

Acknowledgement

The authors would like to thank FAPESP by financial support that permitted the realization of study. Process: 2009/14923-8

21. References

[1] Ávila, F., A., Paulillo, A., C. Schocken-Iturrino, R., P. *et al.,* 2000. Evaluation of efficiency of a probiotic in the controlo f diarrhea and weight gain in calves. Arquivos Brasileiros de Medicina Veterinaria e Zootecnia 41-46.

[2] Batista, C., G., Coelho, S., G., Rabelo, E., *et al.,* 2008. Performance and health of calves fed milk without antimicrobials residue or milk from mastitis treated cows with or without probiotic. Arquivos. Brasileiro de Medicina Veterinária e Zootecnia. 185-191.

[3] Belongia, E.A., Osterholm, N.T., Soler, J.T., *et al.,* 1993 Transmission of *Escherichia coli* O157: H7 infection in Minnesota child day–care facilities. Journal American. Medicine. Association. 269, pp. 883-888.

[4] Beutin, L., Geier, D., Zimmermann, S., *et al.,* 1997. Epidemiological relatedness and clonal types of natural populations of *Escherichia coli* strains producing Shiga toxins in separate populations of cattle and sheep. Applied Environmental Microbiology 63, 2175–2180.

[5] Beutin, L., Kaulfuss, S., Cheasty, T., Brandenburg, B. Zimmermann, S., Gleier, K., Willshaw, G.A., Smith, H.R., 2002. Characteristics and association with disease of two major subclones of Shiga toxin (Verocytotoxin)-producing strains of *Escherichia coli* (STEC) O157 that are present among isolates from patients in Germany. Diagnostic Microbiology Infect Diseases, 44, 337-346.

[6] Buts, J.P., 2004. Exemple dún medicament probiotique: Sacchamoryces boulardii lyophilize. In Rambaud, J.C., Buts, J.P., Corthier, G. and Flourié, B. (eds) Flore microbienne intestinale. John Libbey Eurotext, Montrouge, France, pp.221-244.

[7] Chaucheyras-Durand, F., Fahima, F., Ameilbonne, A., *et al.,* 2010. Fates of acid-resistant and non-acid-resistant shiga toxin-producing *Escherichia coli* strains in rumiant digestive

contents in the absence and presence of probiotics. Applied. Environmental. Microbiology, 640-647.

[8] Chaucheyras-Durant, F., Durant, H., 2010. Probiotics in animal nutrition and health. Beneficial Microbes, 1, 3-9.

[9] China B, Pirson V, and Mainil J. 1996. Typing of bovine attaching and effacing Escherichia coli bymultiplex amplification of virulence-associated genes. Applied. Environmental. Microbiology. 82:3462–3463.

[10] Cross., M., 2002. Microbes versus microbes: immune signals generated by probiotic lactobacilli and their role in protection against microbial pathogens. FEMS, 245-253.

[11] De Vuyst, L., Callewart, R. and Pot, B., 1996. Characterization of the antagonistic activity of Lactobacillus amylovorus DCE 471 and large scale isolation of its bacteriocin amylovorin L471. Systematic and Applied Microbiology 19: 9-20.

[12] Dicks, l.M.T., Botes, M. Probiotic lactic acid bacteria in the gastro-intestinal tract: health benefits, safety and mode of action. 2010. Beneficial Microbes, 1, 11-29.

[13] Food And Agriculture Organization Of The United Nations, World Health Organization. Evaluation of health and nutritional properties of probiotics in food including powder milk with live lactic acid bacteria. Córdoba, 2003. 34p. Available at: http://ftp.fao.org/es/esn/food/ probioreport_ en.pdf>. Accessed 03 Fev 2005.

[14] Fuller, R., 1989. Probiotics in man and animals. Journal Applied Bacteriology Oxford, 66, 365-378.

[15] Gibson, G., R., Roberfroid, M., B., 1998. Dietary modulation of the human colonic microbiota: introducing the concept of prebiotics. Journal Nutrition, 125, 1401-1412.

[16] Guarner, F., Malagelada, J., R., 2003. Gut flora in health and disease. Lancet, London, 360, 512-518.

[17] Hussein, H. S. 2007. Prevalence and pathogenicity of Shiga toxin producing Escherichia coli in beef cattle and their products. Journal of Animal Science, 85, E63–E73.

[18] Isolauri, E., Salminen, S., Ouwehand, A., C., 2004. Probiotics. Best Pract. Research. Clinical of Gastroenterology, 2, 299-313.

[19] Karapetkov, N., Geogieva, Rumyan, N., Karaivanova, E. 2011. Antibiotic susceptibility of different lactic acid bacteria strains, Beneficial Microbes, 2, 335-339.

[20] Karmali, M.A., 1989. Infection by verocytotoxin-producing Escherichia coli. Clinical Microbiology. Review, 2, 15-38.

[21] Kritas, S.K., Govaris, A., Christodoulopopoulos, G., Burriel, A.R. 2006. Effect of Bacillus licheniformis and Bacillus subtilis supplementation of Ewe´s feed on sheep milk production and young lamb mortality. Journal of Veterinary Medicine,53, 170-173.

[22] Lee, Y., K., Nomoto, K., Salminen, S., Gorbach, S., L., 1999. Handbook of probiotics. New York, Wiley, 211pp.

[23] Lema, M., Williams, L., Rao, D.R., 2001. Reduction of fecal shedding of enterohemorrhagic Escherichia coli O157:H7 in lambs by feeding by microbial feed supplement. Small Ruminant Research 39, 31-39.

[24] Posse B., Zutter, L.D., Heyndrickx, M., Herman, L. 2007. Metabolic and genetic profiling of clinical O157 and non-O157 Shiga-toxin-producing Escherichia coli, Institut Pasteur, 158, 591-599.

[25] Puupponen-Pimiä, R., Aura, A., M., Oksmancaldentey, K., M., *et al.*, 2002. Development of functional ingredients for gut health. Trends Food Science Technological, Amsterdam, 13, 3-11.

[26] Ramamurthy, T. 2008. Shiga toxin-producing *Escherichia coli* (STEC): the bug in our backyard. Indian Journal of Medical Research, 128, 233–236.

[27] Roos, T.B., Tabeleao, V.C., Dummer, L.A., *et al.*, 2010. Effect of Bacillus cereus var Toyoi and *Saccharomyces boulardii* on the immune response of sheep to vaccines. Food and Agricultural Immunology, 21,113-118.

[28] Sanders, M., E., Klaenhammer, T., R., 2003. Invited review: the scientific basis of *Lactobacillus acidophilus* NCFM functionality as a probiotic. Journal. Dairy Science, 84, 319-331.

[29] Servin, A.I., 2004. Antagonistic activities of lactobacilli and bifidobacteria against microbial pathogens. FEMS Microbiology Reviews 28:405-440.

[30] Sidjabat, H., Bensink, J., C., 1997. Verotoxin-producing *Escherichia coli* from the faeces of sheep, calves and pigs. Australian Veterinary Journal 75, 292–293.

[31] Thuory, K., M., Probert, H., M., Smejkal, C., W., *et al.*, 2003. Using probiotics and prebiotics to improve gut health. Drug Discovery Today, Haywards Heath,15, 692-700.

[32] Urdahl, A., M., Beutin, L., Skjerve, E., Zimmermann, S., *et al.*, 2003. Animal host associated differences in Shiga toxin-producing *Escherichia coli* isolated from sheep and cattle on the same farm. Journal Applied Microbiology. 92-101.

[33] Wani S.,A, Bhat M., A, Samanta I, Nishikawa Y, and Buchh A., S. 2003. Isolation and characterization of Shiga toxinproducing Escherichia coli (STEC) and enteropathogenic Escherichia coli (EPEC) from calves and lambs with diarrhea in India. Letters. Applied. Microbiology. 37: 121–126.

[34] Willshaw, G.A., Cheasty, T., Smith, H.R., O'Brien, S.J., Adak, G.K., 2001. Verocytotoxin-producing Escherichia coli (VTEC) O157 and other VTEC from human infections in England and Wales: 1995-1998. Journal Medicine Microbiology, 50, 135-142.

[35] Zhao, T., Doyle, M., Harmon, B., *et al.*, 1998. Reduction of carriage of enterohemorrhagic *Escherichia coli* O157:H7 in cattle by inoculation with probiotic bacteria. Journal Clinical Microbiology, 641-647.

Chapter 5

Kefir D'Aqua and Its Probiotic Properties

José Maurício Schneedorf

Additional information is available at the end of the chapter

1. Introduction

Prebiotics are non-digestible molecules produced by probiotic microorganisms [1]. Probiotic microrganisms are generally bacteria or fungi recognized as safe, with their properties based on the production of organic acids, reduction of biogenic amines, digestion/breakdown of carbohydrates and proteins, immunomodulatory and anti-inflammatory responses, reduction of carcinogenic amines, and production of antimicrobial peptides, among others [2]. These days probiotics are mostly consumed as probiotic yogurts and other probiotic dairy products, dietary supplements, spoonable forms, and probiotic cultured drinks for daily dosage packaging, among others. Prebiotics are also claimed to enhance wellbeing through immunomodulatory and metabolic activities, and act as a natural barrier against pathological processes [1]. These molecules are considered to be a targeted for human and animal production and health, and represents a multimillionaire market of the functional foods. Furthermore, the increasing market of prebiotics counts today with a thousands of patented invention, related to isolation, production, preparation, methods of use, or application of newly health enhancing molecules. The global production and consumption of functional foods is a multi-billion industry, with an estimated market size around US$ 60 billion in 2008-9, several times greater than the health treatment costs only in USA in that years, in the order of US$ 832 million (Figure 1). As a comparison, the global market of probiotic products was US$ 15.9 billion in 2008 and US$ 19 billion in 2009, with a compound annual growth rate (CAGR) of 11.7 % (2009-2014). Furthermore, the probiotic market predicted by 2014 for Europe and Asia comprises, respectively, US$ 12.9 billion (11.1 % CAGR), and US$ 8.7 billion. Japan, a global leader of functional foods, devoted US$ 4.5 billion to the study and commercialization of prebiotics, with US$ 1.5 billion verted exclusively for the oligosaccharide commerce in 2009 [3]. The USA have occupied the second position in the last decade, with a commercialization of US$ 110 million for functional oligosaccharides (35 % inulin, 20 % mannan oligosaccharides, and 10 % fructan), and with a CAGR rate of 20 % The European and the U.S. market for prebiotics is projected to reach nearly US$ 1.2 billion and US$225 million, respectively, by the year 2015 [3]. This has reached nearly US$ 21.6 billion in 2010 and is expected to reach US$ 31.1 billion in 2015, and at a CAGR of 7.6 % for the 5-year period.

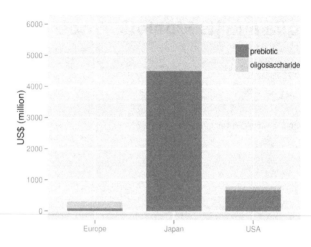

Figure 1. Global market of prebiotics from 2008 to 2010 [3].

2. Studies on water kefir

In general, prebiotics are considered nondigestible but fermentable oligosaccharides, involved on health promotion for the host [4]. Such compounds are known to provide improvements in nutritional status, besides additional health benefits such as protection against carcinogenesis, mutagenesis, prevention of injuries caused by free radicals, control of intestinal flora, gastrointestinal resistance, decrease of blood pressure induced by hypertension, production of β-interferon, cortisol and norepinephrine, increase of phagocytic activity of peritoneal and lung macrophages, increase of IgA cells in these sites, antimicrobial activity, and anti-inflammatory activity, among others [1].   Kefir, an acid-alcoholic fermentation traditionally consumed in Eastern Europe as milky suspensions due its potential health benefits [5], is able to produce peptide and sugar prebiotics (e.g., lactacin, bactericins, KGF, kefiran) [1].

Historically, kefir grains (Figure 2) were considered a gift from Allah among the Muslim people of the northern Caucasian mountains [6]. The word kefir is derived from the Turkish word *keif*, which can be translated to good feeling for the sense experienced after drinkig it, or their promoted health claims. Kefir grains were passed from generation to generation among the tribes of Caucasus being considered a source of family wealth [6]. Kefir grains can be also cultivated in a solution of raw sugar and water (e.g., molasses), known as sugary, water or water kefir. Sugary kefir grains are very similar to milk kefir grains in terms of their structure, associated microorganisms and products formed during the fermentation process, albeit without the characteristic cauliflower look of them. Kefir d'aqua, sugary kefir, or water kefir, is generally a home made fermented beverage based on a sucrose solution with or without fruit extracts. Kefir consists of a gelatinous and irregular grains formed by a consortium of yeasts and lactic acid bacteria embedded in a resilient polysaccharide matrix named kefiran [7]. Since 2002 our research group has dedicated to study the properties and beneficial effects of kefir and kefiran extracts [7, 8] and, more recently, an oligosaccharide isolated from water kefir fermentation, and named aqueous kefir carbohydrate (AK) [9].

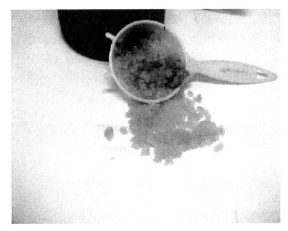

Figure 2. Sample of water kefir grains after souring a molasses solution.

Different from the milky bacteria-encapsulated polysaccharide kefiran, AK seems to be an oligosaccharide isolated from an aqueous fraction of kefir grains [10].

2.1. Kefir characteristics

2.1.1. Microbial strains

Different sets of yeasts and bacteria in water kefir have been identified from several regions and sources, and with both culture-dependent or molecular methods. Notwithstanding, kefir is able to change their bacterial/yeast ratio, even their microbial strains as a function of time, experimental conditions, temperature, and neighboring microorganism, in the inner grain [11]. A typical consortium appears to consist of mostly lactic acid bacteria plus yeasts promoting alcoholic fermentation, together with some acetic acid bacteria (Table 1), possibly oxidizing the ethanol formed [12]. Despite the great microbial diversity found in kefir samples from different regions, there are common strains prevailing in kefir sources from different countries. The most likely strains found in kefir are *Lactobacillus*, *Leuconostoc*, *Kluyveromyces* and *Acetobacter* genus, although the symbiotic 'organism' had also presented some rare microorganisms, such as *Chryseomonas* and *Kloekera* [13].

2.1.2. Growth

Changes in physical, chemical and microbiological parameters during continuous cultures of water kefir has been studied by several authors since 50's [15]. In our lab grains samples grown in molasses solutions at 50 to 200 $g \cdot L^{-1}$ in distilled water have been tested for some parameters, as optima temperature and pH of development, ionic strength, some metabolites (glucose and glicerol), growth changes after freezing even at -70 °C, and bacteria/yeast proportions. The results have shown a maximum temperature of growth about 25 °C, and a continuous pH decrease for the suspensions up to 20 h (from pH 6.1 to pH 4.5). While kefir suspensions presented decreasing levels of glucose (7 times), glicerol increased 3 times during cultivation in molasses at physiological conditions for 7 days. The bacteria/yeast quotient of

Bacteria	
Lactobacillus brevis	*Lactobacillus hilgardii*
Lactobacillus lactis cremoris	*Lactobacillus casei subsp. casei*
Lactobacillus casei subsp. rhamnosus	*Acetobacter aceti*
Lactobacillus casei subsp. Pseudoplantarum	*Lactobacillus plantarum*
Lactobacillus buchneri	*Lactobacillus fructiovorans*
Lactobacillus keranofaciens	*Lactobacillus kefiri*
Lactobacillus collinoides	*Lactococcus lactis subsp. lactis*
Lactococcus lactis subsp. cremoris	*Leuconostoc mesenteroides subsp. mesenteroides*
Leuconostoc mesenteroides subsp. Dextranicum	*Enterobacter hormachei*
Gluconobacter frateuri	*Chryseomonas luteola*

Yeasts	
Saccharomyces bayanus	*Saccharomyces cerevisiae*
Saccharomyces florentinus	*Saccharomyces pretoriensis*
Zygosaccharomyces florentinus	*Candida valida*
Hanseniaspora vinae	*Hanseniaspora yalbensis*
Kloeckera apiculata	*Candida lambica*
Candida colliculosa	*Toruspola delbruechii*
Candida inconspicua	*Candida magnoliae*
Candida famata	*Candida kefyr*
Kluyveromices lactis	*Kluyveromices marxianus*

Table 1. Some microbial strains found in water kefir samples [13, 14].

water kefir showed a prevalence of lactic acid bacteria in the grains (31±8 % greater), whereas yeasts have been mainly found in the suspensions (63±6 % greater). Surprisingly, water kefir grains have been demonstrated a higher resistance against extreme environment conditions. As an example, the grains were able to growth in KCl up to 5 %, or even at temperatures lower than 4 °C. At household conditions of growth, biomass curves of freezed-stored grains have shown an continuous linear trend up to the 5th month of grains storage, and with a decay rate of 4g/day/month. However, a progressive disruption of the overall metabolism of the self-organized grains have been identified under -70 °C freezing. For testing this highly apparent resistance of kefir grains, we had performed some challenges against antibiotics, irradiation and gas treatments, with water kefir.

2.1.3. Resistance

As a well-structured gelatinous grains with diverse microbial strains in their composition, it was hypothesize that the bacteria and yeasts present in kefir could be protected inside the polysaccharide matrix, exhibiting a different resistance under physical and chemical stresses than freely strains in solution. Keeping this in mind it has been tested the colony resistance of kefir against three disordering factors: ultraviolet radiation exposure (UV), antibiotic administration, and gas treatment (oxygen and ozone) [16]. After an exponential growth phase the samples were submitted to UV and chemical treatments. Far UV (15 W D_2) was taken daily in tubes containing the grains during 5, 10, 30 and 60 min, up to 9 days. The growth of grains were followed gravimetrically after cutting dried grains into six layers, from the inner core to the outer shell of the grains. Antibiotic treatment was carried out with 1 mL penicillin G (20 $\mu g \cdot L^{-1}$), 50 mg nystatin (Fungizon) and 1 mL streptomycin (100 $\mu g \cdot mL^{-1}$) dispensed separately in kefir cultures during 12 days at 24 h intervals. Gas treatment was done with continuous ozonization at 1, 5, 10, 30, 60, and 120 min in 0.5 g of kefir starter grains, following cultivation as described. In all these challenges the grains were able to resist against extreme conditions during cultivation. UV treatment, for example, suggested a relative recovery of growth after the irradiation period (Figure 3). This was revealed comparing the slopes of growth curves obtained before the UV irradiation (1.22±0.15 g/day/g of sample), after 7 days treatment (0.30±0.02 g/day/g of sample) and 15 days treatment (0.56±0.07g/day/g of sample). With the antibiotic treatement, a decrease in growth rates was observed 72 h after administration in culture media, with bacteria bringing out more biomass to the grain structure than yeasts. In the other hand, the gas treatment resulted an exponential decay for the growth rate up to 41±23 (oxygen) and 25±8 % (ozone) after 7 days after the exposures. Although these disordering factors were able to decrease kefir growth during the challenges, none of them was able to completely disrupt the grain structure or biomass production after exposures. In conclusion, the ancient culture of symbiotic kefir showed a strong resistance against UV, antibiotic and ozone defiances, allowing a retrieval close to the normal growth after the disturbances.

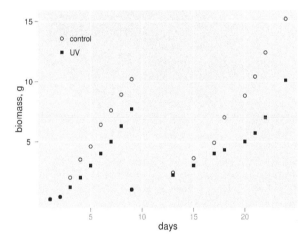

Figure 3. Growth curves of kefir grains submitted to far-UV irradiation up to the 9th day, following normal cultivation with 1 g-starter sample.

2.1.4. Artificial symbiogenesis

The microbial flora present in kefir grains has been studied from a symbiotic community point of view by Linn Margulis since 1995 [17]. Accordingly, it has been stated [18] that separated cultures of microbial kefir grains, either do not grow in milk or have a decreased biochemical activity, which further complicates the study of the microbial population of kefir grains. The mechanism of symbiogenesis of kefir grains from distinct strains of unicellular organisms is unknown, although there are some data about the recover of their structure and probiotic properties from lyophilization, and even so, about the formation of an artificial consortium produced by bits of kefir grains transferred to a yeast extract-sucrose solution [19]. Using a simple approach, we had developed artificial cultures of kefir by trapping their strains in alginate beads [20]. To do so, kefir grains were cultured in 200 g·L^{-1} of molasses solution for 7 days. Then the supernatant was collected, centrifugated at 7000 rpm during 15 min, resuspended into 5 mL of molasses as above, and filtered to avoid minor grain fragments. For cell immobilization 100 mL of a 4 % sodium alginate solution was mixed with the treated kefir suspension and dropped into 1.5 % of a cold calcium chloride solution. The alginate-kefir beads resulted were then continuously cultivated with molasses replacement at 48 h intervals. Strikingly, novel kefir grains had been arisen from solution after three months of cultivation (Figure 4), resembling the ordinary household grains, as monitored by optical microscopy at low resolution, and with the commom budding property exhibited by normal grains (Figure 5).

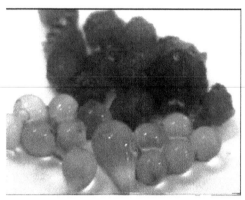

Figure 4. Fresh alginate-kefir beads (botton of the image) and the beads cultured with 48-h medium changes for 96 days.

Antimicrobial activity was chosen as a comparison index for native and artificial grains. The assays were carried out introducing 0.1 mL (3×10^8 cells) of *S. aureus*, *S. tiphymurium*, *E. coli*, and *C. albicans* in 1.5 mL of kefir suspensions, following incubation for 24 h at 35 °C. After this period 0.1 mL of each tube was swabbed in Petri dishes containing the proper culture media and incubated for 24 and 48 h. By counting the colony unit formers (CUF) for native and artificial grains, the antimicrobial activity of kefir exhibited a similar pattern, with total inhibiton for all strains for both kefir types (native and artificial produced). Photomicroscopy showed an increase of grain budding from alginate-kefir beads after the 96th day of incubation, with the novel grains achieving an identical kefir morphology up to 120 days, and presenting a mean diameter of 22±2 mm. These findings indicate a partial maintenance of both structural and probiotic properties of kefir during the grain development unnaturally induced, a high-degree of self-organization for the symbiotic culture. In this goal we also had tested the potential of kefir grains to hold an exogenous strain, trying to incorporate *Saccharomyces cerevisae* on grain development. The procedure, similar to that described above [21], was conducted by adding different amounts *S. cerevisae* in the starter cultures before the shaping of alginate-kefir beads.

The anti-inflammatory activity of this modified grains, as revealed by paw edema assays in rats, showed even higher than native grains (Figure 6). This artificial process of strain internalization for kefir grains suggests a plausible strategy for incorporate some bacteria with specified purposes, e.g., *Lactobacillus acidophilus* for lowering blood cholesterol. In this way, previous studies [6] have demonstrated decreased levels on serum total cholesterol of rats

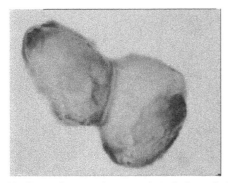 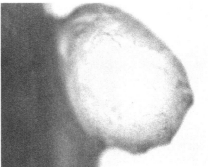

(a) Binary division of grains obtained from the (b) A small kefir grain sprouting from the main body of symbiogenesis produced from alginate-kefir beads cultivated alginate-kefir beads (x15) (x15)

Figure 5. Symbiogenesis of kefir grains anchored to calcium alginate beads and treated with molasses for 3 months. (a) grain division, and (b) grain sprouting [20].

fed with a high-cholesterol diet supplemented with fermented milk produced by modified kefir grains. This modified kefir was obtained from a mixture of 10 types of *Lactobacillus* and *S. cerevisae*. In the other hand, the addition of yeast cells of *S. cerevisae* from a co-culture of *L. kefiranofaciens* and *C. kefyr*, or *T. delbrueckii*, did not showed any enhanced effect on kefiran production [22]. Notwithstanding, when yeast extracts were added to *L. kefiranofaciens* cultures, the authors reported an increase in kefiran production, and suggested the role of yeast extracts as mimicking the actions of yeast cells on *L. kefiranofaciens* in the grains as a typically natural co-culture system.

This property of inherent modulation of kefir strains has been also reported with native grains, whenever they were stored for long periods, or even during their cultivation [23]. In this aim, we have evaluated the bacteriocinin activity of kefir from an adaptative potential of growth against some pathogenic strains [24]. To accomplish this, kefir samples were challenged with *Staphylococcus aureus* or *Escherichia coli*, by pipetting 1 mL of 2×10^9 cells/mL of the strains into 70 mL of kefir culture at each 48 h-medium change (50 $g \cdot L^{-1}$ molasses) for 20 days. Kefir grains was then separated, dried and weighted before the medium changes. Then, 0.1 mL of the supernatant was withdrawn from fermented kefir and seeded on EMB agar (*E. coli*) or manitol agar (*S. aureus*, following incubation at 35.5 °C for 48 h. The same aliquot was also used for disc diffusion antimicrobial assays. Following, 0.3 mL of inoculated kefir was centrifuged, filtered with 0.22 mm Millipore filter, and pipetted into BHI media containing 3.3 mL of each single inoculated bacteria (unitary Mc Farland's scale). The incubation was done at 35.5 °C up to 12 h, and the bacterial growth was monitored spectrophotometrically at 600 nm. After the incubation period, the grains exhibited major morphological changes on their structure for those groups treated with the inoculations. Surprisingly, the filtered kefir sample *S. aureus*-stimulated incubated for 20 days was able to suppress the growth of the same *S. aureus* strains (Figure 7). This finding suggest an epigenetic or adaptative potential for bacteriocinins secretion by kefir to resist to *S. aureus*, as the soured suspension was changed at 48 h-intervals, avoiding the presence of antibiotic molecules previously produced by the symbiotic.

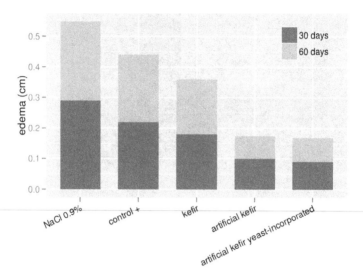

Figure 6. Inhibition of rat paw edema carrageenan-induced (1 mg/paw, 0.1 mL) by kefir suspensions obtained from cultivation of native kefir grains, and those produced by symbiogenesis with or without *S. cerevisae* incorporation. The assays were carried out for 30 and 60 days after obtained the modified grains. Positive control - 10 mg·kg^{-1} indomethacin [20].

2.2. Kefir properties

2.2.1. Suspension, grains and kefiran

2.2.1.1. Aqueous kefiran (AK)

There are several studies pertaining to the claimed health properties of the kefir consortium, but mainly with milky preparations. Accordingly, milky kefir is known to present a large antibacterium spectrum, gastrointestinal improvement and proliferation of normal lactic intestinal flora and bacterial colonization, anti-carcinogenic, wound healing and β-galactosidase activities, immuno-stimulatory, anti-diabetes [25], anti-oxidative [26], anti-lipidemic [27], and anti-allergenic effects, among others [28]. In the same way, although there are a lot of data reported about an exopolysaccharide with prebiotic properties isolated from kefir grains, the literature concerns only on the purified molecule from lacteous sources. In this goal our research group had been studied physical-chemical and prebiotic properties of a variation of the milky kefiran, an oligosaccharide named aqueous kefiran (AK), and fractionated from molasses solution [29] . Isolated AK solutions prepared at 0.1 % had presented a mean yield, instrinsic viscosity, relative density, and electrical conductivity of, respectively, 1.1 g·kg^{-1} of dried grains, 0.297±0.03 dL·g^{-1}, 1.044 g·mL^{-1}, and 2.46 μS·cm^{-1}. Infra-Red spectroscopy (IR) of AK presented strong bands at 3600-3100 (ν O-H) and 10^7 cm^{-1} (ν C-O), suggesting a polyhydroxylated nature of the sample. Minor bands were shown at 2950-2880 (ν C-H), 1470 and 1390 cm^{-1} (δ_x C-H), revealing an aliphatic characteristic of the compound. The composition of monosaccharide residues of AK, as determined from

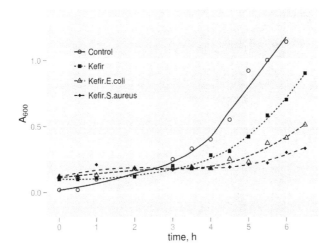

Figure 7. Changes in *S. aureus* growth in the presence of kefir suspensions stimulated for 20 days with *S. aureus* or *E. coli* [24].

thin-layer chromatography and GC, presented mean values of glucose (40 %), ramnose (24 %), galactose (10 %), and arabinose (26 %). From HPLC measurements, the molecular weight of AK was determined as 3534 Da, then suggesting a ten-monomer oligosaccharide structure for the prebiotic. Water kefiran is rarely reported in the related literature as well patent depository banks [30]. Nevertheless, both kefir and kefiran, major milk-based, have been used to obtain technically and commercially feasible biotechnological products, as starter cultures by casein immobilization in cheese production [31], food-grade additive of milk gels for fermented products [10], industrial scale-up of alcoholic fermentation of whey [32], for batch alcoholic fermentation [34], for exploiting waste residues from the citrus industry [33], and for development of multipurpose edible films [35], among others.

2.3. On biological surfaces

2.3.1. Biomimetic membranes

Albeit kefiran has presented diverse prebiotic activities, no direct mechanism of its action on cell membranes have been understood yet. Aiming to help this, the influence of AK on biomimetic membranes composed of l-α-phosphatidylcholine/cholesterol supported bilayer lipid membrane was studied by voltammetry and electrochemical impedance spectroscopy (EIS) [4]. Our findings suggest that kefiran could induce molecular pores at supported bilayer ipid membrane (s-BLM) surfaces up to 5 min at 11.4 μmol·L^{-1}, and with a 34 Å of initial radius. The suggested mechanism (Figure 8) seems to involve some hydrogen bonding between the carbohydrate and the phosphate head group of the phospholipid with a carpet-like model of interaction, and is related to the prebiotic concentration. This results can contribute to disclose direct molecular interactions between prebiotic oligosaccharides and cell surfaces, both related to the biological activity of the prebiotic compound in several experimental models. In this way the prebiotic actitivy of AK could also be related to some metabolic pathways, as enzyme-kinetic or transport systems. Thinking on it, we have evaluated the plausible action of AK on mitochondrial suspensions, as a model of a whole and independent metabolic system.

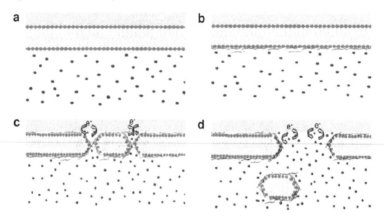

Figure 8. Carpet-like mechanism proposed for water kefiran-membrane interaction. Oligosaccharide molecules line up on the membrane surface (a) until a critical concentration is reached (b) and a detergent-like effect takes place (c). At this stage, oligosaccharides from kefiran and membrane components form aggregates that leave the membrane cause disruption (d) [4].

2.3.2. Mitochondria

Cellular mechanisms of action were investigated to verify the potential activity of water kefiran on the respiratory activity of isolated mitocondria [36]. Samples from rat liver (1200 mg·mL^{-1} protein) were preincubated with kefiran in 20 mM phosphate buffer pH 7.3 containing 70 mM sucrose, 1 mM EDTA, and 5 mM MgCl$_2$. The oxygen consumption of mitochondria was determined by chronoamperometry at 50 rpm stirring suspensions in 2 mL using a Clark-type electrode Pt-Ag/AgCl connected to a potentiostat, and with -600 mV of applied potential. The system was previously calibrated with a N$_2$-saturated solution and baker yeast suspensions. The current signals after successive additions of buffer, mitochondrial samples, 100 mM succinate, 100 μL of kefiran, and 100 mM malonic acid, were obtained during 90 min. After proper digital filtering and signal amplification, the current values obtained were converted to oxygen concentration and flux. The results for organelle suspensions revealed a total inhibition of mitochondrial respiration with 0.2 % kefiran solution. Aiming to assess the prebiotic properties of AK on the mitochondrial respiratory pathways (Complex I and II), mitochondria suspensions (300 mg·mL^{-1} protein) were preincubated with the prebiotic together with different carbon sources (50 mM Glu, 100 mM malate, 50 mM pyruvate, or 100 mM succinate) [37]. After the incubations, it was found a decrease in absorbance values at 340 nm after addition of 2 mM NADH. Furthermore, some changes at 520 nm were also found, after addition of 5 mM potassium ferrycianide in 50 mM KCN solution, using malonic acid (100 mM) and metformin (1 mM) as inhibitory markers for Complex I and II, respectively. The inhibition of Complex I showed values of 53±4 % for kefiran (50 mg·mL^{-1}), whereas the Complex II showed inhibition values of 54±5 % for AK. Moreover, a mitochondrial swelling test also revealed a mean increased value of 13 % for the kefiran tested. These results as a whole point to an inhibitory effect for AK on the oxidative phosphorilation chain of mitochondria.

2.4. On microorganisms

Kefir is well known to resist to a large spectrum of pathological strains, and it seems to be recognized as safe, although its culture contamination has been reported as a source of health impairments. [38]. Antibiotic activity of both kefir and purified AK (50 mg·mL^{-1}) has been evaluated [8] using both the disk diffusion method and susceptibility tests against some well known pathogenic bacteria (*S. pyogenes, S. salivarius, S. aureus, P. aeruginosa, S. tiphymurium, E. coli, L. monocytogenes,* and *C. albicans*). The results of the disc diffusion promoted by kefiran are present at Figure 9. A rapid decrease in surviving pathogens with 0.45 mg·mL^{-1} of kefiran in the susceptibility tests was also observed, whereas the prebiotic was able to produce inhibition haloes about 26±2 mm, greater than those found for oxacilin, ampicillin, ceftriaxone, and azithromycin, at their usual concentrations. In these assays, *S. pyogenes* and *S. tiphymurium* were the most sensible bacteria challenged with kefir in vitro [39], as both strains had their growth completely abolished into Petri dishes, as revealed by CFU counting after 24 h of selective cultivation. *Listeria monocytogenes* also presents a valuable target for testing kefir, due to its commonly contamination in dairy products (milk and home made cheese), and its strong resistance at higher temperatures and osmolarity, together with the survival of strains at low pH medium. In this way, we evaluated MIC and MBC values for kefir suspension (0.1, 1.0 and 1.5 mL) pipetting the aliquots together with 0.1 mL *L. monocytogenes* (3 x 10^8 cell/mL), and following incubation at 35.5 °C for 24 h. After inoculation for 24/48 h, it was found a bacteriostatic property of kefir at 24 h with all aliquots, but a bacteriocidal activity at 48 h with 1.5 mL kefir suspension, suggesting a relative protection of kefir and their prebiotic compounds against *Listeria monocytogenes.* In another work, we tried out antimicrobial activity for both water kefir and its grain extract against *Staphylococcus aureus* [40]. Kefir samples were thawed and continuously cultivated in 100 g·L^{-1} of molasses solutions during 7 days and 24 h of nourish replacement. The grain extract was obtained from 250 g of kefir grains grinded, boiled in distilled water during 1 h and precipitated twice with cold ethanol for 18 h. Antimicrobial activity was carried out against *Staphylococcus aureus* ATCC 6538 through the agar difusion method using paper discs. Suspensions of 0.1 mL of *S. aureus* were innoculated into 25 mL BHI medium and swabbed in Petri dishes. Paper discs containing 0.1 mL of 5, 20 and 50 mg of kefir extract, 0.1 mL of kefir suspension, 0.9% NaCl (negative control), and ampicillin (10 µg, positive control) were transferred to growth dishes following incubation at 35 °C for 24 h. The antimicrobial activity of kefiran extract against *S. aureus* attained similar values for disc haloes with 50 mg/0.1 mL (20±1 and 27±3 mm), and closer to the ampicillin halo (21±0 mm). Although the polysaccharide extracted from kefir grains presented a lower inhibition area for *S. aureus* as compared to ampicillin, the latter drug is known to exhibit some adverse effects such as diarrhoea, sickness, vomit and kidney disorders.

2.5. On animals

Despite the known probiotic and prebiotic effects of kefir and AK, little is reported about their responses in healthy individuals, e.g. a physiological status of animals naturally receiving

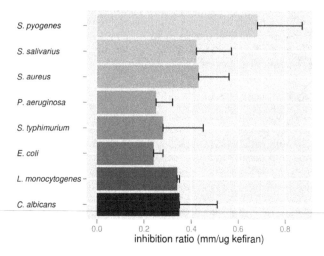

Figure 9. Zone diammeters obtained by disc diffusion of haloes produced from the action of water kefiran against some pathogenic strains.

fermented kefir suspensions [41]. Targeting this, it was evaluated the consumption of kefir suspension by Wistar rats (n=5/group) kept in metabolic cages at room temperature, and with water and commercial diet *ad libitum* [42]. After 30 days no mean difference was observed between the animals receiving daily 1 mL of kefir suspension (50 $g \cdot L^{-1}$ 24 h-fermented) by gavage, and the control group (1 mL NaCl 0.9 %). However, the kefir group of male rats excreted more urine (29±14 %), consumed more ration (22±6 %) and water (18±7), and get more weight (43±16 %) than the female group of kefir.

2.5.1. Anti-inflammatory and antimicrobial activity

2.5.1.1. Rodents

Anti-inflammatory responses of sugary kefir and its derivatives are poorly related in the literature. Notwithstanding, kefir may exert a beneficial effect on acute inflammatory responses, additonally improving the immune status of treated animals. In this sense an ED_{50} value of 12.5 $mg \cdot kg^{-1}$ was found by rat paw edema, together with inhibitions values about 30±4 % and 54±8 %, for carrageenan (Figure 10) and dextran-induced inflammatory process, respectively (n=8/group). However, no changes in vascular permeability was evidenced in that experiments [29]. When compairing with cyproheptadine, a H1-receptor blocker, these results pointed to the antiinflammatory response probably derived from serotonin receptor and arachidonic acid pathways. In another assay, the anti-edematogenic activity of both kefir suspensions and grinded grains were also evaluated with a similar approach through carrageenan, dextran or histamine. Kefir suspensions orally administered 30 min before stimulli were found to be more effective (62 % inhibition) than kefir grains mechanically disintegrated (40 %). The overall data suggest a participation of prostaglandins mediators more than just histamine and serotonine in the anti-inflammatory response as a whole.

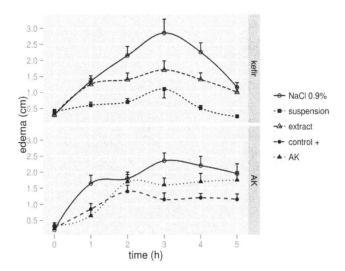

Figure 10. Anti-inflammatory activity of kefir (suspension and extract) and water kefir carbohydrate (AK) on the rat paw edema induced by intraplantar injection of carrageenan (1 μg·mL^{-1}, 1 mL). Positive control - indomethacin, 10 mg ·kg^{-1} [9, 29].

With the use of an analgesia model of acetic acid-induced writhing reflex in mice [43], both kefir grains and their soured suspensions also exhibited an anti-inflammatory response through abdominal contorsions (28±2 % inhibition, n=5/group), whenever the animals were treated *i.p.* with 0.6 % acetic acid (Figure 11).

Following this findings, cicatrizing activities of both kefir and purified kefiran (50 mg·mL^{-1}) were also conducted with rats (n=5/group) [8]. For this test, a 6 mm-punched wound was made on a shaved dorsal area of the animals, following inoculation of *Staphylococcus aureus* at 3 x10^8 cels/mL, and treatment of the animals topically with a 70 % kefir gel made with kefiran up to 7 days. The treatment resulted in a faster reduction of the infected-induced wound diameter, as compared with the control group (Figure 12), and even greater than the group treated with a neomycin-clostebol association at day 7.

The skin samples excised from the animals treated with kefir gel also presented a well developed granulation of the epithelium together with neovascularization areas, suggesting a partial healing in the treated group (Figure 13) [8].

A kefir gel prepared as above was also tested with a prior heat treatment of kefir, aiming do distinguish between probiotic and prebiotic effects of the consortium. In that job, an oitment developed from grinded grains at 70 % was topically used in cicatrizing assays, for testing their microbial resistance against different heat treatments [24]. Cream samples were elaborated with prior treatment of kefir grains by autoclaving (15, 30, and 45 min), or by heating in a water bath at 55 °C, for 15 h. The kefir creams were then applied topically to a 8-mm wonded-induced dorsal area of rats (n=25/group), previously inoculated with *P. mirabilis*, following cicatrizing measurements up to 7 days. The positive control group was

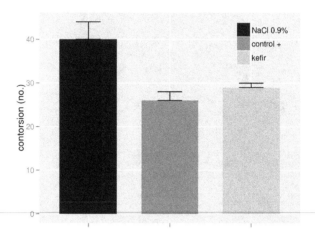

Figure 11. Oral administration of 24h-fermented kefir suspension (1 mL) and indomethacin (10 mg ·kg^{-1}) on the acetic acid-induced writhing reflex in mice, as induced by 0.6% acetic acid [43].

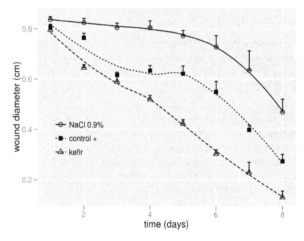

Figure 12. Cicatrizing activity in skin lesions of animals inoculated with 3x10^8 CFU/mL of *S. aureus*. Data represent untreated animals, animals treated with 5 mg ·kg^{-1} of neomycin−clostebol association (positive control), and animals treated with 70% kefir gel [8].

treated with a cream made from a chloramphenicol-colagenase association. IL-1β, TNF-α, and cell blood countings were also determined at the end of the treatments. The main results can be shown at Figure 14. The kefir cream previously treated at 55 °C for 18 h exhibited a similar decrease in dorsal lesion areas as the positive group (chloramphenicol-colagenase association), and even that observed with the untreated kefir group at the 5th and 7th days.

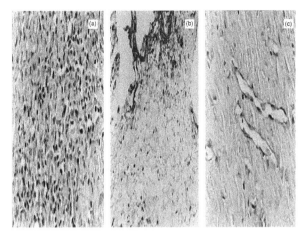

Figure 13. Morphological changes of the skin lesions induced in rats treated with kefir gel 7 days after the abrasions. Haematoxylineosin, 200X. (a) Control rats untreated; (b) rats treated with 5 mg/kg of neomycinclostebol emulsion; (c) rats treated with 70% kefir gel [8].

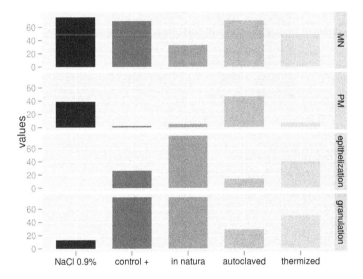

Figure 14. Relative histological findings (MN, PM, epithelization and granulation tissue) from rats infected with *P. mirabilis*, and treated with different preparations of kefir ointments. MN and PM are, respectively, a relative counting for mononuclear and polymorphonuclear cell. The ointments were prepared with native kefir grains, as well with thermized (60 °C, 15 h) and autoclaved grains. Positive control - collagenase-chloramphenicol association [24].

Intriguing, the group treated with autoclaved kefir grains also revealed a meaning decrease of lesion areas, greater than that presented for the negative control group (NaCl 0.9 %).

These findings happened to be so due to a nonproteic molecule taking part in the healing action to the animals, in agreement with the activities of the isolated AK molecule. Furthermore, all tested groups were able to enhance the epithelial tissue proliferation, as compared with the negative control group. In another inflammation model, anti-granuloma assays were also conducted with sugary and milk kefir, together with grinded grains (kefiran extract) and isolated AK. To do this, rats (n=5/group) were challenged with induction of granulomatous tissue by subcutaneously introduction of cotton pellets through abdominal skin incisions, following oral treatment with the agents after 2 h during 7 days [7] (Figure 15).

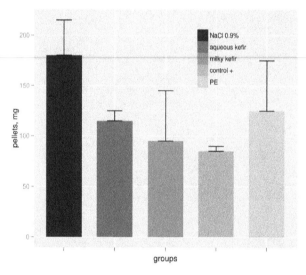

Figure 15. Effect of administration of kefir suspensions in soured milk and molasses (50 g ·L^{-1}), or aqueous polysaccharide extract (PE, 0.1 %, 1 mL), during 6 days, on the formation of granulomatous tissue in rats. Positive control - dexamethasone (0.2 mg ·kg^{-1}) [7].

Both aqueous and milky kefir suspensions (50 g·L^{-1}) showed similar inhibition values (41±3 and 44±6 %, respectively), whereas the isolated kefiran from molasses suspension lead to a smaller inhibition (34±2 %). As kefir grains is known to stimulate innate immune responses against pathogens [8], we had evaluated the immune activity of neutrophils from rats treated with water kefir suspension [44]. Then cytokine TNF-α levels, cell recruiting, cellular metabolism, neutrophils oxygen uptake, H$_2$O$_2$ production, and myeloperoxidase screening, were tested in animals treated with kefir by gavage. (Figure 16). Wistar rats receiving kefir suspension *p.o.* during 7 days revealed meaning differences as compared as those receiving NaCl 0.9 %. In that animals there were a decrease of 30±3 % in neutrophil recruiting from collected peritoneal cells, 32±3 % in peroxyde production stimulated by forbol ester, and 26±1 % in the myeloperoxidase activity. Then, the orally administered suspensions of water kefir was able to decrease general neutrophil activity in treated animals, probably following antioxidative pathways of the metabolism (Figure 17).

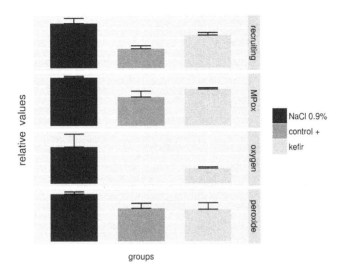

Figure 16. Relative values for neutrophil recruiting, myeloperoxidase index (MPox), oxygen consumption, and H_2O_2 production from peritonal cells isolated from rats treated *p.o* with water kefir suspensions, and during 7 days after stimuli. H_2O_2 release was stimulated by phorbol 12-myristate 13-acetate (PMA). Positive controls - α-tocopherol (H_2O_2 and MPox assays), dexamethasone (cell recruiting) [44].

2.5.1.2. Intestinal motility

Animal digestibility in rats has been also attempted with kefir samples [45]. In that work it was evaluated changes in intestinal motility induced by a sugary kefir suspension daily administered (n=6/group, Wistar rats) during 15 days. After this period, the animals were kept without food during 24 h and treated with water kefir suspension, water, atropine (negative group), or acetylcholine (positive group). Following, the animals received orally 10 % active charcoal after 30 min. The animals were then submitted to euthanasia after 45 min and the intestinal tracts were exposed from the pylorus to cecum. As a result, kefir suspension was able to enhance intestinal transit up to 65±2 % (Figure 18), closer to the acetylcholine group, and greater than the negative groups. These results indicated an improvement of the peristaltic activity of the intestinal tract of the rats treated with kefir, and evoke its plausible use on treating bowel diseases and gut problems.

2.5.1.3. Dogs

Based on the promising findings obtained with rodents, we had inspect some *in vivo* responses of clinically healthy dogs and rabbits treated orally with kefir suspensions. Dogs presenting balanoposthitis (n=5/group), a commom inflammation of the foreskin surfaces of the genital tract of domestic animals, were treated with a 70 % kefir lanette-based ointment, applied daily during 3 days, whereas the positive group was treated with a 0.2 % nitrofurazone solution [46]. After the 25th day, there were more remitted symptoms in the animals treated with kefir cream (62.5 %), as compared as those treated with nitrofurazone solution (37.5 %), a largely compound used in gynaecological infections (Figure 19). Furthermore, the action of

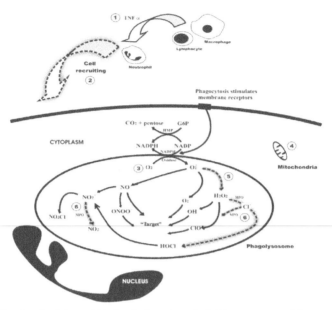

Figure 17. Mapping of cellular and biochemical events evaluated from rat neutrophils treated with water kefir. (Dotted arrows indicates reasonable mechanisms for kefir action). (1) Cellular recruiting; (2) Cellular respirometry; (3) Cellular metabolism; (4) Production of H_2O_2; (5) Identification of the MPO. Hexose monophosphate (HMP); Myeloperoxidase (MPO) [44].

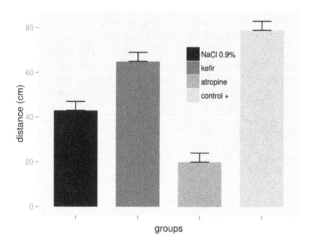

Figure 18. Action of kefir suspension ($8.6 \ g \cdot kg^{-1}$), atropine ($1 \ mg \cdot kg^{-1}$), acetylcholine ($1 \ mg \cdot kg^{-1}$, positive control), and NaCl (0.9 %), orally administered, on the intestinal motility of Wistar rats, as determined by charcoal administration.

the kefir ointment showed more selective for *Staphylococcus* than nitrofurazone, as it was able to decrease 57 % in the frequency of that strains, albeit preserving the naturally-occurring microorganisms of that animals.

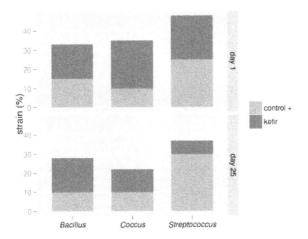

Figure 19. Bacterial counting before and after the treatment of balanoposthitis in dogs with nitrofurazone or kefir gel. Positive control - 0.2% nitrofurazone [46].

2.5.1.4. Lipidemic activity

The intake of soured kefir was tested in the healthy rabbits to identify its plausible effects in serum cholesterol levels. Rabbits (n=10/group) were fed with kefir grains in natura mixed with reconstituted pelletized industrial rations during 30 days, following their growth and serum lipid assessments (total cholesterol, triglycerides, HDL, LDL, and VLDL) [47]. The rabbits who received kefir grains in natura had significantly lesser growth than the control group. Besides, the fraction of total cholesterol and HDL had significant increases, with a mean reduction of the Castelli II index (LDL/HDL ratio) for the kefir group. This datum suggest the increase of total cholesterol as due to the increase of serum HDL, as measured from the rabbit auricular veins. As reported before [27] the total cholesterol levels has been reduced in broiler chicks fed with milk-fermented kefir, in agreement with above findings. In conclusion, these results would suggest that the probiotic can be thought for weight control therapies and prophylactic actions against dyslipidemies.

2.6. On plant

The addition of diverse compounds to plant culture medium has been successfully used for different species in tissue culture techniques. Banana and malt extract, as well as coconut water, e.g., is related to promote the growth of different species of orchids in micropropagation studies [48]. Although the action of kefir in plant physiology is unknown, recent studies demonstrated that kefir was able to induce the synthesis of phytoalexins in soy cotyledons, and also inhibits germination in uredioniospores of *Phakopsora pachyrhizi*, a fungus which cause Asian rust [49]. In this goal, the *in vitro* growth and foliar anatomy of orchids kept in a culture medium with different concentrations of Knudson medium, kefir and sucrose have been evaluated [50]. Biochemical analysis (carotenoids, soluble sugars, chlorophyll, phenolic compounds, and key enzymes of secondary metabolism), foliar anatomy and *in vitro* growth of orchids (*Cattleya walkeriana*) cultivated at different concentrations of Knudson medium, kefir and sucrose, were valued through micropropagation studies. [51].

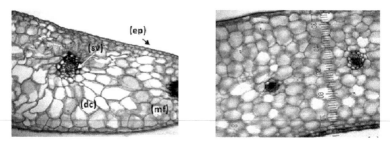

Figure 20. Foliar anatomy of micropropagated orchids (*Cattleya walkeriana*) cultivated *in vitro* with Knudson medium (A), and 25 % Knudson medium and 75 % kefir grains (B). Vascular system (sv), foliar mesophile (mf), epidermis (ep) and cell disorders (dc) [50].

Furthermore, the biochemical data assessed from the micropropagated orchids (Figure 21) evidenced a meaningful increase of the carotene level (up to 24 times greater than control), total phenolic (33 %) and polyphenol oxidase activity (about 3 times greater than control). In this sense, the use of kefir in *in vitro* orchid micropropagation have been promoted more growth, organization and thickness of foliar tissues.

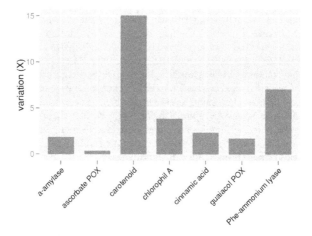

Figure 21. Changes in some compounds and secondary metabolism-key enzymes of micropropagated orchids cultivated with 75 % grinded kefir grains in Knudson medium [51].

The resulted treatment of micropropagated orchids (Figure 20) has been displayed a better organization and larger thickness of the mesophile as observed in culture media at 75 % kefir, when compared with the anatomical development of plants cultivated exclusively in Knudson medium [50].

3. Conclusion

Kefir can be considered an amazing example of coevolution of a microbial consortium. Their grains seems to simulate a multicellular living organism, as they are able to growth, divide, and age. From a survival point of view, kefir is very well adapted to resist to different and even extreme environments, also competing to a large spectrum of microbial strains. As kefir have acquired a strong resistance against several microorganisms, as well to improve the natural immunity of mammals since ancient ages, it is reasonable to think the consortium as a potential naturally-occurring drug able to decrease a large sort of illness afflictions.

Acknowledgements

The author gratefully acknowledge to all the students that have participated on the kefir studies summarized in this work, as well as the following Brazilian research support institutions, Minas Gerais State Research Foundation - FAPEMIG and National Council for Scientific and Technological Development - CNPq.

Author details

José Maurício Schneedorf
Biochemistry Laboratory, Exact Sciences Institute, Federal University of Alfenas, MG, Brazil

4. References

[1] Schneedorf JM., Anfiteatro D. *Kefir, a probiotic produced by encapsulated microorganism and inflammation. In: Carvalho JCT. (ed.). Antiinfammatory phytotherapics (Portuguese)*; Tecmedd; 2004. p 443–467.

[2] Schneedorf JM. *Biochemistry in Agriculture and Poultry (Portuguese)*. Probiotics and Prebiotics. Ed. Ciência brasilis; 2005.

[3] MarketsandMarkets. Probiotic market - advanced technologies and global market (2009 - 2014). 2010. Technical report, Market Publishers.

[4] Barbosa AF., Santos PG., Lucho AS., Schneedorf JM. Kefiran can disrupt the cell membrane through induced pore formation. *Journal of Electroanalytical Chemistry* 2011; 653:61–66.

[5] Schneedorf JM. Como é composto o quefir e quais os seus benefícios para a saúde. *Ciência Hoje* 2006;37:4–5.

[6] Lopitz-Otsoa A., Rementeria F., Elguezabal NR., Garaizar J. Kefir: a symbiotic yeasts-bacteria community with alleged healthy capabilities. *Revista Iberoamericana de Micologia* 2006;2(67-74).

[7] Rodrigues KL, Carvalho JCT., Schneedorf JM. Anti-inflammatory properties of kefir and its polysaccharide extract. *Inflammopharmacology* 2005;13(5-6):485–492.

[8] Rodrigues KL., Caputo LRG., Carvalho JCT., Fiorini JE., Schneedorf JM. Antimicrobial and healing activity of kefir and kefiran extract. *International Journal of Antimicrob Agents* 2005;25(5):404–408.

[9] Moreira MEC., Santos MH., Zollini GP., Wouters ATB., Carvalho JCT., Schneedorf JM. Anti-inflammatory and cicatrizing activities of a carbohydrate fraction isolated from sugary kefir. *Journal of Medicinal Food* 2008;11(2):356–361.

[10] Piermaria J., Delacanal M., Abraham A. Gelling properties of kefiran, a food-grade polysaccharide obtained from kefir grain. *Food Hydrocolloids* 2008;22(8):1520–1527.

[11] Leroi F.,Pidoux M. Detection of interactions between yeasts and lactic acid bacteria isolated from sugary kefir grains. *Journal of Applied Microbiology* 1993;74(1):48–53.

[12] Gulitz A., Stadie J., Wenning M., Ehrmann MA., Vogel RF. The microbial diversity of water kefir. *International Journal of Food Microbiology* 2001;151(3):284–288.

[13] Oliveira RB., Pereira MA., Veiga SMO., Schneedorf JM., Oliveira NMS., Fiorini JE. Microbial profile of a kefir sample preparations: grains in natura and lyophilized and fermented suspension. *Ciência e Tecnologia de Alimentos* 2010;30:1022–1026, 12.

[14] Waldherr FW., Doll VM., Meibner D., Vogel RF. Identification and characterization of a glucan-producing enzyme from lactobacillus hilgardii tmw 1.828 involved in granule formation of water kefir. *Food Microbiology* 2010;27(5):672–678.

[15] Schneedorf JM., Monteiro NML., Padua PI., Bérgamo M. Characterization of a brazilian kefir, a symbiotic culture produced from encapsulated microorganism used in popular medicine. In *Proceedings from XVII Annual Meeting of the Brazilian Federation of Experimental Biology Societies (BA, Brazil); 2002.*

[16] Pichara N., Alves M., Cardoso C., Fiorini JE., Schneedorf JM. Resistance of symbiotic microorganisms against physical and chemical stress. In *Proceedings from XVII Annual Meeting of the Brazilian Federation of Experimental Biology Societies (BA, Brazil); 2001.*

[17] Lynn Margulis. From kefir to death. Brockman J., Matson K. In How things are; William Morrow and Co.; 2011. p69–78.

[18] Koroleva NS. Products prepared with lactic acid bacteria and yeasts. In: Therapeutic properties of fermented milks; Elsevier Applied Sciences Publishers; 1991, p159–179

[19] Pidoux M. The microbial flora of sugary kefir grain (the gingerbeer plant): biosynthesis of the grain fromlactobacillus hilgardii producing a polysaccharide gel. *MIRCEN Journal of Applied Microbiology and Biotechnology* 1989;5(2):223–238.

[20] Rodrigues KL., Fiorini JE., Carvalho JCT., Schneedorf JM. Artificial symbiogenesis developed for kefir grains. In *Proceedings of the XIX Annual Meeting ofthe Brazilian Federation of Experimental Biology Societies (SP, Brazil); 2004.*

[21] Rodrigues KL., Carvalho JCT., Fiorini JE., Schneedorf JM. Modified spreading biofilms. incorporation of saccharomyces cerevisiae in kefir grains. In *Proceedings of the III Research Meeting of Unifenas (MG, Brazil); 2004.*

[22] Taniguchi M., Nomura M., Itaya T, Tanaka T. Kefiran production by *Lactobacillus kefiranofaciens* under the culture conditions established by mimicking the existence and activities of yeast in kefir grains. *Food Science and Technology Research* 2001;7(4):333–337.

[23] Magalhães K., Pereira GM., Dias D., Schwan R. Microbial communities and chemical changes during fermentation of sugary brazilian kefir. *World Journal of Microbiology and Biotechnology* 2010;26:1241–1250. 10.1007/s11274-009-0294-x.

[24] Blanco B. Antimicrobial and cicatrizing activity of a kefir cream submitted to different thermal treatments. Master's thesis, University of Alfenas (Portuguese), Brazil; 2006.

[25] Kwon Y., Apostolidis E., Shetty K. Anti-diabetes functionality of kefir culture-mediated fermented soymilk supplemented with rhodiola extracts. *Food Biotechnology* 2006;20(1):13–29.

[26] McCue PP., Shetty K. Phenolic antioxidant mobilization during yogurt production from soymilk using kefir cultures. *Process Biochemistry* 2005;40(5):1791–1797.

[27] Cenesiz S., Yaman H., Ozcan A., Kart A., Karademir G. Effects of kefir as a probiotic on serum cholesterol, total lipid, aspartate amino transferase and alanine amino transferase activities in broiler chicks. *Medycyna Weterynaryjna* 2008;64(2):168–170.

[28] Sarkar S. Potential of kefir as a dietetic beverage - a review. *British Food Journal* 2007;109(4):280–290.

[29] Moreira MEC., Santos MH., Pereira IO., Ferraz V., Barbosa LC., Schneedorf JM. Anti-inflammatory activity of carbohydrate produced from aqueous fermentation of kefir. *Química Nova* 2008;31:1738 – 1742.

[30] Bruno G. (2011). Use of dried water kefir grains as a carrier of oil-like substances in an inexpensive manner. Patent number DE 102009040624 (B3); 2011.

[31] Dimitrellou D., Kourkoutas Y., Koutinas AA., Kanellaki M. Thermally-dried immobilized kefir on casein as starter culture in dried whey cheese production. *Food Microbiology* 2009;26(8):809–820.

[32] Koutinas AA., Athanasiadis I., Bekatorou A., Psarianos, A., Kanellaki M., Agouridis N., Blekas G. Kefir-yeast technology: Industrial scale-up of alcoholic fermentation of whey, promoted by raisin extracts, using kefir-yeast granular biomass. *Enzyme and Microbial Technology* 2007;41(5):576–582.

[33] Plessas S., Kollopoulos D, Kourkoutas Y., Psarianos C., Alexopoulos A., Marchant R., Banat IM., Koutinas AA. Upgrading of discarded oranges through fermentation using kefir in food industry. *Food Chemistry* 2008;106(1):40–49.

[34] Zajsek K., Gorsek A. Modelling of batch kefir fermentation kinetics for ethanol production by mixed natural microflora. *Food and Bioproducts Processing* 2010;88(1):55–60.

[35] Piermaria JA., Pinotti A., Garcia MA., Abraham AG. Films based on kefiran, an exopolysaccharide obtained from kefir grain: Development and characterization. *Food Hydrocolloids* 2009;23(3):684–690.

[36] Silva GP., Leite LN., Schneedorf JM. Oligosaccharides inhibit rat liver mitochondrial respiration. In *Proceedings from the XXXVIII Annual Meeting of The Brazilian Society for Biochemistry and Molecular Biology (SP, Brazil); 2009.*

[37] Leite LN., Silva AC., Schneedorf JM. Oligosaccharides of prebiotic nature are able to inhibit the oxidative phosphorilation chain in mitochondria. In *Proceedings of the XXXVIII Annual Meeting of The Brazilian Society for Biochemistry and Molecular Biology (SP, Brazil); 2009.*

[38] Gulmez M., Guven A. Survival of escherichia coli o157:h7, listeria monocytogenes 4b and yersinia enterocolitica o3 in different yogurt and kefir combinations as preformentation contaminant. *Journal of Applied Microbiology* 2003;95(3):631–636.

[39] Rodrigues KL., Fiorini JE., Schneedorf JM. Evaluation of antimicrobial activity of kefir in vitro. In *Proceedings of the XVIII Annual Meeting of the Brazilian Federation of Experimental Biology Societies (BA, Brazil); 2002.*

[40] Rodrigues KL., Fiorini JE., Schneedorf JM. Antimicrobial activity of kefir and its polysaccharide matrix against *Staphylococcus aureus*. *In* Proceedings of the Annual Meeting of the Brazilian Society of Biochemistry and Molecular Biology (MG, Brazil); 2003.

[41] Urdaneta E., Barrenetxe J., Aranguren P., Irigoyen, A., Marzo F., Ibá nez F. Intestinal beneficial effects of kefir-supplemented diet in rats. Nutrition Research 2007;27(10):653 – 658.

[42] Dias AB., Cardoso LGV., Carvalho JCT., Schneedorf JM. Physiological parameters in p.o. sub-chronic administration of kefir in rats (portuguese). In Proceedings of the I Research Meeting of Unifenas (MG, Brazil); 2002.

[43] Diniz RO., Garla LK., Carvalho JCT., Schneedorf JM. Study of anti-inflammatory activity of tibetan mushroom, a symbiotic culture of bacteria and fungi encapsulated into a polysaccharide matrix. Pharmacological Research 2003;47(1):49–52.

[44] Zollini GP., Blanco BA., Moreira MEC., Massoco C., Fiorini JE., Schneedorf JM. Neutrophils activity of rats treated with kefir. In Proceedings of the XXVI Annual Meeting of the Brazilian Society for Biochemistry and Molecular Biology (BA, Brazil); 2007.

[45] Cardoso LG., Ferreira MS., Schneedorf JM., Carvalho JCT. Evaluation of a soured kefir on intestinal motility of rats. Jornal Brasileiro de Fitoterapia 2003;1:107–109.

[46] Blanco BA., Zollini PA., Schneedorf JM. Use of a kefir ointment in the treatment of balanoposthitis in dogs. Submmited; 2011.

[47] Bissoli MC. Lipidemic response of rabbits fed with rations supplemented with kefir (master thesis, portuguese). Master's thesis, University of Alfenas, Brazil; 2005.

[48] Chugh S., Guha S., Rao IU. Micropropagation of orchids: A review on the potential of different explants. Scientia Horticulturae 2009;122(4):507–520.

[49] Mesquini KR., Schwan E., Nascimento JF., Bonaldo SM., Pena MIB. Efeito de produtos naturais na indução de fitoalexinas em cotilédones de soja e na germinação de urediniósporos de Phakopsora pachyrhizi. Revista Brasileira de Agroecologia 20007;2:1091–1094.

[50] Silva AB., Schneedorf JM., Silva JAS., Togoro AH. Foliar anatomy and in vitro growth of cattleya at different concentrations of kefir, knudson medium, and sucrose. Bioscience Journal 2011;27:896–901.

[51] Alves MA.,Schneedorf JM. Biochemical and morphological effects induced by kefir in orchid micropropagation. Technical report, Federal University of Alfenas; 2010.

Chapter 6

Indomethacin – Induced Enteropathy and Its Prevention with the Probiotic Bioflora in Rats

Oscar M. Laudanno

Additional information is available at the end of the chapter

1. Introduction

It is already proved that chronic administration of non-steroidal anti-inflammatory drugs (NSAIDs) produce multiple small intestine erosions (SI) with a higher prevalence in the terminal ileum (1) .This new condition is called NSAIDs induced enteropathy. In long term NSAIDs administration studies, almost 60 to 70% of patients were diagnosed through endoscopic capsules as bearing an asymptomatic enteropathy (2); characterized by increased intestinal permeability and mild mucosa inflammation, with hypoalbuminemia and deficient iron anemia(3). It was hypothesized that NSAIDs could act as liposoluble acids interacting with superficial membrane phospholipids, inducing a direct damage on the enterocyte mitochondria during the absorption. The mitochondrial damage could lead to an intracellular energy depletion, calcium efflux and generation of free radicals. The intercellular integrity is disrupted increasing the intestinal permeability, thus making the enterocytes more vulnerable in the lumen content, such as bacteria, bile, enzymes and neutrophile activation (5).

In this hypothesis no prostaglandins are effective, where the NSAIDs COX-1/ COX-2 inhibitors produce gastrointestinal necrosis (6) besides, we were able to prove that COX-3 inhibition with paracetamol simultaneously with COX-1, produce multiple erosions in the small intestine (7), and that paracetamol aggravated the intestinal erosions produced by diclofenac (8). Anyway, the selective COX-1, COX-2 or COX-3 inhibition does not produce gastrointestinal lesions (9).

bioflora is a well known probiotic containing 4 bacteria, i.e., *lactobacillus casei, lactobacillus plantarum, streptococci faecalis* and *bifidobacterium brevis,* with anti-inflammatory effect given either orally or sc, with live or dead bacteria (10, 11); that in stressed rats hindered the bacterial overgrowth, blocking neutrophiles without intestinal bacterial translocation and in other organs, and increase of t lymphocytes (cd4+) (12) the aim of the present study was to study prevention yielded by bioflora in indo induced enteropathy, its probable mechanism induced by the bacterial overgrowth, the neutrophiles, the bacterial translocation and de cd4+ intestinal immunodeficiency.

2. Material and methods

Randomized female Sprague-Dawley rats groups (n=10 each one), 200g, 24h fast, water ad libitum, avoiding coprophagy were submitted to the following experiments: I. 30 mg/kg Indo, SC each12h; 2 days (control). II. 1 ml Bio ($1,3 \times 10^7$ live bacteria), by orogastric gavage in bolus each 12h for 2 days and Indo. The rats were sacrificed by ether overdose, performing laparatomy, total gastrectomy and enterectomy, stomach aperture and small intestine to tabulate the macroscopic necrotic percentage by computerized planimetry. The number of intestinal erosions (mm^2) was quantified, obtaining gastric and intestinal mucosa samples for histochemical examination (myeloperoxydase (MPO)). Bacteriological cultures were performed on mesenteric lymph nodes. Four cm terminal ileum was removed to quantified CD4+ T lymphocytes utilizing immunohistochemical techniques; anti-rat human antibody (Dakko, USA) evaluating each sample through Madsen scale. (13)

Statistics: Student's t test and ANOVA; for the microbiological evaluation of mesenteric lymph nodes exact Fisher's test, and Man-Whitney's test for intestinal cultures; $p < 0.05$ significance was accepted. Drugs: Indomethacin (Sigma Chemical Co. St. Louis, Missouri) and Bioflora probiotic (Laboratorios Sidus).

3. Results

Percentage of macroscopic gastric lesional area is presented in table 1, demonstrating that the Bio-Indo Group provided a marked gastric mucosa protection ($p < 0.001$), and MPO showed also a decrease of neutrophile infiltrate ($p < 0.02$).

In table 2, are shown the erosive intestinal area were Bioflora avoid the occurrence of Indo induced erosions ($p < 0.01$) and MPO reverted also the neutrophile infiltrate.

In table 3 can be observed the significant decrease of the intestinal bacterial overgrowth produced by Bio ($p < 0.01$), as well as the bacterial translocation to the intestinal mesenteric lymph nodes ($p < 0.02$) and the immunohistochemistry of the ileum mucosa. Bio restored the immunity showing a marked increase of T lymphocytes (CD4+). (Figure 1).

4. Discussion

Our results confirmed that the NSAIDs such as Indo produced marked decrease of small intestine immunity due T lymphocytes (CD 4+) effect, that might lead to a secondary bacterial overgrowth, intestinal bacterial translocation with altered intestinal permeability and finally occurrence of intestinal erosions. This could lead to a new hypothesis since the increase of T (CD4+) that impede the bacterial overgrowth and the neutrophile infiltration might protect the defensive barrier avoiding the onset of NSAID enteropathy.

Reuter (14), demonstrated the importance of the enteropathic circulation of NSAIDs, where sulindac, without effect, does not produce a damage to the small intestine; there could be also altered absorption of biliary salts by NSAIDs, and which is most important, loss of integrity of COX-1 and COX-2 (15).

The cycloxygenase inhibition could affect the blood flow of intestinal villi, since it was observed microvascular injury in the jejunal villi as a previous event to the erosion occurrence (16). The eNOS could be administered associated with NSAIDs, since it provides gastrointestinal protection, but not INOS that aggravates ulceration. (17, 18)

Misoprostol in high doses showed a mild increase of the intestinal permeability to Indo (19) although other works do not show such effect (20). Metronidazol that attenuate the intestinal inflammation and hemorrhage was also studied, although it did not modified the intestinal permeability (24). Sulphasalazine was also evaluated showing a slight improvement of the intestinal permeability (22).

There is important to differentiate the NSAIDs induced enteropathy from others such as the one produced in the espondiloarthrosis, especially if NSAIDs are administered, in Crohn's disease (23). Patients with NSAIDs enteropathy must suppress as a first option NSAIDs, since the disease could persist up to a year after therapy discontinuation (24) and any kind of NSAIDs is forbidden, COX-2 included (25) except in patients with chronic joint pain and gastroduodenal ulcer risk that could be treated with naproxen, without cardiovascular risks and with a proton pump blocker such as esomeprazol (26).Briefly, NSAIDs enteropathy presents in its physiopathology a similarity with Chron's disease (27), although attenuated, where the theory of the inflammatory intestinal disease is actually an immunodeficiency with bacteria proliferation on the intestinal mucosa crypts and penetration of the intestinal defensive barrier. This observation Is supported by the fact that a-defensines production is not correlated with the disease severity(28); finally in the NSAIDs mucosa enteropathy a good defense of the intestinal mucosa to avoid bacterial penetration is to treat immunodeficiency, through probiotics prescription Live bacteria could theoretically prevent the damage induced by NSAIDs altering the microbial alteration induced by NSAIDs in the intestinal microbial ecology (30) and by immune function modulation (31). Anyway there were different probiotics that exacerbated the intestinal ulceration, confirmed with the same model of induced Indomethacin enteropathy (32). The Bioflora probiotic provided a marked protection of the gastrointestinal mucosa in the same indomethacin model. The efficacy of the drugs under study, probiotics included, depends also on the inhibition of the pro-inflammatory cytokines activated by the TLR4/D88 mediators, that are important in the intestinal pathology of Crohn's disease and NSAIDs enteropathy development (33, 34).

5. Conclusion

We postulated that NSAID induced lesion in stomach and small intestine, by two mechanism different, in stomach the NSAID inhibited both COX1 and COX2 and provokes depletion of Prostaglandins and gastric necrosis; in contrast, the NSAID in small intestine produced marked decrease of the immunity due T Lymphocytes (CD4T) effect, that lead to a secondary bacterial permeability with the neutrophile infiltration in mucosa intestinal and formation of mesenteric lymph nodes; besides, the inhibition COX3 induce multiple erosions in small intestine. The cyclooxygenase inhibition affect the blood flow of intestinal villi as a previous event to the erosions occurrence. The Probiotics its increased T lymphocytes (CD4T), inhibited the bacterial overgrowth, the neutrophiles, the bacterial translocation and erosions in all the small intestine.

	% gastric necrotic area	MPO mg / protein
INDO	65 ±7 P	410 ±31 P
BIO-INDO	7.5 ±1.3 < 0.001	30 ±7 <0.01

Table 1. Table 1. Gastric necrotic area percent and MPO in the INDO Group (Control) and in the Bio-Indo treated one.

	Erosions in SI mm^2	MPO mg / protein
INDO	380 ±31 P	435 ± 45 P
BIO-INDO	41 ± 6 <0.001	55 ± 11 <0.001

Table 2. Table 2. Number of erosions on the small intestine and MPO, with marked remission in the BIO-INDO group.

	SI Culture CFU		Mesenteric lymph node cultures		CD4+ Ileum	
INDO	7,5 ±3,5 x10^{10}	P	9 (+) 1 (-)	P	0,5 ±0.1	P
BIO-INDO	2,3 ±0,8 x 10^5	<0.01	8 (-) 2 (-)	< 0.01	4 ± 1	< 0.01

Table 3. Prevention of intestinal bacterial overgrowth, bacterial translocation and increased immunity through T lymphocytes T (CD 4+) by Indo and Bio-Indo.

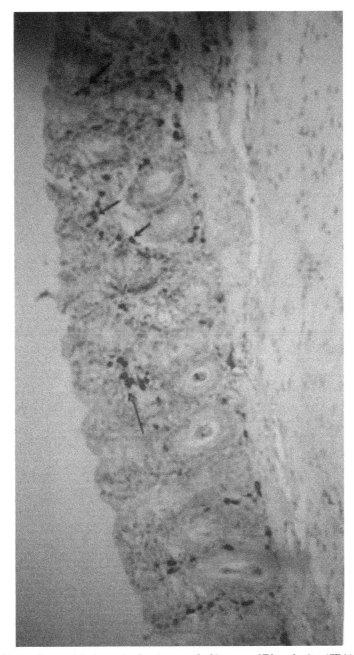

Figure 1. Bioflora Restored the inmunity showing a marked increase of T lymphocites (CD4t)

Author details

Oscar M. Laudanno

Gastroenterologia Experimental. School of Medicina. Rosario. UNR, Argentine

6. References

[1] Adebayo, Bjamason I. Is nosteroidal anti-inflammatory drug. (NSAID) enteropathy clinically more important than NSAID gastropathy? Postgrad Med y 2006; 82: 186 -191.

[2] Bjamason I, Haylar 7, Macpherson AJ, Russell AS. Side-effects of NSAIDs on the small and large intestine in humans. Gastroenterology 1993; 104: 1832 - 1847.

[3] Bjamason I, Zanelli, Prouse P, et al. Blood and protein loss via small intestinal inflammation induced by NSAIDs. Lancet 1987; 2: 711 -714.

[4] Somasundaram S, Simpson RJ, Watts J, et al. Uncoupling of intestinal mitochondrial oxidative phosphorylation and inhibition of cyclooxygenase are required for the development of NSAID-enteropathy in the rat. Aliment Pharmacol Therap 2000; 14: 639 - 650.

[5] Bjamason I, Zanelli G, Smith T, et al. NSAID drug induced inflammation in humans. Gastroenterology 1987;93:480-489.

[6] Wallace JL, Mc Knight W, Reuter BK, et al. NSAID-induced gastric damage in rats: requirement for inhibition of both cyclooxygenase 1 and 2, Gastroenterology 2000; 119: 706 - 714.

[7] Laudanno OM. COX.1 - COX.2 simultaneous inhibitory mechanism in gastric injury and COX.2 - COX.3 in small intestine injury. The trends in COX.2 Inhibitory Research Editor: Maynard J Howardell. Nova Science Publisher, Inc. 2006; Chapter 3. 41 -46.

[8] Laudanno OM, San Miguel P, Cesolari J. Paracetamol amplifica las erosiones intestinales inducidas por Diclofenac, en ratas. Mecanismo COX-3. 2002; Arg Gasfroent pg 9 (GP - 033).

[9] Laudanno OM, Piombo G, Cesolari J, et al. AINEs inhibidores selectivos COX.1 o COX.2, sin dano gastrointestinal, en ratas. Medicina 2001; 61: 684 (A).

[10] Laudanno OM, Cesolari J, Arramberry L, et al. Bioflora prevents intestine ulcers produced by Diclofenac, in rats. BIOCELL 2003; 27 (2): 227 A.

[11] Laudanno OM, Vasconcellos L, Catalano J, Cesolari J. Anti-inflammatory effect of Bioflora probiotic administered orally or subcutaneously with live or dead bacteria, Dig Dis Sci 2006; 51: 2180 - 2183.

[12] Laudanno OM, Cesolari J, Godoy A. Bioflora probiotic in immunomodulation and prophylaxis of the intestinal bacterial translocation in rats. Dig Dis Sci 2008; 53; 2067; 2070.

[13] Madsen KL, Doyle JS, Jewell LD, et al. Lactobacilli species prevents colitis in interleukin 10 gene-deficient mice. Gastroenterology 1999; 116: 1107 - 1114.

[14] Reuter BK, Daries NM, Wallace JL. NSAID enteropathy in rats: role of permeability, bacteria, and enterohepatic circulation. Gastroenterology 1997; 112: 109- 117.

[15] Sigthorsson G, Simpson RJ, Walley M. COX.1 and COX.2, intestinal integrity and pathogenesis of NSAID-enteropathy in mice. Gastroenterology 2002; 122: 1913 - 1923.

[16] Kelly DA, Piasecki C, Anthony A, et al. Focal reduction of villous blood flow in early indomethacin enteropathy: a dynamic vascular study in the rats. Gut 1998; 42: 366 -373.

[17] Ohno R, Yokota A, Tanaka A, et al. Induction of small intestinal damage in rats following combined treatment with cyclooxygenase-2 and nitric-oxide synthase inhibitors. JPharmacol Exp Ther 2004; 310: 821 - 827.

[18] Tanaka A, Kumikata T, Mizoguchi H, et al. Dual action of nitric oxicle in pathogenesis of indomethacin-induced small intestinal ulceration in rats. J Physiol Pharmacol 1999; 50: 405-417.

[19] Efarrnasson I, Smethust P, Clurk P, et al. Effect of prostaglandin on indomethacin induced increased intestinal permeability in man. Scand J Gastroent. 1989; 164:97-112.

[20] Jorchirs RT, Hunt RH. Increased bowel permeability so (51 Cr) EDTA in con 50 is caused by repar or is not presented by cytoprotection. Arch Rheum 1998; 31: R11.

[21] Bjamason I. Smethurst P, Price A, Gumpel MJ. Metronidazole reduces intestinal inflammation and blood loss in NSAID-induced enteropathy. Gut 1992; 33: 1204 - 1208.

[22] Bjamason I, Zanelli G, Pyouse P, et al. Treatment of nonsteroidal anti-inflammatory drug induced enteropathy Gut 1990; 31: 777 - 780.

[23] Smale S, Sigthorsson G, Bjamason I. Epidemology and diferential diagnosis of NSAID-induced injury to the mucosa of small intestine. Best Pract Res Clin Gastroenterol 2001; 15: 723 - 738.

[24] Laine L, Smith R, Mink, et al. Systematic review: the lower gastrointestinal adverse effects of nonsteroidal anti-inflammatory drugs. Aliment Pharmacol Ther 2006; 24: 751 - 767.

[25] Brophy JM. Cardiovascular effects of cyclooxygenase-2 inhibitors. Curr Opin Gastroent. 2007; 23 (6): 617 - 624.

[26] Chan FKL. The David Y. Graham Lecture: Use of Nonsteroidal Antiinflammatory Drugs in a COX-2 Restricted Environment. Am J Gastroent. 2008; 103 (1) 221 - 227.

[27] Fortum PJ, Hawkey CJ. Non steroidal inflammatory drug and the small intestine. Curr Opin Gastroent. 2007; 23: 134-141.

[28] Wehkamp J, Harder J, Weichenthal M, et al. NOD2 (CARD 15) mutations in Crohn's disease are associated with diminished mucosal alfa-defensin expression. Gut 2004; 53: 1658-1664.

[29] Boirivant M, Strober W. The mechanism of action of probiotics. Curr Open Gastroent 2007; 23: 679 - 692.

[30] Collins MD, Gibson GR. Probiotics, prebiotic and symbiotics: approaches for modulating the microbial ecology of the gut. Am J Clin Nutr 1999; 69: 10525 - 10527 S.

[31] Erick KL, Hubbard NE. Probiotics immunomodulation in health and disease. J Nutr 2000; 21: 426 - 430.

[32] Amil R, Guer MS, Butler RN, et al. Lactobacillusrhammonosus exacerbates intestinal ulceration in a model of indomethacin-induced enteropathy. Dig Dis Sci 2007;57:1247-1252.

[33] Scarpignato C. NSAID-induced intestinal damage; are luminal bacteria the therapeutic target? Gut 2008; 57:145-148.

[34] Wantabe T, Higuchi K, Kobala A, et al. Non-steroidal anti-inflammatory drug-induced small intestinal damage is Toll-like receptor 4 dependent. Gut 2008; 57: 181 - 187.

Chapter 7

Use of Yeast Probiotics in Ruminants: Effects and Mechanisms of Action on Rumen pH, Fibre Degradation, and Microbiota According to the Diet

Frédérique Chaucheyras-Durand, Eric Chevaux,
Cécile Martin and Evelyne Forano

Additional information is available at the end of the chapter

1. Introduction

The valorization of fibrous feed sources by ruminants is possible thanks to their unique digestive system involving an intensive preliminary ruminal fermentation step prior to a more classical enzymatic phase. The reticulo-rumen hosts a highly specialized anaerobic microbial community responsible for fibre breakdown, which is influenced by biochemical and microbial characteristics of the rumen environment. In particular, the role of the different microbial species involved in pH regulation and the influence of feed management are presented in section 2. Indeed, intensive farming pratices may disturb the microbial balance due to an excessive high fermentable carbohydrate supply required to sustain high animal performance, and it can turn into metabolic disorders that are likely to impact animal health as reviewed in section 3. This is one area where yeasts probiotics can help the ruminant and the feed nutritionist optimizing the cows nutrition owing to an increasingly well understood proper mode of action. Section 4 reports the positive effects these feed additives, under the form of active dry yeast, have on rumen fermentation, feeding behaviour and feed efficiency, as well as tips to properly assess these effects.

Once the optimal rumen conditions are set up (section 6), fibre will be efficiently digested. It becomes then interesting to dive into the world of the fibrolytic microbiota in section 5 to truly percieve the unicity of the fibre rumen degradation process, bearing in mind that the nature of fibre will impact its digestibility and subsequent animal production response. In addition to its role on rumen pH stabilization that directly affects the fibrolytic microflora, yeast probiotics represent a valuable tool to optimize cow nutrition as detailed in section 7.

However, section 8 will emphasize the yeast strain effect and the need of a viable feed additive to be able to offer a comprehensive solution to ruminants' diet formulation. Finally, besides the clearly established benefits on rumen management and fibre degradation, live yeast as probiotics are also currently being assessed in other promising fields of applications (section 9).

2. Rumen pH: A key parameter linked to rumen function

Due to intense microbial activity, fermentation of feedstuffs in the reticulo-rumen produces a wide range of organic acids. Some of these acids can accumulate and reduce ruminal pH if rumen buffering systems are unable to counteract their impact. Low rumen pH for prolonged periods can negatively affect feed intake, microbial metabolism, and nutrient degradation, and leads to acidosis, inflammation, laminitis, diarrhea and milk fat depression. High yielding dairy cows and fattening beef cattle fed diets rich in readily fermentable starch or sugars at high feed intake levels are particularly susceptible to acidosis, and goats, sheep and other ruminants are also prone to the disease. It is now recognized that subacute ruminal acidosis (SARA) affects from 10% to 40% of dairy cattle in a herd, resulting in large financial losses and major concern for animal welfare reasons. Therefore, rumen pH regulation is a key determinant in the maintenance of an optimal rumen function.

2.1. How to measure rumen pH accurately

Common field techniques for pH measurement have been relied on collection of samples by rumenocentesis or oral stomach tubing [1,2]. Rumenocentesis has proven to be a more reliable technique for the determination of ruminal pH than oral stomach tubing because saliva contamination is often associated with the stomach tubing technique [3,4]. If rumenocentesis may be done with minimal disturbance [5], frequent sampling raises ethical issues and is not without risk for the animal health. Enemark et al. [2] conducted a study to evaluate the potential of biochemical markers in blood, feces, and urine to predict ruminal pH. They concluded that no peripheral markers could properly predict ruminal pH. A permanent surgical modification, such as rumen cannulation, and the use of an external data logger connected to a pH probe immerged into the rumen [3,6] have been successful in well controlled research studies to monitor rumen pH kinetics, which allow to better characterize microbial fermentations and predict acidosis situations. Recently, telemetric boluses able to measure and record rumen pH in cattle continuously have been developed by different companies. When interrogated by wireless, the bolus transmits the recorded data to an operator standing beside the cow with a receiving station. These rumen pH boluses methods offer a simple, accurate and long lasting measurement of pH in intact cattle [7]. They have been successfully applied in controlled animal studies and offer the opportunity to link pH kinetics to measurements in field situations, but clarifications are still needed about the location of the probes (reticulum, rumen) and thereby the representativeness of the measure, their calibration, long-term measure accuracy, and life time. Moreover, the cost of these systems are still high and the current proposed boluses are not yet applicable to non cannulated small ruminants.

2.1.1. Microbial mechanisms which lead to pH modulation and acidosis

Rumen microbial populations hydrolyze and ferment dietary compounds into volatile fatty acids (VFAs), whose amounts drive pH evolution. Moreover, lactic acid is a common product of carbohydrate fermentation, produced by bacterial species such as *Streptococcus bovis*, *Selenomonas ruminantium*, *Mitsuokella multiacidus*, *Lachnospira multipara* or *Lactobacillus sp*. *S. bovis* is considered as a major contributor in lactate production from high fermentable diets. Indeed, it is able of very rapid growth, is acid-resistant and produces extracellular and intracellular amylases which hydrolyze raw starch and soluble starch, respectively [8]. Moreover, it has been shown that *S. bovis* produces mainly L-lactate under moderately acidic pH but shifts its metabolism towards D-Lactate production when the pH decreases [9], this latter isoform being more toxic as it is less efficiently re-utilized by the microbiota and the animal tissues. *Megasphaera elsdenii* is considered as the predominant lactate-utilizing bacterial species in the rumen and can be found in large numbers in the rumen of cereal grain-fed cattle [10]. *Selenomonas ruminantium* subsp *lactylitica* is another important lactate-utilizing species. Contrary to *S. ruminantium*, *M. elsdenii* is not submitted to catabolite repression by soluble sugars [11] and ferments lactate to propionate via the acrylate pathway [10]. It exhibits also a lactate racemase activity which is involved in the conversion of D- into L-lactate, which is more easily metabolized. Nevertheless, with high amounts of readily fermentable carbohydrates, or during adaptation from forage to concentrate diets, acid overload of the rumen is possible and may lead to a strong decline in rumen pH, which may trigger acidosis in cattle [1]. Indeed, as rumen pH falls, lactate producers may outnumber lactate utilizers, leading to an accumulation of this metabolite in the rumen. Due to the low pK_a (3.7) of lactic acid compared to the pK_a of the major VFAs (4.8-4.9 for acetate, propionate and butyrate), even low amounts of lactic acid may play a major role on the onset of acidosis. If rumen pH continues to fall, *Lactobacilli* may replace *S. bovis*, initiating a spiraling effect with excessive D-lactate accumulation [9].

Thanks to their capacity to engulf and slowly ferment starch granules into VFAs (particularly butyrate), rumen protozoa can compete with lactate-producing amylolytic bacteria and lactic acid can be actively taken up by entodiniomorphid ciliates [12]. Overall these processes have a beneficial effect on pH stabilization and may participate to limit the severity of acidosis.

2.1.2. Effect of the diet on rumen microbiota, microbial fermentations and pH evolution

The effect of a diet shift (from high forage to high concentrate) on the composition of the rumen microbiota has been extensively studied, in particular since the last 10 years because of the development of culture-independent techniques quantifying microbial abundance and assessing population dynamics. Tajima et al. [13] have shown that a diet shift from high forage to high grain in steers induced profound changes in bacterial abundances, an increase in *S. bovis* and *Prevotella ruminicola* 16S *rrs* gene copy numbers and a decline in fibrolytic *Fibrobacter succinogenes* population densities being measured. Using quantitative PCR, Mosoni et al. [14] measured significant decrease in *F. succinogenes, Ruminococcus albus* and *R. flavefaciens* 16S *rrs* gene copy numbers/g of rumen contents in sheep fed 50% concentrate 50% hay, compared with a 100% hay diet. In lambs, the effect of hay *vs* concentrate diet fed at weaning was studied on abundance of different species of the rumen microbiota [15]. Whereas abundance of total bacteria, measured by qPCR, was significantly higher with concentrate diet than with hay diet, the relative abundance of the fibrolytic species *F. succinogenes* and that of methanogens were significantly lowered in the presence of concentrate. *R. flavefaciens* abundance was 2.5-fold lower with the concentrate diet. The rumen microbiome of dairy cows in which subacute ruminal acidosis (SARA) had been induced with either grain or alfalfa pellets has also been analysed [16]. T-RFLP analysis indicated that the most predominant shift during SARA was a decline in Gram-negative *Bacteroidetes* organisms. However, the proportion of *Bacteroidetes* was greater in alfalfa pellet-induced SARA than in mild or severe grain-induced SARA. This shift was also evident from real-time PCR data for *P. albensis, P. brevis,* and *P. ruminicola,* belonging to the phylum *Bacteroidetes.* The real-time PCR analysis also indicated that in severe grain-induced SARA, *S. bovis* and *Escherichia coli* were dominant, *M. elsdenii* dominated in mild grain-induced SARA, and *P. albensis* was abundant in alfalfa pellet-induced SARA. Comparing 16S rRNA gene libraries of hay *vs* high grain-fed beef cattle, Fernando et al. [17] reported significantly higher numbers of bacteria of the phylum *Fibrobacteres* in libraries of hay-fed cattle whereas the libraries of grain-fed animals contained a significantly higher numbers of bacteria of the phylum *Bacteroidetes.* Real-time PCR analysis revealed increases in *M. elsdenii, S. bovis, S. ruminantium,* and *P. bryantii* populations during adaptation to the high-grain diet, whereas the fibre-degrading *Butyrivibrio fibrisolvens* and *F. succinogenes* populations gradually decreased as the animals were adapted to the high-concentrate diet. All together, these studies indicate a negative effect of low pH on cellulolytic bacteria. Indeed, they cannot grow with a low intracellular pH, and an increase in pH gradient leads to an entry of undissociated VFAs in the cells and an accumulation of dissociated anions in the intracellular compartment induces severe toxicity for the bacteria [18].

An increase in the percentage of rapidly degradable starch in the diet generally favors the development of protozoa as soon as the rumen pH is not below 5.5 [19]. The genus *Entodinium* can then represent up to 95% of the total ciliate community. When rumen pH is below 5.5, ciliate protozoa populations are decreased and defaunation can even be observed transiently [20].

A low rumen pH has also a strong impact on rumen fungi. Indeed, the production of zoospores by *Caecomyces* have been sharply decreased *in vitro* at pH 5.5. Zoospore numbers were below 10^3/ml or even not detected in animals fed diets inducing low rumen pH [21]. Moreover, the presence of large amounts of soluble sugars, as with high concentrate diets, may induce saturation of the spore adhesion sites and reduce fungal colonization [22].

Changes in the structure of the rumen microbiota are generally accompanied with modifications of fibrolytic activities. Indeed, compared with a forage diet, cereal grain supplementation induces a decrease in specific and total polysaccharidase activities of the solid-associated microorganisms, whereas the response of glycosidase activities is more variable [19]. A relationship between the decrease in polysaccharidase activities (xylanase, avicelase) of these microorganisms and the decrease in ruminal fibre degradation rate has been found by several authors [23-25]. Low pH seems to be more detrimental to growth and survival of cellulolytic microorganisms than to microbial cellulases whose activities are generally optimal at moderately acidic pH (between 5.5 and 6.0) [18]. However, Martin et al. [23] have quantified cellulase and hemicellulase activities and 16S rRNA of cellulolytic bacteria in rumen contents of cows fed a 40% barley diet, and found that cereal supplementation modified the activity but not the abundance of cellulolytic bacterial community.

Sauvant et al. [26] summarized studies conducted on 14 feedstuffs and showed that a strong relationship exists between rumen pH values induced *in vitro* by each feedstuff's fermentation and its percentage of Dry Matter (DM) degradation (Figure 1), indicating that the nature of the feedstuff impacts on its acidogenic potential. Indeed, rapidly degradable starch (as in barley or wheat) will more strongly impact rumen pH than slowly degradable starch (as in corn or sorghum).

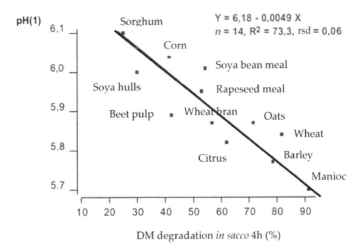

Figure 1. Relationships between acidogenic potential of feedstuffs and their degradation *in sacco*. From [26].

For example, when comparing wheat and corn supplementation in beef steers, mean pH was less and time below pH 6.2 was greater for the wheat based diet than for the corn based diet, which was linked to a higher lactate and VFA concentration [27]. The effect of 3 dietary challenges differing by the nature and degradation rate of their carbohydrates (wheat, corn or beet pulp) was investigated on rumen pH kinetics and fermentation profile in sheep [28]. Mean ruminal pH was significantly less for wheat than for corn and beet pulp at 4.85, 5.61, and 6.09, respectively. This was correlated with a change in the fermentation profile: ruminal lactic acidosis was induced by wheat, whereas butyric and propionic SARA were respectively provoked by corn and beet pulp after the 3 day challenge.

The particle length of forages can greatly affect rumen pH. Indeed, physically effective Neutral Detergent Fibre (peNDF) represents the physical characteristics of fibre by accounting for particle length and NDF content, which promote chewing and the flow of salivary buffers to the rumen [29]. Yang and Beauchemin [30] compared rumen pH response when short (7.9 mm) or long (19 mm) cut alfalfa silage was included in either high or low concentrate diets. They showed that increasing peNDF intake reduced ruminal acidosis; mean ruminal pH and the duration that pH remained below 5.8 were highly correlated to intake of long particles.

3. Impact of a lowered rumen pH on rumen efficiency and animal productivity

3.1. Consequences of a low rumen pH: acidosis, inflammation, rumen wall integrity and impact on animal health

Acute acidosis occurs after the consumption of an excessive quantity of readily fermentable carbohydrates that rapidly alters ruminal function and can have irreversible metabolic consequences. Ruminal perturbations include an increased concentration of lactate (up to 100mM) and a decrease in VFA concentration after 8 to 24h, this latter being the result of poor microbial activity and/or of quicker absorption of the VFA from the rumen to the blood in response to pH fall [31]. Rumen pH values can then drop under 5.0 and trigger metabolic acidosis with an accumulation of D-lactate in the bloodstream. SARA is probably more difficult to characterize because biological parameters in the rumen fluctuate within physiological limits and are difficult to maintain [31]. This unstable state may reflect the oscillatory behavior of the ruminal microbial population in response to diet-based fermentative jolts. According to Kleen and Canizzo [32], the exact definition of SARA remains debatable, but it is certain that SARA is present in a large number of dairy herds. SARA is characterized by a drop of ruminal pH to non-physiological levels; pH values of 5.5 and 5.8 and the duration per day below these threshold values are used to define individuals or groups experiencing SARA or being at risk for SARA. SARA is frequent in high producing cattle and has wide-reaching economic consequences, as it has been estimated to cost \$1.12 /d per cow in USA [33]. In Europe, field studies data indicate that SARA prevalence would range between 10 and 30% in dairy herds [32]. In these studies, the pH thresholds of 5.5 and 5.8 were generally used, rumenocentesis being the reference method for collecting rumen fluid.

The microbial dysbiosis occurring in the rumen during acidosis may trigger the release of potential harmful molecules which may impact the animal health. Indeed, due to an increase of the death and lysis of Gram-negative bacteria under low pH, free lipopolysaccharide (LPS) concentration is increased in the rumen fluid and translocation of this endotoxin can occur across the rumen mucosa [34]. Endotoxin release can trigger an inflammatory response, with an increase in acute phase protein concentrations in peripheral blood [34-37]. Endotoxin is suggested to be involved in metabolic disorders such as laminitis, abomasal displacement, fatty liver or sudden death syndrome [38].

Moreover, the low pH of rumen digesta may have a negative impact on rumen wall integrity. Repeated aggressions by fermentation acids may cause papillar atrophy, diffuse areas of acute or chronic lesions, scars resulting from severe local rumenitis, perforations and mucormycosis which are at the origin of pain, discomfort, as well as erratic feed intake and alteration of rumen function [39].

Low ruminal pH is often associated with increased occurrence of bloat, which is characterized by an accumulation of gas in the rumen and reticulum. Indeed, frothy bloat is caused by entrapment of gas produced from fermentation of readily digestible feeds (high digestible legumes or cereals). Bloat can impair both digestive and respiratory function, and can occur both in cattle raised on pasture or in confinement [40]. Abscessed livers are generally considered to be associated with both acute and subacute ruminal acidosis. Ulcerative lesions, hairs, and other foreign objects that become embedded in the ruminal epithelium can provide routes of entry into the portal blood for microbes that cause liver abscesses [41]. *Fusobacterium necrophorum* (and/or *F. funduliforme*), a commensal rumen Gram-negative species, has been identified as a causative agent of liver abscess; as it is able to use lactate as its major substrate, and its population increases in the rumen of cattle fed high-grain diets [42]. Diarrhea has been very frequently associated with ruminal acidosis and microbial dysbiosis [1]. Changes in fecal consistency, color, brightness, and odour are generally observed; presence of undigested whole grains and large size particles is also a sign of rumen dysfunction [43].This phenomenon may be linked to excessive hindgut fermentation because too much readily fermentable carbohydrates reach the post-ruminal compartments [36] but also the increase in osmolarity of the digesta would lead to soften the fecal mass [43].

Under low rumen pH conditions, erratic feed intake is generally observed but a decrease in intake, mostly on acidogenic feed, has also been reported [44]. In fattening bulls fed high concentrate diets, it has been observed that animals change their feeding behavior to counteract acidosis by spreading their meals over the day [45]. A 10-30% increase in water intake was observed in sheep submitted to acidotic challenges [46]. Water intake could represent a means to dilute acidity but also to reduce rumen fluid viscosity. An increase in salt licking has been also measured in the same study and in goats fed with high concentrate diets [47]. Licking would favor salivary bicarbonate production. Animals under acidosis would also be able to modify their dietary choice to optimize their digestive comfort. Acidosis and low rumen pH conditions may also have consequences on social behavior. For example, sheep undergoing successive acidotic challenges were more active and more aggressive towards each other, spent more time standing, adopted alarm postures more often, and reacted more slowly to hot stimulus during the acidosis bouts [46]. These discomfort signs would not be only linked to rumen pH evolution but to the set up of an inflammatory status in the rumen triggered by changes in microbiota balance.

3.2. Effect of rumen pH on milk yield and quality

From a dietary standpoint, rumen pH is a function of the dry matter intake (DMI) where it becomes below 6 when DMI exceeds 3.8% body weight, i.e. high producing animals with elevated nutritional requirements are more at risk [26]. The quality of the ingested feed directly matters too where pH turns out below 6 when the rumen digested starch accounts for more than 40% of the diet DM [26].

Cows fed high-concentrate diet (nadir 75:25 concentrate:forage ratio) will have a lower ruminal pH, acetate, and butyrate concentrations, whereas propionate concentration will go up. When the rumen acidity is alleviated with a buffer, total VFA production increases, and so does milk production and milk fat content, especially for high concentrate fed cows. Milk fatty acid profile gives also a good insight of what happened in the rumen and more trans 10-11 C18:1 is well correlated to a depressed milk fat due to its inhibitory effect on de novo fatty acids synthesis in the mammary gland [48]. In addition, the stage of lactation may modulate the animal sensitivity to high-concentrate diet with a better resistance to less optimal rumen fermentation conditions for late lactation cows [49]. However, not only the forage:concentrate ratio matters on rumen pH but the nature or technological process of the grains [50] and the frequency of distribution of the concentrate [51] also do.

High fibre diets will not sustain an elevated production of propionate that will negatively impact the milk lactose synthesis and overall milk yield. The cow will thus mobilize her body fat reserves (ketone bodies metabolized in the liver from butyrate) to compensate for this lack of energy.

4. Benefits of using yeast probiotics to control pH stability

4.1. Targets

pH evolution is the result of impaired microbial balance and animal compensation mechanisms. Strategies aiming to induce beneficial effects on the balance of the rumen microbiota and thereby stabilize rumen pH can represent interesting means to reduce the risk of acidosis. This may be achieved by targeting microbial populations involved in massive release of fermentation acids, and/or those implicated in lactic acid removal.

4.2. How best measuring a probiotic effect on animal performance?

Two types of experimental design are basically available to the scientist: contemporaneous or crossover. Parallel designs (i) can be completely randomized design with only one explanatory variable or (ii) randomized complete block design in presence of 2 factors where the experimenter divides animals into subgroups called blocks (eg. sex, origin, size…) such that the variability within blocks is less than the variability between blocks. In crossover design, each experimental unit receives two or more treatments through time, and as the comparison of treatments is made within subjects, each subject acts as its own control which increases statistical power to detect a direct treatment effect [52] and makes it more efficient than the randomized complete block design. However, there are limitations important to bear in mind amongst with a carryover effect is likely to occur between periods, the latter being able to vary between treatments.

The particular nature of probiotics as live microorganisms impacting the rumen flora balance and fermentations make their comparative assessment critical when using experimental design encompassing a carry-over effect. The inclusion of a washout period between successive treatments is a good way of minimizing the remanent treatment effect over time, but there is good evidence suggesting that the 15-28 days usually applied are not long enough.

Indeed, in a complete rumen content transfer study between two cows, Weimer et al. [53] showed that it could last up to 65d for the bacterial community composition to reach back its original profile. A measurement of methanogens population dynamics over time [54] indicated that 4 weeks were not enough to adapt from the dietary shift of grazing to concentrate. These recent microbial studies support questioning about the relevance of crossover type of designs in assessing probiotics effect on rumen parameters [55]. However, it would not be fair omitting to report studies where such a design allowed displaying significant probiotic effects, but the inconsistence or absence of response with a latin-square design may also be due to the tested probiotic strains themselves or to the too short adaptation period.

4.3. Experimental proofs

Stabilization of ruminal pH in the presence of yeast probiotics has been reported by several authors [56-59]. In a meta-analysis, Sauvant et al. [26] concluded that yeast supplementation increased ($P<0.05$) rumen pH *in vitro*, but did not find any significant *in vivo* effect neither on pH, nor on VFAs or lactate. However, the authors admitted that the studies selected for the meta-analysis had used different strains of *S. cerevisiae*, or yeast culture which is defined to be mainly composed by dead cells and fermentation products. More than an increase in mean rumen pH, reductions in duration within a day under a certain pH threshold, as well as in area under the pH curve have been measured in the presence of live yeast probiotics [56, 59]. A recent study conducted in a commercial dairy herd [60] compared sodium bicarbonate and live yeast supplementation in 2 pens of 60 cows on milk production and feed efficiency and rumen pH was monitored every 5 min during 5 weeks in 4 cows equipped with a pH probe. Sodium bicarbonate is very often used as an efficient buffer to overcome pH fall in dairy cows. Mean pH remained consistently higher for the live yeast supplemented cows when compared to the control group cows (6.22 vs 6.03). In addition, live yeast supplemented cows spent less time below a pH threshold of 5.6.

4.4. Modes of action on rumen microbiota and lactate accumulation

Effects of live yeasts have been studied on lactate-metabolizing bacteria. *In vitro*, one strain of *S. cerevisiae* was able to outcompete *S. bovis* for the utilization of sugars; due to a higher affinity of the yeast cells for sugars, the reduction in quantity of fermentable substrate available for the bacterial growth consequently limited the amount of lactate produced [61]. Dead cells had no effect on lactate production. Moreover, stimulation of growth and metabolism of lactate-utilizing bacteria, such as *M. elsdenii* or *S. ruminantium*, was observed *in vitro* in the presence of different live yeasts [61-64] through a supply of different growth factors such as amino acids, peptides, vitamins, and organic acids, essential for the lactate-fermenting bacteria. The impact of yeast probiotics on ruminal lactate concentration has been confirmed in *in vivo* studies. In sheep receiving a live yeast product during their adaptation to a high-concentrate diet, ruminal lactate concentration was significantly lower compared to control animals. Consequently, rumen pH was maintained at values compatible with an efficient rumen function, as shown by higher fibrolytic activities in the rumen of the supplemented animals [24, 65]. In dairy cows, reductions in ruminal lactate concentrations have also been observed with yeast probiotics [66-67].

According to the composition of the diet, the fermentation pattern can be shifted to butyric orientated acidosis [28]. Brossard et al. [6,12] reported the pH stabilising effect of one strain of *S. cerevisiae* in sheep fed a high-wheat diet under a butyric latent acidosis. Authors suggested that this strain could act by stimulating ciliate Entodiniomorphid protozoa, which are known to engulf starch granules very rapidly and thus compete effectively with amylolytic bacteria for their substrate [68]. In addition, starch is fermented by protozoa at a slower rate than by amylolytic bacteria and the main end-products of fermentation are VFAs rather than lactate, which may explain why these ciliates had a stabilizing effect in the rumen by delaying fermentation.

When ruminants encounter successive acidotic bouts, it is not well known whether live yeast supplementation could alter rumen microbiota and fermentations. Indeed, the severity of acidosis may change with repeated challenges, partly because of modifications in feeding behavior [69], and because of possible shifts in rumen microbial communities leading to selection of the most acid resistant species. Studies in sheep submitted to acidotic challenges showed that cellulolytic bacterial culturable population was greatly decreased after a first acidotic challenge but that after 3 challenges, the level of population came back to normal [70]. However, it is probable that this population, enumerated in a filter paper-based medium, had encountered profound changes in its structure and/or diversity. In this study, with repeated challenges, a positive evolution of rumen pH parameters were observed in live yeast supplemented animals which was accompanied with decreased numbers of lactate producing bacteria and a beneficial effect on bacterial diversity which was maintained at a higher level [71].

Provided an adequate balance between soluble nitrogen and carbohydrate supply, it is likely that live yeast probiotics can enhance microbial growth; indeed, more digested carbohydrates would be incorporated into microbial mass thanks to an optimized fermentation coupling and not "wasted" under the form of VFAs, thereby the risk of acidosis would be reduced [72].

4.5. Beneficial consequences of yeast probiotics on rumen fermentations, feeding behavior, feed efficiency, and animal production

Bach et al. [56] reported that the supplementation of live yeast increased average rumen pH and average maximum pH by 0.5 units, and average minimum pH by 0.3 units in loose-housed lactating cows (Figure 2). In this study, a significant change was observed in the eating behavior of the animals. Cows supplemented with live yeast had a shorter inter-meal interval (3.32h) than unsupplemented cows (4.32h). This change in feeding behavior could help in rumen pH recovery, or the beneficial effect of live yeast on pH stabilization could induce a change in eating behavior.

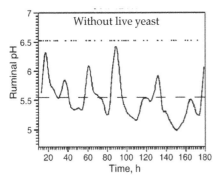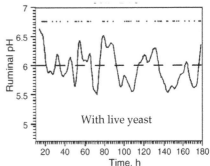

Figure 2. Ruminal pH pattern (solid line) during the 8 days of sampling as affected by live yeast supplementation. The dashed line depicts average ruminal pH. The dots indicate the beginning of a meal. From [56], example shown with one cow.

A meta-analysis conducted on all types of yeast (including live yeast and yeast culture) and all types of dairy ruminants (cows, goats, ewes) [58] concluded that the addition of yeast improved milk yield by 1.2 g/kg body weight. In their multi-analysis reporting data collected from 14 dairy cow trials fed the same live yeast strain, De Ondarza et al. [73] found that live yeast improved (P < 0.0001) milk yield by 1.15 kg/day. The effect was slightly greater for cows in early lactation (<100 Days In Milk, DIM) than for cows >100 DIM, suggesting that animal performance is improved when the acidosis risk is high, notably at critical periods of the lactation cycle.

The effect of yeast probiotics on DM intake shows either no effect [73] or a significant increase in DMI [58]. Live yeast supplementation seems to have an effect on intake pattern rather than on intake *per se* [56]. As a result, feed efficiency is generally improved in the presence of live yeast [73,74]. Milk composition is generally not or only slightly affected by yeast supplementation. Milk fat and protein percentages have been found to be slightly but significantly lower in the presence of live yeast [73], but due to the increase in milk yield, yields of milk fat and true protein were higher than in control cows.

5. Fibre digestion in the rumen: a key process in ruminant nutrition

By symbiosis with specific micro-organisms, ruminants possess a unique ability to use plant cell wall components as energy and nutrient sources and thereby convert plant biomass into milk, meat, wool and hides. A large proportion of energy intake of ruminant comes in the form of structural complex polysaccharides (cellulose, hemicelluloses, pectins), which are mainly present in the plant cell walls. Indeed, the rumen harbors an abundant and diversified community of bacteria, fungi and protozoa able to thoroughly hydrolyze plant cell wall polysaccharides. Effective degradation is the result of microbial adhesion to plant tissue and production of active enzymatic machinery well adapted to plant cell wall breakdown.

5.1. Relation between fibre digestion and intake and productivity

Digestion of fibre is the result of the competition between rates of passage and degradation and the ruminal passage rate (%/h) depends on fibre particles size and digestibility [75]. Reducing particle size will increase DMI but the effect on total digested fibre is also related to the quality of the roughage and its nature: legumes NDF is quicker digested than perennial grass NDF despite a higher lignification, but less resistance to breakdown [76]. Particle size also affects the reticulo-omasal passage kinetics along with the intrinsic fragility of the fibre, its density and shape. The importance of particle size on forage rumen degradation has been recently highlighted [77] as the adjustment parameter to increase the available surface area for attachment of ruminal fibrolytic bacteria and protozoa without negatively affecting cellulolytic activity and other fermentation processes in the rumen.

Fibre occupies space and limit intake by filling the rumen as they are hollow and therefore fill a bigger volume than their mass indicates. In addition, a fraction of the dietary fibre will remain undigested or slowly degraded and will accelerate the rumen filling [78] reducing thus the entrance of other important ingredients to meet the animal nutritional requirements. Knowing that feed intake is the main predictive variable of milk yield [79], the increase of dietary forage will lead to a milk yield reduction besides isonitrogenous rations [80]. Rinne et al. [81] also concluded to a linear decrease of milk yield when the corn silage NDF content increased due to later harvest.

5.2. How to measure fibre digestion

Different methods can be used to measure fibre digestion in the rumen. This compartment is mostly targeted because in general the proportion of fibre which is digested in the hindgut is small. However, the contribution of the large intestine to plant cell wall digestion may increase with the proportion of cereal in the diet [82].

Degradation of dry matter, and NDF fraction of raw materials or more complex mixture of ingredients can be assessed with various *in vitro* techniques requiring mixed rumen contents [83,84], *in situ* (nylon bags) kinetics [82,85] or rumen evacuation [86] in rumen cannulated animals, or in non cannulated ruminants (total fecal collection). The measurement of particle sizes in the fecal material using the Penn State forage and total mixed ration particle separator can be of interest to estimate fibre digestibility [60].

Fibre degrading functional groups can be enumerated on complex culture media in which a source of polysaccharide is added as sole energy source. Measurement of fibrolytic activities can be performed on pure cultures as well as on rumen contents samples. After extraction of ruminal microbial enzymes, activities are measured against various polysaccharides and the concentration of reducing sugars released after enzyme action is determined [19]. PCR-based techniques using specific primer sets are powerful to quantify absolute or relative abundance of targeted fibrolytic species within a complex sample [14,87,88], or to specifically detect and quantify *in vivo* the expression of cellulase or hemicellulase genes from selected microorganisms [89].

5.3. Microbial communities involved in fibre degradation in the rumen

In the rumen, degradation and fermentation of plant cell wall polysaccharides is achieved by bacteria, protozoa and fungi. The different fibrolytic species, or even strains, are specialized to a various extent in the degradation of specific substrates. The overall effective degradation is the result of these different capacities, related to substrate composition and to interactions existing between these communities and also between the fibrolytic and the non-fibrolytic microorganisms within the ecosystem.

In the Bacteria domain, the cellulolytic function is covered by a very limited number of cultivated species. These species are established a few days after birth in the newborn ruminant, although no solid feed penetrates into the rumen [90]. Indeed, from one week of age, the size of the cellulolytic bacterial community is close to that found in adult animals. Cellulolytic bacteria are unable to properly colonize the rumen in absence of a complex and diversified bacterial fermentative community [91,92]. In young lambs kept without contact with their dams or other adults, cellulolytic bacteria were not detected in the rumen during three months after birth, which suggests the essential role of newborn-dam contacts in the transmission of rumen microbiota and rumen maturation [92].

The concentration of fibrolytic bacteria is generally close to 10^9 culturable cells/g of rumen content. Quantitative PCR studies have shown that the main cellulolytic species *Fibrobacter succinogenes*, *Ruminococcus flavefaciens* and *Ruminococcus albus* represent 1-5% of the total bacteria [14, 93] but recent data suggest that these bacteria account for about 50% of the total active cellulolytic bacteria [94]. *F. succinogenes* is very active on crystalline cellulose and hemicelluloses (xylans). However, it is only able to use products of cellulose hydrolysis [94]. *R. albus* and *R. flavefaciens* are active on cellulose, xylans and pectins. Other species are considered as secondary fibrolytic species such as *Butyrivibrio fibrisolvens* and *P. ruminicola*, because they are not able to breakdown the cellulose polymer. However, they possess high carboxymethylcellulose-, xylan- and pectin-degrading activities and probably play an important role in overall fibre digestion [95,96].

The enzymatic equipment of the three main cellulolytic species has been well studied since the last 20 years. In the database CAZy (Carbohydrate Active enZymes, http://www.cazy.org ;

[97]) are referred protein sequences involved in carbohydrate binding and hydrolysis. The recent whole genome sequencing programs confirm that a huge number of genes is involved in fibre breakdown in each bacterial cell, demonstrating great functional redondancy, which is essential for the good functionning of the ecosystem. Genome sequences of strains belonging to *F. succinogenes, R. flavefaciens, R. albus, P. ruminicola,* and *P. bryantii* are now available. From these genome sequences, 183 putative CAZymes have been found for *F. succinogenes,* and more than 140 for *R. flavefaciens* and *R. albus* [98].

Efficacy of fibrolytic bacteria to degrade plant cell wall components are explained by their adhesion capacities and the production of a well adapted enzymatic equipment. Bacteria use different strategies to colonize plant material: for example, *Ruminococci* exhibit several structures on their cell surface, such as type IV pili and components of glycocalyx. Moreover, they produce an elaborate cellulosomal enzyme complex that is anchored to the bacterial cell wall [99,100]. In *F. succinogenes,* attachment to the substrate is mediated by fibro-slime proteins and type IV pilin structures attached to the outer membrane; 13 cellulose binding proteins anchored on the outer membrane seem to be important in effective adhesion to crystalline cellulose [101].

Ciliate protozoa also participate to fibre degradation. Characterization of their ability to directly process plant material have been addressed by diverse strategies, such as direct, biochemical detection of specific fibrolytic enzymes in extracts derived from individual protozoan species [102], or by molecular cloning studies to directly identify protozoal genes encoding enzymes capable of degrading cellulose or hemicellulose [103]. Among protozoa, only Entodiniomorphs (*Polyplastron, Eudiplodinium, Epidinium)* are considered as cellulolytic. Their abundance is between 10^4 and 10^6 cells/g of rumen content. Ciliates are able to engulf whole plant particles, and digest plant polymers in digestive vacuoles. They synthesize a well adapted enzymatic equipment composed of cellulases and hemicellulases [104,105]. Up to now, about a dozen of fibrolytic genes have been identified in the various protozoa species. An activity-based metagenomic study of a bovine ruminal protozoan-enriched cDNA expression library identified four novel genes possibly involved in cellulose and xylan degradation [106]. Several studies have reported that defaunation, i.e. removal of protozoa, can have a negative effect on fibre degradation in the rumen [107,108]. Mosoni et al. [88] showed that long term defaunation had rather a beneficial effect on the abundance of fibrolytic bacterial species *R. flavefaciens* and *R. albus,* quantified by qPCR, but not on that of *F. succinogenes,* which is the most efficient in low digestible plant cell wall degradation, which could explain at least in part, the observed negative effect on fibre digestion.

Anaerobic fungi are also involved in digestion of plant material. They represent a very homogenous phylogenetic group (phylum *Neocallimasticota*) and a very specialized functional group as all species are fibrolytic [109]. The fungal biomass is estimated to represent between 5 and 10% of the total microbial mass. During their life cycle, flagellatted zoospores alternate with filamentous sporangia which are tightly attached to plant tissues, thanks to their cellulosome-like complexes [110]. Rumen fungi produce a very efficient set of cellulases and hemicellulases, whose specific activities are higher than that of bacteria [111]. They also possess esterase activities which contribute to the cleavage of ester bridges which link phenolic compounds of lignin to structural carbohydrates [112,113]. Moreover, thanks to the development of a rhizoidal network they are able to weaken and even disrupt plant tissue which enhances accessibility to digestible structures [114]. Studies carried out with gnotoxenic lambs harbouring or not fungi confirmed their important role in fibre breakdown in the rumen [115].

6. Limiting factors in fibre digestion

6.1. Animal characteristics

A cow chews during eating and rumination to reduce feed (forage) particle sizes and allow the best fermentation process possible via a better distribution of feedstuff and bacteria in the rumen as well through rumen pH maintenance (high buffer capacity of the saliva). Indeed, this first step of the digestive process stimulates saliva production (274 ml/ min chewing and 6g sodium bicarbonate/ liter of saliva) and rumen motility. With an average daily time spent eating, ruminating and resting of 1/3, a production of up to 150 l of saliva per day is achieved. However, about half of the saliva will be produced during rumination, whereas eating will account for 20% and resting 30% [116].

The chewing responses to forage fragility and digestibility have been described [117]: at equal particle size, a low NDF Digestibility (NDFD) rate and less fragile forage increase by about 30 min/day the chewing time when compared to a high NDFD and fragile hay, whereas fragility appears less related to chewing when forage NDFD is similar. These results suggest that increased dietary physically effective NDF may affect chewing activity either through prolonging chewing time or increasing chewing rate. In addition, longer particle size will promote salivation and thus a shorter time with rumen pH<5.8 [118].

From a species standpoint, chewing activity is highly related to the intake capacity and body weight. Animals with a greater intake capacity seem to chew feed more efficiently (i.e. goat, sheep), while heavier animals (cows) can cope with relatively more fibre, because rumination capacity is in line with body size [119].

6.2. Composition of the diet and structure of fibre

Many biotic and abiotic factors may limit the efficacy of fibre degradation in the rumen which may be driven by changes in fibre colonization efficacy. For example, the chemical composition of the plant material modulates the rate and extent of fibre digestion [120]. Digestibility of forage fibre (cell walls) has long been known to be negatively associated with lignin concentration. This relationship between lignin and fibre digestibility is very strong for a same forage compared according to different maturity stages, but it is less clear when comparing different forages harvested at a similar maturity stage, so with similar lignin concentrations [121]. To explain the observed variation in fibre digestibility of forages with similar lignin concentrations, composition of lignin and chemical cross-linking of lignin to cell wall polysaccharides have been suggested as involved additional factors. For example, cross-linking of lignin and arabinoxylans may limit cell wall digestibility by placing lignin in very close proximity to the polysaccharides and preventing physical access by hydrolytic microbial enzymes [120]. The slow entrance of microbial cells into some plant cell tissues such as sclerenchyma and also their slow diffusion capacities down the lumina represent also an important limitation factor for totally efficient fibre digestion [122].

Several studies have shown that the feed particle size may influence the degradation rate of fibre fractions as well as the bacterial colonization of the feed particles. Witzig et al. [123] investigated the effect of the forage source and particle size on the composition of the ruminal *Firmicutes* community assessed by qPCR and Fluorescent In Situ Hybridization *in vitro*. They found that *Ruminococcus albus* was more abundant on short particle size of forage, whereas the xylanolytic *Roseburia* sp. was favored by coarse particle grass silage based diets, and that abundance of *Clostridium* cluster XIV was higher with increasing grass silage proportion in the diet.

6.3. Characteristics of the rumen environment

As described earlier in this chapter, it has been demonstrated that a diet rich in readily fermentable carbohydrates can adversely alter the structure and/or activities of fibre-degrading community, because of a decline in ruminal pH and acidosis occurrence. As a consequence, ruminal digestion of NDF is decreased [124] (Figure 3).

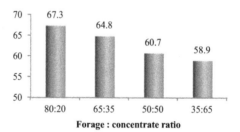

Figure 3. Effect of forage:concentrate ratio on apparent rumen NDF digestibility (%) in cows. From [124].

It is generally admitted that most of fibre-degrading microorganisms are sensitive to oxygen because most of them lack detoxification enzymes necessary for removal of reactive oxygen species. The presence of dissolved oxygen in the rumen ecosystem has been demonstrated [125,126] and oxygen regularly enters the rumen due to feed and water uptake and mastication, which can be illustrated by a greater post-feeding redox potential as measured in dairy cows by Marden et al. [57,127]. Newbold et al. [128] measured the concentration of cellulolytic bacteria in Rusitec in which either normal or low O_2 concentrations had been maintained. Oxygen concentration significantly influenced cellulolytic bacteria, whose numbers were increased by almost 15-fold when low O_2 concentrations were applied in the fermenters. Adhesion of cellulolytic bacteria to cellulose has been shown to be inhibited in the presence of oxygen *in vitro* [129].

6.4. Physiology of fibrolytic microorganisms and microbial interactions

Among biotic factors, the existence of a complex set of interactions between fibrolytic microbes and the other actors of feed digestion does impact fibre degradation. For example, synergistic cross feeding interactions have been described between cellulolytic and non cellulolytic species which lead to a global improvement in degradation [130]. A relevant example is the interaction between proteolytic bacteria and cellulolytic bacteria, the former releasing ammonia, used as preferential nitrogen source for the latter, and the latter releasing soluble sugars from cellulolysis, which will be metabolized by proteolytic bacteria. Moreover, hydrogen transfer between fibre degrading organisms and hydrogen consuming methanogens is necessary for an optimal functioning of fibre degradation mechanisms. Indeed, methanogens help to reduce the hydrogen partial pressure and thereby avoid the inhibition of ferredoxine oxidoreductase which has an essential role on NADH re-oxidation [130]. The result of this interaction is a gain in energy for both partners and an increase in fibre digestion. On the opposite, competition mechanisms have been described between cellulolytic bacterial species for adhesion on cellulose [131,132]. Secretion of inhibitory peptides by *Ruminococcus* strains have been shown *in vitro* to impact growth of rumen fungi [133]. Finally, the physiology of the microorganisms plays also an essential role on overall fibre digestion. Indeed, there are great differences between species regarding their preference and affinity for substrates, their energy requirements, or their capacity to resist to environmental stresses.

7. Benefits of using yeast probiotics to promote fibre digestion

7.1. Targets

To optimize fibre digestion, there is a need to minimize the indigestible fibre fraction, maximize rate of fibre digestion, and maintain a ruminal environment that promotes the population of fibre-digesting bacteria. The indigestible fibre in forages (iNDF) is related to lignin concentration, but also contains structural carbohydrates (cellulose and hemicellulose) which are 'trapped' with lignin. Whereas lignin, of which biochemical degradation process involves oxidative pathways, is considered not digested in the animal gastro-intestinal tract, the release of the carbohydrates bound to lignin would be interesting in terms of increasing feed value of the forage.

To achieve these goals with probiotics, several strategies may be developed depending on the dietary conditions of the animals. Indeed, indirect or direct effects can be sought. Indirect benefits could be mediated through pH stabilization effects (see section 4), or modification of the environment of the microbiota which will definitely sustain or promote fibre-degrading microbiota and their action on plant cell walls. Direct effect of probiotics on fibrolytic microorganisms can also be wished to exist, as nutritional requirements for peptides, amino acids, ammonia, organic acids or branched chain fatty acids have been described for bacteria and fungi and the supply of these components might be achieved through the use of probiotics.

7.2. Experimental proofs

Using different methods, it has been reported that live yeast supplementation improves rumen fibre digestion *in vivo* [85,134-137], although this has not always been observed [138].

7.3. Modes of action on rumen microbiota

In vitro, the potential of probiotic yeasts to enhance growth and activity of fibre-degrading rumen microorganisms has been established. Fungal zoospore germination and cellulose degradation were increased in the presence of a strain of *S. cerevisiae* [139]; the authors suggested that yeasts could enhance fungal colonization of plant cell walls, which was confirmed recently [136]. The effectiveness of some yeast strains to stimulate growth or/and activities of fibrolytic bacteria has also been demonstrated. *In vitro,* a *S. cerevisiae* strain stimulated growth of *Fibrobacter succinogenes* S85 and reduced the lag time for growth of *Ruminococcus albus* 7, *Ruminococcus flavefaciens* FD1, and *Butyrivibrio fibrisolvens* D1 [140]. Callaway and Martin [141] showed that the same yeast could accelerate the rate, but not the extent, of cellulose filter paper degradation by *F. succinogenes* S85 and *R. flavefaciens* FD1. *In vivo*, in gnotoxenic lambs harbouring three species of bacteria (*F. succinogenes, R. albus,* and *R. flavefaciens*) as sole cellulolytic organisms, cellulolytic bacteria became established earlier and remained at a high and stable level even after a stressful period (lambs were fitted with a rumen cannula) in the lambs receiving a probiotic yeast daily [137]. Ciliate protozoa, which are not able to establish unless bacterial communities have previously colonized the rumen [142], appeared more rapidly in the rumen of conventional lambs in the presence of live yeasts [143].This supports the hypothesis that live yeast supplementation accelerates maturation of the rumen microbial ecosystem. Fibre degradation processes would thereby be set up more efficiently in the early age of the animal, as shown by the increase in polysaccharidase and glycoside-hydrolase activities in the presence of yeast in the rumen of gnotoxenic lambs [137].

There are some evidence that live yeast additives indirectly promote fibre degradation or fibrolytic microbial activities by stabilizing rumen pH in case of ruminal acidosis (see section 4). Greater polysaccharide-degrading activities of the solid-associated bacterial fraction in rumen-cannulated adult sheep fed a high-concentrate diet were measured in the presence of yeasts [144]. The proportions of 16S rRNA of *F. succinogenes, R. albus,* and *R. flavefaciens* have been shown to increase in the rumen of sheep receiving another yeast product [145]. A 2 to 4-fold increase in the number of 16S rRNA gene copies of *R. albus* and *R. flavefaciens* was also measured with real-time PCR in rumen contents of sheep receiving a high-concentrate diet and a live yeast probiotic [14].

Guedes et al. [85] reported that a live yeast strain increased NDF degradation of different corn silage samples incubated *in sacco*. In their study, cows were fed with grass silage-corn silage based diet and the rumen pH was not indicative of SARA situation. However, it is noteworthy that a yeast effect was observed on pH and lactate concentration but the authors suggested that the yeast efficacy was not only attributable to a pH stabilization effect. Using the same technique, Chaucheyras Durand et al. [136, unpublished] have studied the effect of the same yeast strain on fibre degradation of different substrates and followed the kinetics of colonization by fibre-degrading bacteria and fungi using qPCR in rumen cannulated cows. In this study, the diet offered to the cows was composed of grass silage and hay and was not at risk regarding SARA. Results showed that the supplementation of 10^{10} cfu/day/cow of the yeast additive promoted colonization of fibrous substrates by cellulolytic bacteria (*F.succinogenes, R.flavefaciens, B.fibrisolvens*) and fungi but that the degree of stimulation was depending on the nature of the substrate, and on the microbial species targeted. It was noticed that feedstuffs with highest levels of lignin and thereby with less easily accessible digestible carbohydrates were better degraded in the presence of yeast, suggesting a particularly marked impact on the microbial breakdown of lignin-polysaccharide linkages. The same strain of *S. cerevisiae* significantly improved NDF degradation of 40 corn silages samples incubated *in sacco* in rumen cannulated cows, with differences in the degree of improvement according to the degradability of the corn silage [85]. Indeed, the yeast probiotic increased NDF degradation of the low digestible corn silages more strongly than that of the high digestible corn silages (Figure 4). These results suggest that live yeast could help to reduce indigestible NDF by promoting the action of bacteria and fungi involved in the hydrolysis of lignin-polyholoside bonds (Figure 5).

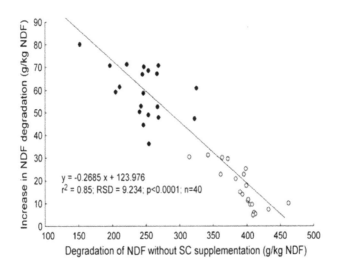

Figure 4. Figure 4. Effects of supplementation with a yeast probiotic (*Saccharomyces cerevisiae* CNCM I-1077) on fibre (NDF) degradation of maize silages after 36h of incubation in the rumen of cows: open circles, high fibre degradation group , full circles, low fibre degradation group. From [85].

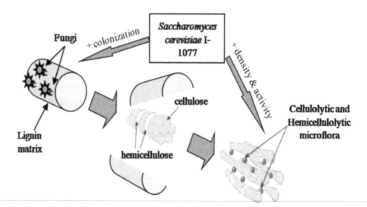

Figure 5. A proposed scheme for mode of action of *Saccharomyces cerevisiae* CNCM I-1077 on fibre degrading communities.

In the study of Chaucheyras-Durand et al. [136, unpublished], a positive effect of live yeast was demonstrated for the first time on *Butyrivibrio fibrisolvens* abundance on fibrous substrates. The hemicellulose fraction of forages consumed by ruminants consists mainly in xylan substituted with acetyl, arabinosyl, and glucuronyl residues. Xylan is also cross-linked via ferulic and p-coumaric acids which are esterified to the arabinose side chains. It is supposed that the ester linkages between these phenolic acids and polysaccharides provide a steric hindrance to the degradation of fibre by rumen microbiota. Consequently, the promotion of *B. fibrisolvens*, that possesses ferulic and p-coumaric acid esterases which hydrolyze these ester linkages [146] appears particularly interesting.

One of the main factors implicated in the beneficial effect of live yeasts on fibre-degrading bacteria is probably the capacity of yeast cells to scavenge oxygen. Indeed, although the rumen environment is known to be strictly anaerobic, dissolved oxygen can be detectable *in situ*; as high as 16 liters of oxygen can enter an ovine rumen daily during feed and water intake, rumination or salivation [147]. Most of ruminal microorganisms are considered to be highly sensitive to oxygen, but this is particularly true for fibre-degrading organisms. Respiratory-deficient mutants of *S. cerevisiae* were unable to stimulate bacterial numbers in rumen-simulating fermenters, whereas the wild-type parent strains, able to consume oxygen, did effectively stimulate bacterial activities [128]. Other studies have reported that redox potential of rumen fluid was lowered in the presence of live yeasts in lambs [143], in sheep [148] and in cows [57] suggesting that live yeast cells could create more favorable environmental conditions for growth and activities of the cellulolytic microbiota. Due to the fact that live yeasts could release vitamins or other growth factors to closely associated bacterial cells [149], yeast impact could also be mediated through the interplay between different bacterial species (i.e. non cellulolytic species) and would not only be explained by a direct effect on oxygen consumption.

7.4. Consequences on rumen fermentations, feed efficiency, and animal production

The beneficial effects on fibre digestion can be partly at the origin of the increase in dry matter intake often observed with yeast supplementation [149], but more generally a better fibre digestion is recognized to benefit the animal rumen health and its function by improvement of feed efficiency. The study carried out by Bitencourt et al. [150] did support this assumption with cows fed a corn silage, soybean meal, citrus pulp and steam-flaked corn based TMR. The diet NDF digestibility was improved by 11.3% in presence of 10^{10} cfu/day of the live yeast and the milk production tended to be improved by 0.9 kg/d. Cows were not in SARA situation (6.43<pH<6.5). In De Ondarza et al. multi-analysis [73], live yeast effect was particularly strong in low yielding cows. In addition, feed efficiency of the supplemented animals was improved which illustrates a better use of the diet. When targeting the cows fed diet above 30% NDF, feed efficiency was higher than the overall mean and the live yeast treated animals gained an extra 40g of milk per kg DMI. The shorter intervals between meals of live yeast fed cows reported in [56] strongly suggests the fact that the TMR digestibility was improved as the meal size and length were not affected by the treatment. As mentioned earlier, improvement of rumen pH for the cows receiving the live yeast at the same dose than the previously cited studies would also support a higher activity of the cellulolytic flora and thus explain the higher meal frequency.

8. Importance of yeast viability and strain selection

A better understanding of the modes of action of live yeast probiotics is important to further select of new yeast strains acting on specific key target microorganisms and areas of ruminal fermentation. Therefore, strain selection process is obviously critical in terms of safety; chosen organisms should be on the GRAS (Generally Recognized As Safe) list, or sufficient evidence would have to be provided to guarantee their innocuity for the animal, consumer and environment. Moreover, strain selection is important as different probiotics clearly exhibit markedly different effects on digestive microbiota of the same targeted organism. Dose response effects have also been reported for a same strain within the same experiment [63,85], suggesting that an optimal concentration of live cells has to be defined precisely according to the product application.

Efficacy of probiotics is strongly related to cell viability and metabolic activity [151], therefore, stability within the rumen is also an important consideration. Although yeast strains cannot properly colonize the rumen for a long period of time, certain strains can remain metabolically active in rumen fluid for more than 24 h [152] and live cells may be recovered from the faeces of treated animals up to several days after their initial incorporation in the diet. One objective when selecting a new probiotic strain will then be to assess its capacity to persist for a long time at a significant concentration in the targeted digestive compartment. Production, storage, and delivery protocols for yeast products should be designed to maintain yeast cell viability. High temperature storage, or in the presence of components such as minerals acting as oxidizing agents, may compromise viability [153]. The most common and officially recognised method for quantification of viable yeast probiotics is the colony forming unit (CFU) plate counting technique. Although it is perfectly adapted to take into account cells which have the capacity to multiply in optimal environmental conditions, it has long been recognized that microbial cells may exist in a latent state, in which they will not form colonies on nutrient media but may have other measurable activity [154]. For example, throughout alcoholic fermentation, *Saccharomyces cerevisiae* cells have to cope with stress conditions that could affect their viability and thereby enter into a Viable But Not Culturable (VBNC) state [155,156]. Further methodological developments would be necessary in order to take into account this status, which would improve our understanding on adaptive responses of probiotic yeasts to digestive conditions.

9. Conclusions and future work

Yeast probiotics benefit from a natural and well-accepted image by the consumer, as they are not involved in health disorders and do not have any detrimental impact on environment. Moreover, yeasts have been used for a long time in human nutrition. More and more well controlled research studies indicate that they can be useful to positively balance the rumen microbiota, stabilize rumen pH, and promote microbial degradation of plant cell walls. Thanks to their action, improvement in animal production and health can be obtained and in that sense one can expect a promising future for these additives in ruminant nutrition. As particularly shown for fibre degradation, the nature of dietary ingredients has a great influence in the rumen response to yeast probiotics. More research is needed to enlarge the efficacy data base using various diets and raw materials, which in term would lead to elaboration of predictive tools applicable on farms.

In the context of a high feed cost, fermentation aids such as live yeast represent a valuable nutritional tool which allows increasing the forage portion of the diet and consequently limiting the costly sources of energy. In addition, current intensive farming practices require high levels of fermentable carbohydrates which put the animal at risk of developing metabolic disorders. In that sense, yeast probiotics become even more relevant when the digestive microbiota is challenged, for example during a feed transition (weaning, grazing, step up feeding programs) or during periods of stress (hot temperature, transportation). In these particular conditions, higher yeast doses appear to better support rumen challenges. As differences have been reported in terms of response of the ruminal microbiota to different yeast additives (strain and capacity to retain metabolic activity), it is important to focus on the way the yeast strain is selected. Future research will also need to address the behavior of the yeast cells in the digestive environment. Indeed, identification of specific metabolic and physiologic characteristics exhibited by the yeast strains would allow a better understanding of their interactions within the animal gut and will help to further select more targeted additives for improved benefits in ruminant nutrition.

During plant cell wall breakdown and fermentation, most of cellulolytic bacteria, with the exception of *Fibrobacter succinogenes*, produce a lot of hydrogen, which is used to reduce carbon dioxide by *Archaea* methanogens to produce methane. This hydrogen transfer is important for a good functioning of the rumen ecosystem, but at the same time methane formation represents a loss of energy (10-12% of the metabolizable energy of the host animal) and this gas being a potent greenhouse gas, it should be decreased [157]. Studies with gnotobiotically-reared lambs have shown that animals inoculated with *F. succinogenes* were less prone to produce methane than lambs inoculated with *Ruminococci* and fungi, without significant modifications of rumen fibre degradability and volatile fatty acid concentrations [158]. The use of microbial solutions to promote *F. succinogenes* would then appear interesting to be able to mitigate methane emissions by cattle.

It is noteworthy that the increase in feed efficiency reported in presence of yeast probiotics has already an indirect effect on polluting outputs as it will decrease the amount of output/kg of milk/meat produced, but targeting microorganisms directly involved in these fermentative processes may be of interest.

Biohydrogenation mechanisms would also be a good target as they appear to be involved in milk fat depression which is very commonly observed in high-yielding cows, at risk for SARA. Under certain conditions, rumen microbial biohydrogenation results in the formation of fatty acids that are potent inhibitors of milk fat synthesis, i.e. trans10,cis12-CLA, and of possibly related intermediates from linolenic acid and other polyunsaturated fatty acids [48]. It has been shown that *Butyrivibrio sp.*is able to produce mainly trans-11,vaccenic acid via cis9, trans11-CLA instead of trans10,cis12-CLA from linolenic acid. By increasing the *Butyrivibrio* sp. population so that they utilize more linolenic acid at the expense of the organisms which form the detrimental isomer trans10,cis12 CLA, the potential exists to avoid a decrease in milk fat content. Stabilising ruminal pH through the addition of live yeasts should be beneficial for improved growth of these organisms which are sensitive to low pH. Moreover, promising data have been recently obtained that show a stimulation of *B. fibrisolvens* colonization on plant cell walls.

Yeast probiotics which have a good survival beyond the rumen may have interesting effects on intestinal homeostasis, and could thereby positively influence immune system and animal health. Indeed, certain strains of *Saccharomyces* may reduce pathogen load or their effects through competitive exclusion, cell binding or degradation of the toxins produced by intestinal pathogens. The beneficial effect that live yeast can have on pH regulation could also limit the release of inflammatory molecules, such as lipopolysaccharide or biogenic amines, and counteract the set up of acid-resistance mechanisms which may increase the virulence of certain pathogens. It has been reported that acidification of the rumen environment may increase mycotoxin absorption at low pH and decrease microbial detoxication mechanisms [159], so a better control of rumen pH by probiotic yeast may also aid in decreasing mycotoxin animal exposure.

Author details

Frédérique Chaucheyras-Durand
Lallemand Animal Nutrition, Blagnac, France
and INRA UR 454 Microbiologie, Saint-Genès Champanelle, France

Eric Chevaux
Lallemand Animal Nutrition, Blagnac, France

Cécile Martin
INRA UMR 1213 Herbivores, Saint-Genès Champanelle, France

Evelyne Forano
INRA UR 454 Microbiologie, Saint-Genès Champanelle, France

10. References

[1] Nocek JE. Bovine acidosis: implications on laminitis. Journal of Dairy Science 1997;80 1005-1028.

[2] Enemark JM, Jorgensen RJ, Kristensen NB. An evaluation of parameters for the detection of subclinical rumen acidosis in dairy herds. Veterinary Research Communications 2004;28 687-709.

[3] Nocek JE, Kautz WP, Leedle JA, Allman JG. Ruminal supplementation of direct-fed microbials on diurnal pH variation and in situ digestion in dairy cattle. Journal of Dairy Science 2002;85(2) 429-433.

[4] Duffield TF. Monitoring strategies for metabolic diseases in transition dairy cows. Médecin Vétérinaire du Québec 2004;34(1/2) 34-35.

[5] Mialon MM, Deiss V, Andanson S, Anglard F, Veissier I. An assessment of the impact of rumenocentesis on pain and stress in cattle and the effect of local anaesthesia. The Veterinary Journal 2012 http://dx.doi.org/10.1016/j.tvjl.2012.02.019.

[6] Brossard L, Martin C, Chaucheyras-Durand F, Michalet-Doreau B. Protozoa involved in butyric rather than lactic fermentative pattern during latent acidosis in sheep. Reproduction Nutrition Development 2004;44 195-206.

[7] Mottram T, Lowe J, McGowan M, Phillips N. Technical note: A wireless telemetric method of monitoring clinical acidosis in dairy cows. Computers and Electronics in Agriculture 2008;64 45-48.

[8] Stewart CS, Flint HJ, Bryant MP. The rumen bacteria. In : Hobson PN, Stewart CS (eds.) The rumen microbial ecosystem. London: Chapman & Hall; 1997. p10-72.

[9] Russell JB, Hino T. Regulation of lactate production in *Streptococcus bovis*: a spiraling effect that contributes to rumen acidosis. Journal of Dairy Science 1985;68 1712-1721.

[10] Counotte GHM, Prins RA, Janssen RHA, Deie MJA. Role of *Megasphaera elsdenii* in the fermentation of DL-[2-C^{13}]lactate in the rumen of dairy cattle. Applied and Environmental Microbiology 1981;42(4) 649-655.

[11] Russell JB, Baldwin RL. Substrate preferences in rumen bacteria: evidence of catabolite regulatory mechanisms. Applied and Environmental Microbiology 1978;36(2) 319-329.

[12] Brossard L, Chaucheyras-Durand F, Michalet-Doreau B, Martin C. Dose effect of live yeasts on rumen microbial communities and fermentations during butyric latent acidosis in sheep: new type of interaction. Animal Science 2006;82 1-8.

[13] Tajima K, Aminov RI, Nagamine T, Matsui H, Nakamura M, Benno Y. Diet-dependent shifts in the bacterial population of the rumen revealed with real-time PCR. Applied and Environmental Microbiology 2001;67 2766-2674.

[14] Mosoni P, Chaucheyras-Durand F, Béra-Maillet C, Forano E. Quantification by real-time PCR of cellulolytic bacteria in the rumen of sheep after supplementation of a forage diet with readily fermentable carbohydrates. Effect of a yeast additive. Journal of Applied Microbiology 2007;103 2676–2685.

[15] Yáñez-Ruiz DR, Macías B, Pinloche E, Newbold CJ. The persistence of bacterial and methanogenic archaeal communities residing in the rumen of young lambs. FEMS Microbiology Ecology 2010;72(2) 272-278.

[16] Khafipour E, Li S, Plaizier JC, Krause DO. Rumen microbiome composition determined using two nutritional models of subacute ruminal acidosis. Applied and Environmental Microbiology 2009;75(22) 7115-7124.

[17] Fernando SC, Purvis HT 2nd, Najar FZ, Sukharnikov LO, Krehbiel CR, Nagaraja TG, Roe BA, Desilva U. Rumen microbial population dynamics during adaptation to a high-grain diet. Applied and Environmental Microbiology 2010;76(22) 7482-7490.

[18] Russell JB, Wilson DB. Why are ruminal cellulolytic bacteria unable to digest cellulose at low pH? Journal of Dairy Science 1996;79 1503-1509.

[19] Martin C, Fonty G, Michalet-Doreau B. Factors affecting the fibrolytic activity of the digestive microbial ecosystems in ruminants. In: Martin SA (ed.) Gastrointestinal Microbiology in Animals. Trivandrum: Research Signpost; 2002. p1-17.

[20] Goad DW, Goad CL, Nagaraja TG. Ruminal microbial and fermentative changes associated with experimentally induced subacute acidosis in steers. Journal of Animal Science 1998;76 234-241.

[21] Grenet E, Breton A, Barry P, Fonty G. Rumen anaerobic fungi and plant substrates colonization as affected by diet composition. Animal Feed Science and Technology 1989;26 55-70.

[22] Fonty G, Grenet E. Effects of diet on the fungal population of the digestive tract of ruminants. In: Mountfort DO, Orpin CG (eds.) Anaerobic fungi: biology, ecology and function. New York: Marcel Dekker; 1994. p 229-239.

[23] Martin C, Millet L, Fonty G, Michalet-Doreau B. Cereal supplementation modified the fibrolytic activity but not the structure of the cellulolytic bacterial community associated with rumen solid digesta. Reproduction Nutrition Development 2001;41 413-424.

[24] Michalet-Doreau B, Morand D, Martin C. Effect of the microbial additive Levucell SC CNCM I-1077 on microbial activity in the rumen during the stepwise adaptation of sheep to high concentrate diet. Reproduction Nutrition Development 1997;supplEE5 81.

[25] Nozière P, Besle JM, Michalet-Doreau B. Effect of barley supplement on microbial fibrolytic enzyme activities and cell wall degradation rate in the rumen. Journal of Science of Food and Agriculture 1996;72 235-242.

[26] Sauvant D. Le contrôle de l'acidose ruminale latente. INRA Productions Animales 2006;19(2) 69-78.

[27] Philippeau C, Martin C, Michalet-Doreau B. Influence of grain source on ruminal characteristics and rate, site, and extent of digestion in beef steers. Journal of Animal Science 1999;77 1587-1596.

[28] Lettat A, Nozière P, Silberberg M, Morgavi DP, Berger C, Martin C. Experimental feed induction of ruminal lactic, propionic, or butyric acidosis in sheep. Journal of Animal Science 2010;88(9) 3041-3046.

[29] Mertens DR. Creating a system for meeting the fiber requirements of dairy cows. Journal of Dairy Science 1997;80(7) 1463-1481.

[30] Yang WZ, Beauchemin KA. Altering physically effective fiber intake through forage proportion and particle length: digestion and milk production. Journal of Dairy Science 2007;90(7) 3410-3421.

[31] Martin C, Brossard L, Doreau M. Mécanismes d'apparition de l'acidose ruminale latente et conséquences physiopathologiques et zootechniques. INRA Productions Animales 2006;19 93-108.

[32] Kleen JL, Cannizzo C. Incidence, prevalence and impact of SARA in dairy herds. Animal Feed Science and Technology 2012;172 4-8.

[33] Stone WC. The effect of subclinical acidosis on milk components. Cornell Nutrition conference for feed manufacturers. Cornell University, Ithaca NY 1999. p40-46.

[34] Emmanuel DG, Jafari A, Beauchemin KA, Leedle JA, Ametaj BN. Feeding live cultures of *Enterococcus faecium* and *Saccharomyces cerevisiae* induces an inflammatory response in feedlot steers. Journal of Animal Science 2007;85 233-239.

[35] Gozho GN, Krause DO, Plaizier JC. Ruminal lipopolysaccharide concentration and inflammatory response during grain-induced subacute ruminal acidosis in dairy cows. Journal of Dairy Science 2007; 90(2) 856-866.

[36] Plaizier JC, Krause DO, Gozho GN, McBride BW. Subacute ruminal acidosis in dairy cows : the physiological causes, incidence and consequences. Veterinary Journal 2008;176(1) 21-31.

[37] Khafipour E, Krause DO, Plaizier JC. A grain-based subacute ruminal acidosis challenge causes translocation of lipopolysaccharide and triggers inflammation. Journal of Dairy Science 2009;92(3) 1060-1070.

[38] Zebeli Q, Metzler-Zebeli BU. Interplay between rumen digestive disorders and diet-induced inflammation in dairy cattle. Research in Veterinary Science 2012; doi : 10.1016/j.rvsc.2012.02.004.

[39] Thompson P, Hentzen A , Schultheiss W. The effect of rumen lesions in feedlot calves : which lesions really affect growth? In: Proceedings from the 4th Schering Plough Ruminant day, 2006; University of Pretoria, Pretoria, South Africa, p23-27.

[40] Wang Y, Majak W, McAllister TA. Frothy bloat in ruminants: Cause, occurrence, and mitigation strategies Animal Feed Science and Technology 2012;172(1/2) 103-114.

[41] Vasconcelos JT, Galyean ML. ASAS centennial paper: Contributions in the Journal of Animal Science to understanding cattle metabolic and digestive disorders. Journal of Animal Science 2008;86(8) 1711-1721.

[42] Tadepalli S, Narayanan SK, Stewart GC, Chengappa MM, Nagaraja TG. *Fusobacterium necrophorum*: A ruminal bacterium that invades liver to cause abscesses in cattle. Anaerobe 2009;15(1/2) 36-43.

[43] Kleen JL, Hooijer GA, Rehage J, Noordhuizen JP. Subacute ruminal acidosis (SARA): a review. Journal of Verterinary Medecine A : Physiology, Pathology, Clinical Medicine 2003;50(8) 406-414.

[44] Commun L, Alves de Olivera L. L'acidose subclinique chez les ruminants. Conséquences comportementales et indicateurs physiologiques périphériques. Journées Nationales des GTV Nantes 2009;1091-1100.

[45] Mialon MM, Martin C, Garcia F, Menassol JB, Dubroeucq H,Veissier I, Micol D. Effects of the forage-to-concentrate ratio of the diet on feeding behaviour in young Blond d'Aquitaine bulls. Animal 2008;2 1682–1691.

[46] Commun L, Silberberg M, Mialon MM, Martin C, Veissier I. Behavioral adaptations of sheep to repeated acidosis challenges. Animal 2012. In press.

[47] Desnoyers M, Duvaux-Ponter C, Rigalma K, Roussel S, Martin C, Giger-Reverdin S. Effect of concentrate percentage on ruminal pH and time-budget in dairy goats. Animal 2008;2 1802-1808.

[48] Kennelly JJ, Robinson B, Khorasani GR. Influence of carbohydrate source and buffer on rumen fermentation characteristics, milk yield, and milk composition in early-lactation holstein cows. Journal of Dairy Science 1999;82 2486–2496.

[49] Khorasani GR, Kennelly JJ. Influence of carbohydrate source and buffer on rumen fermentation characteristics, milk yield, and milk composition in late-lactation holstein cows. Journal of Dairy Science 2001;84 1707–1716.

[50] Offner A, Bach A, Sauvant,D. Quantitative review of *in situ* starch degradation in the rumen. Animal Feed Science and Technology 2003;106(1-4) 81–93.

[51] Yang CM, Varga GA. Effect of three concentrate feeding frequencies on rumen protozoa, rumen digesta kinetics and milk yield in dairy cows. Journal of Dairy Science 1989;72 950-957.

[52] Diaz Uriarte R. Incorrect analysis of crossover trials in animal behaviour research. Animal Behavior 2002;63(4) 815-822.

[53] Weimer PJ, Stevenson DM, Mantovani HC, Man SLC. Host specificity of the ruminal bacterial community in the dairy cow following near-total exchange of ruminal contents. Journal of dairy Science 2010;93 5902–5912.

[54] Williams YJ, Popovski S, Rea SM, Skillman LC, Toovey AF, Northwood KS, Wright ADG. A vaccine against rumen methanogens can alter the composition of archaeal populations. Applied Environment Microbiology 2009;75(7) 1860–1866.

[55] Beauchemin KA , Yang WZ, Morgavi DP, Ghorbani GR, Kautz W, Leedle JAZ. Effects of bacterial direct-fed microbials and yeast on site and extent of digestion, blood chemistry, and subclinical ruminal acidosis in feedlot cattle. Journal of Animal Science 2003;81 1628-1640.

[56] Bach A, Iglesias C, Devant M. Daily rumen pH pattern of loose-housed dairy cattle as affected by feeding pattern and live yeast supplementation. Animal Feed Science and Technology 2007;136 156-163.

[57] Marden JP, Julien C, Monteils V, Auclair E, Moncoulon R, Bayourthe C. How does live yeast differ from sodium bicarbonate to stabilize ruminal pH in high-yielding dairy cows? Journal of Dairy Science 2008;91(9) 3528-3535.

[58] Desnoyers M, Giger-Reverdin S, Bertin G, Duvaux-Ponter C, Sauvant D. Meta-analysis of the influence of *Saccharomyces cerevisiae* supplementation on ruminal parameters and milk production of ruminants. Journal of Dairy Science 2009; 92 1620-1632.

[59] Thrune M, Bach A, Ruiz-Moreno M, Stern MD, Linn JG. Effects of *Saccharomyces cerevisiae* on ruminal pH and microbial fermentation in lactating dairy cows. Journal of Dairy Science 2007;90(Suppl. 1) 172.

[60] De Ondarza MB, Hall T, Sullivan J, Chevaux E. Effect of live yeast supplementation on milk yield, milk components, and rumen pH in dairy cows. Journal of Dairy Science 2012; E-suppl. In press.

[61] Chaucheyras F, Fonty G, Bertin G, Salmon JM, Gouet P. Effects of a strain of *Saccharomyces cerevisiae* (Levucell SC), a microbial additive for ruminants, on lactate metabolism *in vitro*. Canadian Journal of Microbiology 1996;42 927-933.

[62] Nisbet DJ, Martin SA. Effect of a *Saccharomyces cerevisiae* culture on lactate utilization by the ruminal bacterium *Selenomonas ruminantium*. Journal of Animal Science 1991;69 4628-4633.

[63] Newbold CJ, McIntosh FM, Wallace RJ. Changes in the microbial population of a rumen-simulating fermenter in response to yeast culture. Canadian Journal of Animal Science 1998;78 241-244.

[64] Rossi F, Luccia AD, Vincenti D, Cocconcelli PS. Effects of peptidic fractions from *Saccharomyces cerevisiae* culture on growth and metabolism of the ruminal bacteria *Megasphaera elsdenii*. Animal Research 2004;53 177-186.

[65] Michalet-Doreau B, Morand D. Effect of yeast culture, *Saccharomyces cerevisiae* CNCM I-1077, on ruminal fermentation during adaptation to high-concentrate feeding. In: 4èmes Rencontres autour des Recherches sur les Ruminants, Paris. 1997; 4 p121.

[66] Williams PEV, Tait CA, Innes GM, Newbold CJ. Effects of the inclusion of yeast culture (*Saccharomyces cerevisiae* plus growth medium) in the diet of dairy cows on milk yield and forage degradation and fermentation patterns in the rumen of steers. Journal of Animal Science 1991;69 3016-3026.

[67] Marsola RS, Favoreto MG, Silvestre FT, Shin JC, Walker N, Adesogan A, Staples CR, Santos JEP. Effect of feeding live yeast on performance of holstein dairy cows during summer. Journal of Dairy Science 2010;93 E-Suppl1 432.

[68] Owens FN, Secrist DS, Hill WJ, Gill DR. Acidosis in cattle: a review. Journal of Animal Science 1998;76(1) 275-286.

[69] Dohme F, DeVries TJ, Beauchemin KA. Repeated ruminal acidosis challenges in lactating dairy cows at high and low risk for developing acidosis: ruminal pH. Journal of Dairy Science 2008;91 3354-3367.

[70] Chaucheyras-Durand F, Silberberg M, Commun L, Martin C, Morgavi DP. Repeated ruminal acidotic challenges in sheep: effects on pH and microbial ecosystem and influence of active dry yeasts. Microbial Ecology 2009;57 564-565.

[71] Silberberg M, Chaucheyras-Durand F, Commun L, Richard-Mialon MM, Martin C, Morgavi DP. Repeated ruminal acidotic challenges in sheep: effects on pH and microbial ecosystem and influence of active dry yeasts. Journal of Animal Science 2009;87(E-Suppl) 280.

[72] Chaucheyras-Durand F, Walker ND, Bach A. Effects of active dry yeasts on the rumen microbial ecosystem: past, present and future. Animal Feed Science and Technology 2008;145 5-26.

[73] De Ondarza MB, Sniffen CJ, Dussert L, Chevaux E, Sullivan J, Walker ND. Case study: Multiple-Study analysis of the effect of live yeast on milk yield, milk component content and yield, and feed efficiency. The Professional Animal Scientist 2010;26 661–666.

[74] Moallem U, Lehrer H, Livshitz L, Zachut M, Yakoby S.. The effects of live yeast supplementation to dairy cows during the hot season on production, feed efficiency, and digestibility. Journal of Dairy Science 2009; 92 343-351.

[75] Huhtanen P, Asikainen U, Arkkila M, Jaakkola S. Cell wall digestion and passage kinetics estimated by marker and in situ methods or by rumen evacuations in cattle fed hay 2 or 18 times daily. Animal Feed Science and Technology 2007;133(3-4) 206–227.

[76] Oba M, Allen MS. Evaluation of the importance of the digestibility of neutral detergent fiber from forage: Effects on dry matter intake and milk yield of dairy cows. Journal of Dairy Science 1999;82(3) 589–596.

[77] Zebeli Q, Aschenbach JR, Tafaj M, Boguhn J, Ametaj BN, Drochner W. Invited review: Role of physically effective fiber and estimation of dietary fiber adequacy in high-producing dairy cattle. Journal of Dairy Science 2012;95(3) 1041–1056.

[78] Mertens DR. Challenges in measuring insoluble dietary fiber. Journal of Animal Science 2003;81(12) 3233-3249.

[79] Hristov AN, Price WJ, B. Shafii B. A meta-analysis examining the relationship among dietary factors, dry matter intake, and milk and milk protein yield in dairy cows. Journal of Dairy Science 2004;87(7) 2184–2196.

[80] West JW, Mandebvu P, Hill GM, Gates RN. Intake, milk yield, and digestion by dairy cows fed diets with increasing fiber content from bermudagrass hay or silage. Journal of Dairy Science 1998;81(6) 1599–1607.

[81] Rinne M, Huhtanen P, JaakkolaS. Digestive processes of dairy cows fed silages harvested at four stages of grass maturity. Journal of Animal Science 2002;80(7) 1986-1998.

[82] Martin C, Philippeau C, Michalet-Doreau B. Effect of wheat and corn variety on fiber digestion in beef steers fed high-grain diets. Journal of Animal Science 1999;77 2269-2278.

[83] Hall MB, Mertens DR. In vitro fermentation vessel type and method alter fiber digestibility estimates. Journal of Dairy Science 2012;91 301-307.

[84] Spanghero M, Berzaghi P, Fortina R, Masoero F, Rapetti L, Zanfi C, Tassone S, Gallo A, Colombini S, Ferlito JC. Technical note: precision and accuracy of in vitro digestion of neutral detergent fiber and predicted net energy of lactation content of fibrous feeds. Journal of Dairy Science 2010;93(10) 4855-4859.

[85] Guedes CM, Gonçalves D, Rodrigues MAM, Dias-da-Silva A. Effect of yeast Saccharomyces cerevisiae on ruminal fermentation and fiber degradation of maize silage in cows. Animal Feed Science and Technology 2008;145 27-40.

[86] Towne G, Nagaraja TG, Owensby C, Harmon D. Ruminal evacuation's effect on microbial activity and ruminal function. Journal of Animal Science 1986;62 783-788.

[87] Koike S, Kobayashi Y. Development and use of competitive PCR assays for the rumen cellulolytic bacteria: Fibrobacter succinogenes, Ruminococcus albus and Ruminococcus flavefaciens. FEMS Microbiology Letters 2001;204 361-366.

[88] Mosoni P, Martin C, Forano E, Morgavi DP. Long-term defaunation increases the abundance of cellulolytic ruminococci and methanogens but does not affect the bacterial and methanogen diversity in the rumen of sheep. Journal of Animal Science 2011;89(3) 783-791.

[89] Béra-Maillet C, Mosoni P, Kwasiborski A, Suau F, Ribot Y, Forano E. Development of a RT-qPCR method for the quantification of *Fibrobacter succinogenes* S85 glycoside hydrolase transcripts in the rumen content of gnotobiotic and conventional sheep. Journal of Microbiological Methods 2009;77(1) 8-16.

[90] Fonty G, Chaucheyras-Durand F, Forano E. Structuration de l'écosystème ruminal chez le nouveau-né: influence de facteurs écologiques. Journées Nationales GTV:conference proceedings, May 13-15, 2009, Nantes, France. p205-214.

[91] Fonty G, Gouet P, Jouany JP, Senaud J. Ecological factors determining establishment of cellulolytic bacteria and protozoa in the rumen of meroxenic lambs. Journal of General Microbiology 1983;129 213-223.

[92] Fonty G, Senaud J, Jouany JP, Gouet P. Establishment of the microflora and anaerobic fungi in the rumen of lambs. Journal of General Microbiology 1987;133 1835-1843.

[93] Weimer PJ, Waghorn GC, Odt CL, Mertens DR. Effect of diet on populations of three species of ruminal cellulolytic bacteria in lactating dairy cows. Journal of Dairy Science 1999;82(1) 122-134.

[94] Kong Y, Xia Y, Seviour R, He M, McAllister T, Forster R. In situ identification of carboxymethyl cellulose-digesting bacteria in the rumen of cattle fed alfalfa or triticale. FEMS Microbiology Ecology 2012;80(1) 159-167.

[95] Suen G, Weimer PJ, Stevenson DM, Aylward FO, Boyum J, Deneke J, Drinkwater C, Ivanova NN, Mikhailova N, Chertkov O, Goodwin LA, Currie CR, Mead D, Brumm PJ. The complete genome sequence of *Fibrobacter succinogenes* S85 reveals a cellulolytic and metabolic specialist PLoS One 2011;6(4) DOI 0.1371/journal.pone.0018814.

[96] Dodd D, Mackie RI, Cann IK. Xylan degradation, a metabolic property shared by rumen and human colonic Bacteroidetes. Molecular Microbiology 2011;79(2) 292-304.

[97] Henrissat B, Davies GJ. Glycoside hydrolases and glycosyltransferases. Families, modules, and implications for genomics. Plant Physiology 2000;124(4) 1515-1519.

[98] Flint HJ, Scott KP, Duncan SH, Louis P, Forano E. Microbial degradation of complex carbohydrates in the gut. Gut Microbes 2012;3(4) 1-18.

[99] Miron J, Ben-Ghedalia D, Morrison M. Invited review: adhesion mechanisms of rumen cellulolytic bacteria. Journal of Dairy Science 2001;84(6) 1294-1309.

[100] Flint HJ, Bayer EA. Plant cell wall breakdown by anaerobic microorganisms from the Mammalian digestive tract. Annals of New York Academy of Sciences 2008;1125 280-288.

[101] Ransom-Jones E, Jones DL, McCarthy AJ, McDonald JE. The Fibrobacteres: an important phylum of cellulose-degrading bacteria. Microbial Ecology 2012;63(2) 267-281.

[102] Williams AG, Coleman GS. Hemicellulose-degrading enzyme in rumen ciliate protozoa. Current Microbiology 1985;12(2) 85-90.

[103] Devillard E, Newbold CJ, Scott KP, Forano E, Wallace RJ, Jouany JP, Flint HJ.A xylanase produced by the rumen anaerobic protozoan *Polyplastron multivesiculatum* shows close sequence similarity to family 11 xylanases from gram-positive bacteria. FEMS Microbiology Letters 1999;181(1) 145-152.

[104] Béra-Maillet C, Devillard E, Cezette M, Jouany JP, Forano E. Xylanases and carboxymethylcellulases of the rumen protozoa *Polyplastron multivesiculatum,*

Eudiplodinium maggii and *Entodinium* sp. FEMS Microbiology Letters 2005;244(1) 149-156.

[105] Devillard E, Béra-Maillet C, Flint HJ, Scott P, Newbold CJ, Wallace RJ, Jouany JP, Forano E. Characterization of XYN10B, a modular xylanase from the ruminal protozoan *Polyplastron multivesiculatum*, with a family 22 carbohydrate-binding module that binds to cellulose. Biochemical Journal 2003;373 495-503.

[106] Findley SD, Mormile MR, Sommer-Hurley A, Zhang XC, Tipton P, Arnett K, Porter JH, Kerley M, Stacey G. Activity-based metagenomic screening and biochemical characterization of bovine ruminal protozoan glycoside hydrolases. Applied and Environmental Microbiology 2011;77(22) 8106-8113.

[107] Jouany J P, Demeyer DI, Grain J. Effect of defaunating the rumen. Animal Feed Science and Technology 1988;21 229–265.

[108] Eugène M, Archimède H, Sauvant D. Quantitative meta-analysis on the effects of defaunation of the rumen on growth, intake and digestion in ruminants. Livestock Production Science 2004;85 81-97.

[109] Orpin CG, Joblin KN. The rumen anaerobic fungi. In : Hobson PN, Stewart CS (eds.) The rumen microbial ecosystem. London, Chapman & Hall;1997. p140-195.

[110] Nagy T, Tunnicliffe RB, Higgins LD, Walters C, Gilbert HJ, Williamson MP. Characterization of a double dockerin from the cellulosome of the anaerobic fungus *Piromyces equi*. Journal of Molecular Biology 2007;373(3) 612-622.

[111] Akin DE, Borneman WS. Role of rumen fungi in fiber degradation. Journal of Dairy Science 1990;73(10) 3023-3032.

[112] Ljungdahl LG. The cellulase/hemicellulase system of the anaerobic fungus *Orpinomyces* PC-2 and aspects of its applied use. Annals of New York Academy of Sciences 2008;1125 308-321.

[113] Qi M, Wang P, Selinger LB, Yanke LJ, Forster RJ, McAllister TA. Isolation and characterization of a ferulic acid esterase (Fae1A) from the rumen fungus *Anaeromyces mucronatus*. Journal of Applied Microbiology 2011;110(5) 1341-1350.

[114] Fonty G, Chavarot M, Lepetit J, Canistro J, Favier R. Mechanical resistance of wheat straw after incubation in cultures of ruminal cellulolytic microorganisms. Animal Feed Science and Technology 1999;80(3/4) 297-307.

[115] Fonty G, Williams AG, Bonnemoy F, Withers SE, Gouet P. Effect of anaerobic fungi on glycoside hydrolase and polysaccharide depolymerase activities, *in sacco* straw degradation and volatile fatty acid concentrations in the rumen of gnotobiotically-reared lambs. Reproduction Nutrition Development 1995;35 329-337.

[116] Maekawa M, Beauchemin KA, Christensen DA. Chewing activity, saliva production, and ruminal pH of primiparous and multiparous lactating dairy cows. Journal of Dairy Science 2002;85(5) 1176–1182.

[117] Grant R. Forage fragility, fibre digestibility and chewing response in dairy cattle. Proceedings of 2010 Tri-State Dairy Nutrition Conference, Fort-Wayne, Indiana, USA, 20-21 April. 22pp.

[118] Beauchemin KA, Yang WZ. Effects of physically effective fiber on intake, chewing activity,and ruminal acidosis for dairy cows fed diets based on corn silage. Journal of Dairy Science 2005;88(6) 2117-2129.

[119] De Boever JL, Andries JI, De Brabander DL, Cottyn BG, Buysse FX. Chewing activity of ruminants as a measure of physical structure — A review of factors affecting it. Animal Feed Science and Technology 1990;27(4) 281–291.

[120] Varga GA, Kolver ES. Microbial and animal limitations to fiber digestion and utilization. Journal of Nutrition 1997;127(5 Suppl) 819S-823S.

[121] Jung HG, Mertens DR, Phillips RL. Effect of reduced ferulate-mediated lignin/arabinoxylan cross-linking in corn silage on feed intake, digestibility, and milk production. Journal of Dairy Science 2011;94(10) 5124-5137.

[122] Weimer PJ. Why don't ruminal bacteria digest cellulose faster? Journal of Dairy Science 1996;79(8) 1496-1502.

[123] Witzig M, Boguhn J, Kleinsteuber S, Fetzer I, Rodehutscord M. Influence of the maize silage to grass silage ratio and feed particle size of rations for ruminants on the community structure of ruminal Firmicutes *in vitro*. Journal of Applied Microbiology 2010;109(6) 1998-2010.

[124] Moorby JM, Dewhurst RJ, Evans RT, Danelón JL. Effects of dairy cow diet forage proportion on duodenal nutrient supply and urinary purine derivative excretion. Journal of Dairy Science 2006;89(9) 3552-3562.

[125] Scott RI, Yarlett N, Hillman K, Williams TN, Williams AG, Lloyd D. The presence of oxygen in rumen liquor and its effects on methanogenesis. Journal of Applied Bacteriology 1983;55 143-149.

[126] Hillman K, Lloyd D, Williams AG. Use of a portable quadrupole mass spectrometer for the measurement of dissolved gas concentrations in ovine rumen liquor in situ. Current Microbiology 1985;12 335-340.

[127] Marden JP, Bayourthe C, Enjalbert F, Moncoulon R. A new device for measuring kinetics of ruminal pH and redox potential in dairy cattle. Journal of Dairy Science 2005; 88(1) 277-281.

[128] Newbold CJ, Wallace RJ, McIntosh FM. Mode of action of the yeast *Saccharomyces cerevisiae* as a feed additive for ruminants. British Journal of Nutrition 1996;76(2) 249-261.

[129] Roger V, Fonty G, Komisarczuk-Bony S, Gouet P. Effects of physicochemical factors on the adhesion to cellulose Avicel of the rumen bacteria *Ruminicoccus flavefaciens* and *Fibrobacter succinogenes subsp. succinogenes*. Applied and Environmental Microbiology 1990; 56 3081-3087.

[130] Fonty G, Forano E. Les interactions microbiennes impliquées dans la cellulolyse ruminale. Comptes Rendus de l'Académie d'Agriculture de France 1998;84(1) 135-148.

[131] Chen J, Weimer P. Competition among three predominant ruminal cellulolytic bacteria in the absence or presence of non-cellulolytic bacteria. Microbiology 2001;147 21-30.

[132] Mosoni P, Fonty G, Gouet P. Competition between ruminal cellulolytic bacteria for adhesion to cellulose.Current Microbiology 1997;35(1) 44-47.

[133] Bernalier A, Fonty G, Bonnemoy F, Gouet P. Inhibition of the cellulolytic activity of *Neocallimastix frontalis* by *Ruminococcus flavefaciens*. Journal of General Microbiology 1993;139(4) 873-880.

[134] Plata PF, Mendoza MGD, Barcena-Gama JR, Gonzalez MS. Effect of a yeast culture (*Saccharomyces cerevisiae*) on neutral detergent fiber digestion in steers fed oat straw based diets. Animal Feed Science and Technology 1994;49 203-210.

[135] Miranda RLA, Mendoza MGD, Barcena-Gama JR, Gonzalez MS, Ferrara R, Ortega CME, Cobos PMA. Effect of *Saccharomyces cerevisiae* and *Aspergillus oryzae* cultures and NDF level on parameters of ruminal fermentation. Animal Feed Science and Technology 1996;63 289-296.

[136] Chaucheyras-Durand F, Ameilbonne A, Walker ND, Mosoni P, Forano E. Effect of a live yeast, *Saccharomyces cerevisiae* I-1077 on *in situ* ruminal degradation of alfalfa hay and fibre-associated microorganisms. Journal of Animal Science 2010;88(E-Suppl. 2) 145.

[137] Chaucheyras-Durand F, Fonty G. Establishment of cellulolytic bacteria and development of fermentative activities in the rumen of gnotobiotically-reared lambs receiving the microbial additive *Saccharomyces cerevisiae* CNCM I-1077. Reproduction Nutrition Development 2001;41 57-68.

[138] Angeles SC, Mendoza GD, Cobos MA, Crosby MM, Castrejon FA. Comparison of two commercial yeast cultures (*Saccharomyces cerevisiae*) on ruminal fermentation and digestion in sheep fed on corn-stover diet. Small Ruminant Research 1998;31 45-50.

[139] Chaucheyras F, Fonty G, Bertin G, Gouet P. Effects of live *Saccharomyces cerevisiae* cells on zoospore germination, growth, and cellulolytic activity of the rumen anaerobic fungus, *Neocallimastix frontalis* MCH3. Current Microbiology 1995;31 201-205.

[140] Girard ID, Dawson KA. Effect of a yeast culture on growth characteristics of representative ruminal bacteria Journal of Animal Science 1995;73 264.

[141] Callaway TS, Martin SA. Effects of a *Saccharomyces cerevisiae* culture on ruminal bacteria that utilize lactate and digest cellulose. Journal of Dairy Science 1997;80 2035-2044.

[142] Fonty G, Senaud J, Jouany JP, Gouet P. Establishment of ciliate protozoa in the rumen of conventional and conventionalized lambs: influence of diet and management conditions. Canadian Journal of Microbiology 1988;34 235-241.

[143] Chaucheyras-Durand F, Fonty G. Influence of a probiotic yeast (*Saccharomyces cerevisiae* CNCM I-1077) on microbial colonization and fermentation in the rumen of newborn lambs. Microbial Ecology in Health and Disease 2002;14 30-36.

[144] Jouany JP, Mathieu F, Senaud J, Bohatier J, Bertin G, Mercier M. The effect of *Saccharomyces cerevisiae* and *Aspergillus oryzae* on the digestion of the cell wall fraction of a mixed diet in defaunated and refaunated sheep rumen. Reproduction Nutrition Development 1998;38 401-416.

[145] Chaucheyras F, Millet L, Michalet-Doreau B, Fonty G, Bertin G, Gouet P. Effect of the addition of Levucell SC on the rumen microflora of sheep during adaptation to high starch diets. Reproduction Nutrition Development 1997; EE 5 (suppl) 82.

[146] McSweeney CS, Dulieu A, Bunch R. *Butyrivibrio* spp. and other xylanolytic microorganisms from the rumen have cinnamoyl esterase activity. Anaerobe 1998;4(1) 57-65.

[147] Newbold CJ. Microbial feed additives for ruminants. In: Wallace RJ, Chesson A (eds.) Biotechnology in animal feeds and animal feeding. Weinheim: VCH;1995. p259-278.

[148] Mathieu F, Jouany JP, Sénaud J, Bohatier J, Bertin G, Mercier M. The effect of *Saccharomyces cerevisiae* and *Aspergillus oryzae* on fermentations in the rumen of faunated and defaunated sheep; protozoal and probiotic interactions. Reproduction Nutrition Development 1996;36(3) 271-287.

[149] Jouany JP. Optimizing rumen functions in the close-up transition period and early lactation to drive dry matter intake and energy balance in cows. Animal Reproduction Science 2006;96 250-264.

[150] Bitencourt LL, Pereira MN, de Oliveira BML, Silva JRM, Dias Júnior GS, Lopes F, de Melo RCM, Siécola Júnior S. Response of lactating cows to the supplementation with live yeast. Journal of Dairy Science 2008;91(E-suppl1) 264.

[151] Chaucheyras-Durand F, Fonty G. Effects and modes of action of live yeasts in the rumen. Biologia (Bratislava) 2006;61(6) 741–750.

[152] Durand-Chaucheyras F, Fonty G, Bertin G, Theveniot M, Gouet P. Fate of Levucell SC I-1077 yeast additive during digestive transit in lambs. Reproduction Nutrition Development 1998;38 275-280.

[153] Sullivan ML, Bradford BJ. Viable cell yield from active dry yeast products and effects of storage temperature and diluent on yeast cell viability. Journal of Dairy Science 2011;94(1) 526-531.

[154] Davey HM. Life, death and in between: meanings and methods in microbiology Applied and Environmental Microbiology 2011;77(16) 5571-5576.

[155] Zuzuarregui A, Monteoliva L, Gil C, del Olmo ML. Transcriptomic and proteomic approach for understanding the molecular basis of adaptation of *Saccharomyces cerevisiae* to wine fermentation. Applied and Environmental Microbiology 2006;72(1) 836-847.

[156] Andorra I, Esteve-Zarzoso B, Guillamon JM, Mas A. Determination of viable wine yeast using DNA binding dyes and quantitative PCR. International Journal of Food Microbiology 2010;144(2) 257-262.

[157] Morgavi DP, Forano E, Martin C, Newbold CJ. Microbial ecosystem and methanogenesis in ruminants. Animal 2010;4(7) 1024-1036.

[158] Chaucheyras-Durand F, Masséglia S, Fonty G, Forano E. Influence of the composition of the cellulolytic flora on the development of hydrogenotrophic microorganisms, hydrogen utilization, and methane production in the rumens of gnotobiotically reared lambs. Applied and Environmental Microbiology 2010;76(24) 7931–7937.

[159] Boudra H. Mycotoxins: an insidious menacing factor for the quality of forages and the performances of the ruminants. Fourrages 2009;199 265–280.

Variations on the Efficacy of Probiotics in Poultry

Luciana Kazue Otutumi, Marcelo Biondaro Góis,
Elis Regina de Moraes Garcia and Maria Marta Loddi

Additional information is available at the end of the chapter

1. Introduction

In face of the current debate about the use of antibiotics as growth promoters, due to the probable relationship with resistance to antibiotics used in human medicine, the presence of antibiotic residues in products of animal origin intended for human consumption and the emergent demand from consumer market for products free from additive residues, it was necessary to search for alternative products that could replace antibiotics used as promoters, without causing losses to productivity or product quality.

An alternative is the use of probiotics, which are products made from living micro-organisms or their L-forms (without cell wall). The micro-organisms included as probiotics are usually assumed to be non-pathogenic components of the normal microflora, such as the lactic acid bacteria. However, there is good evidence that non-pathogenic variants of pathogenic species can operate in much the same way as traditional probiotics. For example, avirulent mutants of *Escherichia coli*, *Clostridium difficile*, and *Salmonella* Typhimurium can also protect against infection by the respective virulent parent strain (Fuller, 1995).

In poultry, the early use of probiotics was instituted by Nurmi & Rantala (1973). In their experiments, the authors observed that the intestinal contents of normal adult birds, orally administered to chicks with one day of age, altered their sensitivity to infection by *Salmonella spp.*

From there, several studies have been made and continue being developed with the use of probiotics. Inconsistent results from the use of probiotics in animal production have been a constraint for the promotion of their use. Variations in the efficacy of probiotics can be due to the difference in microbial species or micro-organism strains used, or with the additive preparation methods (Jin et al., 1998a). However, other factors can justify the variations in the results of probiotic use in poultry, such as origin species, probiotic preparation method, survival of colonizing micro-organisms to the gastrointestinal tract conditions, environment where the birds are raised, management (including the application time and application route of the probiotic), the immunologic status of the animals, the lineage of the poultry evaluated, as well as age and concomitant use or not of antibiotics.

Thus, the aim of this review is to discuss the use of probiotics in poultry, with emphasis on the type of probiotic and micro-organisms used, action mechanism and its relation with the variations on the results of poultry survey.

2. Type of probiotic and micro-organisms used

There are several types of probiotics available in the market to be used in poultry, with a range of micro-organisms present and, therefore, with different metabolic activities and action modes. Also, they present variations as to the capacity of colonizing the intestine or not, which justifies variations on the results of their use.

Bacillus, Bifidobacterium, Enterococcus, E. coli, Lactobacillus, Lactococcus, Streptococcus, Pediococcus species, and a range of yeast species and non-defined mixed cultures have been used (Fuller, 1992; Patterson & Burkholder, 2003; Kabir et al., 2004; Mountzouris et al., 2007). However, even those belonging to the same species can have different strains and even these different strains from the same species can have different metabolic activities. These bacteria are used alone or in combination (Miles, 1993; Montes & Pugh, 1993).

Non-defined mixed cultures, known as competitive exclusion cultures, are normally related to the treatment of one-day chicks with an indefinite microbiota derived from adult animals resulting in resistance to colonization against pathogenic micro-organisms.

Among the colonizing species, *Lactobacillus sp., Enterococcus sp.* and *Streptococcus sp.* are worth mentioning, and among the non-colonizing species, *Bacillus spp.* (spores) and *Saccharomyces cerevisiae (*Žikić et al., 2006 apud Perić et al., 2009*).*

Another characteristic of probiotics is that some micro-organisms are constituted by micro-organisms normal to the intestinal microbiota of poultry, and others by bacteria different from the ones from the digestive tract. According to Kabir (2009) the most commonly used species are: *Lactobacillus bulgaricus, Lactobacillus acidophilus, Lactobacillus casei, Lactobacillus helveticus, Lactobacillus lactis, Lactobacillus salivarius, Lactobacillus plantarum, Streptococcus thermophilus, Enterococcus faecium, Enterococcus faecalis, Bifidobacterium spp.* and *Escherichia coli,* and except for *Lactobacillus bulgaricus* and *Streptococcus thermophilus*, all the remaining ones are intestinal strains.

Recently, emphasis has been given to the selection, preparation and application of probiotic strains, especially lactic acid bacteria (Wang & Gu, 2010).

Natural adaptation of lactic acid bacteria to intestinal environment and the lactic acid produced by them have provided advantages for these organisms over other micro-organisms used as probiotic (Guerra et al., 2007).

3. Action mechanisms

The action mechanisms of probiotics (Fig. 1) on the immune system of broiler mucosa are not completely clear. However, it is admitted that probiotics have immune-modulating effects (Cotter, 1994; Erickson & Hubbard, 2000; Edens, 2003; Loddi, 2003; Ng et al., 2009).

According to (Erickson & Hubbard, 2000 and Menten & Loddi, 2003), the bacterium genera present in probiotics that are directly related to the increase in immunity of poultry are *Lactobacillus* and *Bifidobacterium*, mainly when related to diseases affecting the gastrointestinal tract. However, other genera have been related (Hakkinen & Schneitz, 1999; Yurong et al., 2005; Hong et al., 2005).

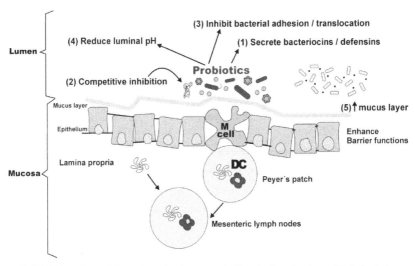

Figure 1. Inhibition of enteric bacteria and enhancement of barrier function by probiotic bacteria. Schematic representation of the crosstalk between probiotic bacteria and the intestinal mucosa. Antimicrobial activities of probiotics include the (1) production of bacteriocins/defensins, (2) competitive inhibition with pathogenic bacteria, (3) inhibition of bacterial adherence or translocation, and (4) reduction of luminal pH. Probiotic bacteria can also enhance intestinal barrier function by (5) increasing mucus production (Adapted Ng et al., 2009).

The immune-modulating effect in poultry happens in two ways: (a) from the microbiota, in which the probiotic migrates along the wall of the intestine and is multiplied to a limited extension, or (b) the antigen released by the dead organisms are absorbed and thus stimulate the immune system (Havenaar & Spanhaak, 1994).

According to Loddi (2003) and Nunes (2008), antigens (lipopolysaccharides and peptidoglycans) are constantly released in intestinal lumen. On the other hand, this release is increased during infectious processes, once these components are fundamental in the development and maintenance of local immune response (Hamann et al., 1998; Loddi, 2003), since they have chemotactic effect on epithelial cells and cells related to mucosa immunity, and induce changes in the intestinal epithelium of the host.

The chemotactic effect is accomplished by mediators such as cytokines, metaloproteins (elastase and cathepsin), prostaglandins, oxygen and nitrogen reactive metabolites, elevating the production of IgA, IgM and IgG immunoglobulins, activating differentiation and proliferation of NK (Natural Killer), CD_3, CD_4 and CD_8 lymphocytes, increasing the migration of lymphocyte T and the production of interferon (Fuller 1989; Jin et al., 1997; Erickson & Hubbard, 2000; Edens, 2003; Loddi, 2003; Zhang et al., 2007; Neurath, 2007; Ng et al., 2009).

The changes induced by probiotics in the intestinal epithelium are accentuated by the decrease in luminal pH, antimicrobial activity and secretion of antimicrobial peptides inhibiting bacterial invasion and blocking the adhesion to epithelial cells. In this sense, they improve the intestinal barrier elevating the production of cytokines (TNF-α, IFN-γ, IL-10 and IL-12) (Arvola et al., 1999), which in turn, induce the secretion of IgA in the intestinal mucosa, causing the release of mucins (Gupta & Garg, 2009).

Mucins, the layer of glycoproteins that when in contact with water, form a film that lubricates and protects the intestinal epithelium against pathogens, forming a physical barrier between the epithelium and the content from the intestinal lumen (Oliveira-Sequeira et al., 2008), keeping the bacteria in a safe place in the intestinal lumen (Mattar et al., 2002).

Studies suggest that the inhibiting effect of bacterial translocation by *Lactobacillus casei* GG *in vivo* and *in vitro* could be related with the regulation of the MUC- 2 gene, which promotes the expression of mucin by goblet cells (Mattar et al., 2002).

In the intestine, probiotics interact with enterocytes, goblet cells, M cells from Peyer's patches, isolated follicles that are extended through the mucosa and submucosa in the small intestine, forming GALT (Gut Associated Lymphoid Tissue) and immune cells among them, intraepithelial lymphocytes. These interactions result in an increase in the number of IgA-producing cells accompanied by the production of secretory IgM and IgA that are particularly important to the immunity of the mucosa, contributing to the barrier against pathogenic micro-organisms (Szajewska et al., 2001).

Thus, in the modulation of the immune response, the suppression of potential pathogens has been observed (Majarmaa, 1997), through the increase of intestinal motility (Gupta & Garg, 2009), increase in the population of intraepithelial lymphocytes in the intestinal epithelium (Dalloul et al., 2003), removal of pathogens (Patterson & Burkholder, 2003), modification of intestinal microbiota (Shane, 2001; Salzman et al., 2003), and increase in the height of intestinal villi (Iji et al., 2001). Added to these effects, the capacity of bacterial groups to develop a fimbria network that blocks the linking location of some enteric pathogens.

Another relevant aspect is related to different bacterial genera, which colonize and are developed, producing an almost permanent exclusion environment, known as competitive exclusion mechanism, which represents the competition for adhesion locations to the membrane of goblet cells, enteroendocrine cells and enterocytes in the intestinal mucosa, which promote a status of physical barrier to the mucosa by creating a special integrity system, preventing intestinal pathogens from becoming established (Rantala & Nurmi, 1974; Soerjadi et al., 1982; Salminen & Isolauri, 1996). Therefore, a mechanism proposal was described by Revolledo et al. (2006) for poultry receiving supplementation of competitive exclusion products, probiotics or immunostimulants (Fig. 2).

As well as this mechanism, there is an antagonist effect through the secretion of substances that inhibit the growth and development of pathogenic bacteria (Fig. 1), such as bacteriocines, organic acids and hydrogen peroxide (Patterson & Burkholder, 2003; Oumer et al., 2001; Mazmanian et al., 2008). As well as these, other benefits from the use of probiotics are: increase of enzymatic activity inducing absorption and nutrition (Hooper et al., 2002; Timmerman et al., 2005) and inhibition of procarcinogenic enzymes (Gill, 2003).

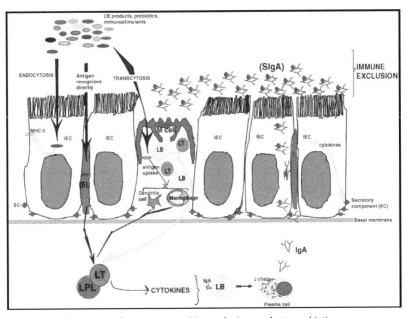

Figure 2. Proposed interactions between competitive exclusion products, probiotics or immunostimulants, and avian intestinal immunity. SIgA =secretory IgA; CE=competitive exclusion; IEC =intraepithelial cell; IEL=intestinal intraepithelial lymphocyte; LPL=lamina propria lymphocytes (activated T lymphocytes); dendritic cell or macrophage =antigen-presenting cells (APC); LB=B lymphocyte; LT=T lymphocyte; M cells =cells for the transport of antigens from the intestinal lumen into the gut-associated lymphoid tissue; SC =secretory component; endocytosis =process in which a substance gains entry into a cell without passing through the cell membrane; transcytosis=process of transport of substances across an epithelium layer by uptake on one side of the epithelial cell into a coated vesicle that might then be sorted through the *trans*-Golgi network and transported to the opposite side of the cell.

Proposed Mechanisms. Antigen uptake: 1. Antigen can be recognized directly by IEL, signals are sent to LT in the lamina propria. 2. When antigen is taken in by M cells using transcytosis process, there are 2 possible mechanisms to stimulate the immune response: a) antigen is directly taken in by macrophages or dendritic cells, which are able to process and present to LT in the lamina propria, or b) antigen activates B cells, which stimulate LT in the lamina propria. 3. Antigen uptake can be made by IEC using endocytosis process. The IEC are able to act as APC and process the antigen, antigen is presented to LT in the lamina propria. SIgA production: activated LT (LPL) produces cytokines, which stimulate LB activation, and finally plasma cells, produce IgA. The IgA acquires the secretory component on the IEC and is able to internalize into IEC; finally SIgA is available in the intestinal lumen to exert surface protection. (Revolledo et al., 2006).

4. Variations on the efficacy of probiotics in poultry

As described before, there is a large range of micro-organisms used as probiotics, with variations in species and strains of the same species, and therefore, they present variations in its metabolic activity and justify variations in the results of their use. However, other factors can justify the variations in the results of using probiotics in poultry, such as the origin species, probiotic preparation method, survival of colonizing micro-organisms in the gastrointestinal tract conditions, the environment where the birds are raised, management (including probiotic application time and application route), the immunologic state of the animals, the lineage of poultry evaluated, as well as age and concomitant use of antibiotics.

Fuller (1986) emphasizes that the specificity of adhesion of lactobacilli (one of the most used probiotic genre in poultry) to epithelial cells is specific host and if the colonization is reached, it is essential to administer bacteria that have been originated form the host species for which they are being given.

On the other hand, it is worth mentioning that there are probiotics presenting efficacy even though they have not been isolated from the original host species. As an example, one can mention the works developed by Impey et al. (1984) and Schneitz & Nuotio (1992) showing that the natural microbiota of chicken (Broilact®) and turkeys provide reciprocal protection for chicks and poults.

Regarding the probiotic preparation method, Fuller (1975) reports that even the carbohydrate source used in the growth media during the preparation of probiotic can affect the micro-organism's ability in adhering to the intestinal epithelium of poultry and the adhesion capacity also changed during its growth cycle. Therefore, notes that even if two strains are identical, the form which they have been prepared can cause variations in the result (Fuller, 1995).

Several beneficial effects of the use of *Lactobacillus* as probiotics are reported in literature in relation to the productive performance of poultry (Kalbane et al., 1992; Nahashon et al., 1996; Jin et al., 1998a; Kalavathy et al., 2003; Schocken-iturrino et al., 2004). Thus, studies on the proteomics of *Lactobacillus* have been made with the objective of allowing its better growth and/or survival by means of appropriate preservation methods (De Angelis & Gobbetti, 2004) to obtain a better performance with its use.

In a study developed by Desmond et al. (2001), the authors have shown that in order to increase the viability of probiotic strains of *Lactobacillus paracasei* NFBC 338 during spray-drying, a pre-stressing of the culture by exposure to temperature of 52°C for 15 minutes increased in 700 fold the survival of the strain (in reconstituted skimmed milk) during caloric stress and 18 fold during spray drying when compared to non-adapted cells, demonstrating that the probiotic preparation method can aid for a larger survival time and consequent results obtained.

It is important to mention that as well as the genetic variation among species, other environmental factors during the preparation of probiotics (pH, water activity, salts and preservative content) influence in the resistance of *Lactobacillus* to caloric stress and spray drying (Casadei et al., 2001; Desmond et al., 2001).

Also, for a micro-organism to be selected to be used as probiotic, it is necessary that it can be able to overcome some barriers that would be harmful to its survival in the gastrointestinal tract. Mills et al. (2011) report that before probiotic bacteria can start to perform its physiological role in the intestine, they should support a number of tensions to ensure it reaches the target site in sufficient number to elucidate its effect. According to the authors, first the bacterium must be processed in an appropriate manner to allow oral consumption and be able to resist the inhospitable conditions imposed during its passage through the gastrointestinal tract.

In order to be in a highly viable state during processing, storage and intestinal transit, bacteria go through adverse conditions including temperature, acidity, bile, exposure to osmotic and oxidative stress both in the production matrix and during intestinal transit (Corcoran et al., 2008). Thus, the benefit from the use of probiotics is the result of the growth of organisms and generation of some beneficial functions in the intestinal tract (Jin et al., 1998a), being that the efficacy in the use of *Lactobacillus* as probiotics depends not only in the proliferation of bacteria in the intestinal tract, but also that they survive through the stomach.

This is due to the fact that every food ingested (including the probiotics provided in feed) is submitted to a gastric pH ranging between 2 and 4 that can cause the death of bacteria going through the stomach in 10 to 100 fold (Fuller, 1986).

Regarding the nutritional status of the animals, studies have shown that improvements in the performance of broilers have been seen when feed does not contain all nutrients in appropriate quantities.

In research developed by Dilworth & Day (1978), the authors verified that the effect of supplementation with *Lactobacillus spp.* on the growth of body mass and feed conversion in broilers is significantly greater when the methionine, cystine and lysine levels in the feed are reduced.

Likewise, Kos & Wittner (1982) have not found improvement in the growth and feed conversion of broilers by the addition of probiotics in feed containing all nutrients in appropriate quantities.

Equally, Mikulec et al. (1999) demonstrated the favorable influence that probiotics have on the growth of body mass and improvement in feed conversion of broilers when the level of crude protein in the diet was not efficient.

Regarding the environment where the animals are raised, studies have demonstrated influence of environmental stress on the results of probiotic research.

According to Weinack et al. (1985), the physiological stress induced by high or low environmental temperatures or withdrawal of food and water interfere either with the colonization of protective micro-organisms or reduces the protection provided by the probiotic.

However, Fuller (1986) reports that the stressor agent must be present before any effect of the probiotic supplement can be observed and that there will only be stimulus to growth it the depressor agent is present, that is, the author emphasizes that for the evidence of improvement on the performance of animals, the breeding environment must not be free from challenges. In experimental conditions, the absence of beneficial results can be justified by this statement.

Montes & Pugh (1993) reported similar results and showed that in birds, the best results with the use of probiotics happened when the birds were submitted to stress conditions, being by the increase or decrease of temperature, transportation, vaccination and overcrowding. In these conditions, an imbalance in the intestinal microbiota is created and the body defense mechanisms are decreased (Jin et al., 1997), which by the supplementation of probiotics, such problems would be minimized, evidencing differences in the performance results.

In literature, several treatment methods using probiotics are described, such as through feed, addition to drinking water, spraying on the birds, inoculation via cloaca or in embryonated eggs (*in ovo*), through the litter used, in gelatin capsules and intra-esophagus (Schneitz, 1992; Ziprin et al., 1993).

This way, the administration route of probiotics can determine an improvement or worsening in the intestinal colonization capacity by the bacteria present in the product used. Direct inoculation in esophagus/crop (intra-esophageal) is the most efficient (Stavric, 1992), although in practical terms it has little viability.

One justification for the absence of results with the use of probiotics in drinking water can be the presence of residual chlorine and the fact of the product becoming inefficient before all chicks have received the micro-organisms in the appropriate dose (Seuna et al., 1978), and sometimes, chicks do not drink water before feeding, which makes the protection uneven within the herd (Schneitz et al., 1991).

Also, according to Siriken et al. (2003), the duration of treatment can be an important factor in the effect of a probiotic on the intestinal microbiota, once probiotics can be given only once or periodically, in weekly or daily intervals. Despite the little knowledge regarding the minimum required dose to evidence the effects of probiotics, experiments in mice, humans and pigs have indicated that the effect decreases when the probiotic is discontinued (Cole & Fuller, 1984; Goldin & Gorbach, 1984).

Lan et al. (2005) reported that for the microbiota to be established in the small intestine and in the caecum, it is necessary approximately two and from six to seven weeks, respectively.

Particularly for controlling the population of *Escherichia coli*, Fuller (1977) reports that such control is dependent on the presence of sufficient number of *Lactobacillus* and that from the results of *in vitro* tests, it seems to be necessary at least 10^7 colony forming units per gram (CFU/g).

Currently, the modern broiler and turkey lineages present high weight gain capacity. However, when compared with lineages of slower growth, they are more susceptible to infectious diseases (Korver, 2012).

According to the same author, modern broilers and turkeys present a depressed systemic innate immune response to allow fast growth, once the deviation of nutrients to the development of systemic inflammatory response is minimum, and despite presenting better immunity mediated by cells, there is evidence of increase in the mortality among fast-growth poultry when compared with slow-growth ones, which might justify differences in the effects between the different bird lineages.

Regarding age, the paper by Mohan et al. (1996) found that beneficial effects of probiotics were seen during the initial growth phase, happening before 28 days and not after 49 days of age.

Certainly, during the initial stages of life, the intestinal microbiota is in an unstable condition, and the micro-organisms given orally probably find a niche where they can occupy (Fuller, 1995). Therefore, Siriken et al. (2003) reported that the existence of an intestinal microbiota at the time of administration and the health of the host must be considered when a probiotic is supplemented for the suppression of pathogenic bacteria.

It should also be noticed that some micro-organisms that can act as probiotics do not resist the action of some antibiotics or anticoccidial used in the feed of birds (Jin et al., 1997, 1998a; Tournut, 1998).

Other factors that might justify the variations in the effects of probiotics in poultry are: variations in the persistence of administered strains (relative intestinal concentration) (Siriken et al., 2003; Huyghebaert et al.,2011), stability during the manufacturing of feed (Huyghebaert et al., 2011), absence of statistical analysis of data in previous studies, experimental protocols not clearly defined, micro-organisms not identified (Simon et al., 2001), viability of organisms not verified (Fuller, 1995; Simon et al., 2001), as well as the fact that in many studies, the origin of micro-organisms in probiotics was not reported (Siriken et al., 2003).

A study performed by Weese (2002) with eight veterinary and five human probiotics showed that only three from the eight veterinarian products provided data regarding its content; the majority of the products had less quantity than the one declared and five products lacked one or more strains declared; and three products had different strains from the ones declared in the package.

Similar work was developed by Lata et al. (2006), where it was verified that among the five probiotics evaluated, four presented information on validity date, species and amount of bacterium per gram of product. The three products containing *Enterococcus faecium* in its composition presented the amount of bacteria as declared in its label. However, the presence of *Lactobacillus sp.* was also found, which was not specified in the labels. In the product containing *Bacillus subtilis* and *Lactobacillus paracasei* in its composition, only *Bacillus subtilis* was found in amounts lower than the one declared.

With all these possible variations, it is not surprising that probiotics not always grant the desired result, but the fact that significant results are obtained show that the correct use of probiotics, under appropriate conditions and using the correct administration method, justify the fact that probiotics are an efficient food supplement in animal breeding.

5. Research results from the use of probiotics in poultry

5.1. Performance of poultry

Using two commercial probiotics, the first composed with Bacillus subtilis (150 g/ton feed) and the second with Lactobacillus acidophilus and casei, Streptococcus lactis and faecium, Bifidobacterium bifidum and Aspergillus oryzae (1 kg/ton feed) for broilers in the period of one to 14 days of age, Pelicano et al. (2004) observed an improvement in feed conversion up to 21 days of age in animals receiving probiotics, regardless of the composition, in relation to the group without any addition. However, there were no significant differences for the total breeding period (1-42 days), demonstrating that the period of treatment with probiotic might influence the performance results.

Improvement in the performance of broilers has been reported by several researchers (Dilworth & Day, 1978; Jin et al., 1996; Mohan et al., 1996; Yeo & Kim, 1997; Santoso et al. 1995; Jin et al., 1998a; Cuevas et al., 2000; Fritts et al.,2000; Kabir et al., 2004; Huang et al., 2004; Schocken-Iturrino et al., 2004; Gil de los Santos et al., 2005; Mountzouris et al., 2007; Rigobelo et al., 2011).

On the other hand, works performed by (Loddi et al. 2000; Lima et al. 2003; Willis & Reid, 2008) have not shown any benefit for the use of probiotics in any breeding phase of broilers.

In Japanese quails (*Coturnix coturnix japonica*), Sahin et al. (2008) evaluated the effect of different concentrations (0.5, 1 and 1.5 g/Kg feed) of a symbiotic (probiotic + prebiotic) on the diet of animals and have not found differences among the treatments in relation to body weight gain, feed conversion rate and carcass yield.

In a similar way, Otutumi et al. (2010) evaluated the effect of including a probiotic based on *Lactobacillus spp*. added through drinking water and feed to meat quails in the period of one to seven days of age on the performance in the period of one to 35 days of age and have not found differences in weight gain, feed conversion and carcass yield. However, the animals receiving the probiotic presented lower feed consumption (P<0.05), without affecting weight gain.

Yang (2009) compiled several studies with diverging results regarding the performance of broilers with the use of probiotics (Table 1).

Faria Filho et al. (2006) performed a meta-analysis study resulting from 35 tests involving probiotics in Brazil between 1995 and 2005. Based on the results, the authors concluded that the usage of probiotics is a viable technique for improvement on the development of broilers.

Item	Control	Probiotics	Improvement (%)	Reference
BWG (g/bird)[1]	1892	1920	+1	Liu et al (2007)
FCR (g/g)[2]	1.75	1.74	0	
BWG (g/bird)	2216	2237	+1	Mountzouris et al (2007)
FCR (g/g)	1.81	1.78	+2	
BWG (g/bird)	2784	2720	-2	
FCR (g/g)	1.62	1.63	0	Murry et al (2006)
Mortality (%)	7.02	4.76	+32	
ADG (g/bird)[3]	49.99	49.65	0	
FCR (g/g)	1.93	1.87	+3	Timmerman et al (2006)
Mortality (%)	8.84	7.27	+18	
BWG (g/bird)	2151	2251	+5	Kalavathy et al (2003)
FCR (g/g)	1.96	1.78	+9	
BWG (g/bird)	1379	1545	+12	
FCR (g/g)	2.08	2.17	-4	Zulkifli et al (2000)
Mortality (%)	1.7	2.2	-29	
BWG (g/bird)	1290	1388	+8	
FCR (g/g)	2.27	2.1	+7	Jin et al (1998b)
Mortality (%)	6.7	5.3	+21	

Table 1. Growth performance and/or mortality rate of birds to probiotic supplementation.

Eggs production has been also investigated in relation to probiotic application. Davis and Anderson (2002) reported that a mixed cultures of *Lactobacillus acidophilus*, *L. casei*,

---

[1] BWG = Body Weight Gain.
[2] FCR = Feed Conversion Ratio.
[3] ADG = Average daily gain.

Bifidobacterium thermophilus and *Enterococcus faecium,* improved egg size and lowered feed cost in laying hens. Moreover, probiotics increase egg production (Kurtoglu et al., 2004; Yörük et al., 2004; Panda et al., 2008) and quality (Kurtoglu et al., 2004; Panda et al., 2008) of chickens.

In laying Japanese quails, Ayasan et al. (2005) observed improvement in the feed conversion efficiency, while reducing egg shell thickness but not affected on feed intake, egg production, egg shell weight, egg shape index and numbers of eggs after six weeks of application of 120 ppm probiotic based on *Yucca schidigera* in feed.

5.2. Exclusion of pathogens and immunity

One of the action mechanisms of the previously mentioned probiotics was the competitive exclusion, which plays an important role in the prevention of enteric colonization by pathogenic micro-organisms, among them, *Salmonella* spp.

According to Scanlan (1997), three mechanisms present an important role in the prevention of enteric colonization of chicks by *Salmonella* spp. previously supplemented by competitive exclusion cultures: a) the micro-organisms constituting the competitive exclusion culture establish an enteric flora before exposure to *Salmonella* spp.; b) the micro-organisms from the inoculated flora compete with *Salmonella* spp. for essential nutrients, and c) the beneficial micro-organisms produce concentrations of volatile fatty acids that lower the intestinal pH and are bacteriostatic for *Salmonella* spp.

Several authors (Hinton & Mead, 1991; Stavric, 1992; Blankenship et al., 1993) reported that these exclusion cultures seem to be more effective against the colonization by *Salmonella* in the cecum. However, some authors have reported their inefficacy (Stavric et al., 1991).

Table 2 shows that in several works there was a high percentage of reduction in the colonization by *Salmonella spp* with the use of probiotics in broilers.

Researchers	Probiotic	Treatment with probiotic	Reduction (%) in the colonization[4]
Menconi et al. (2011)	Lactic acid bacteria	1 h post challenge	95% SH[5]
Knap et al. (2011)	*Bacillus subtilis*	Diet (1 to 42 days of age)	58% SH[6]
Higgins et al. (2010)[7]	Lactic acid bacteria	1h post challenge	4 -76% SE[5]
Higgins et al (2007)	Lactic acid bacteria	1 h post challenge	60 -72% SE[5] 92-96% ST[5]

Table 2. Effectiveness of probiotics in the prevention of *Salmonella* colonization in broiler chicken.

[4] SE = *Salmonella* Enteritidis; ST = *Salmonella* Typhimurium; SH = *Salmonella* Heidelberg.
[5] 24 h after treatment, cecal tonsil.
[6] 42 days of age – drag swabs.
[7] Data related to experiments 1, 2 & 3.

Mountzouris et al. (2010), studying inclusion levels of a probiotic composed by *Lactobacillus reuteri, Enterococcus faecium, Bifidobacterium animalis, Pediococcus acidilactici* and *Lactobacillus salivarius,* found that the inclusion of 10^9 and 10^{10} CFU/kg feed provided benefit in modulation of the composition of cecal microflora. Particularly, they reduced the concentration of coliforms in the cecum (log CFU/g of wet digesta) at 14 and 42 days of age in broilers. Also, the authors have found an increase in the concentration of *Bifidobacterium* and *Lactobacillus* at 42 days of age. Thus, the supplementation of probiotic in the indicated concentrations has been efficient as modulation of beneficial microbiota and reducing the studied pathogens.

According to Leandro et al. (2010), the early use of probiotics establishes a balance in microbial flora against pathogenic bacteria, thus, using probiotic constituted by *Enterococcus faecium, Lactobacillus case, L. plantarum* inoculated *in ovo* at the dose of 10^6 CFU/g per egg has avoided the colonization of the gastrointestinal tract of broilers challenged with 0.1 mL aqueous solution containing 1.36×10^6 CFU *Salmonella* Enteritidis, inoculated via crop. Therefore, broilers challenged early (post eclosion) and not receiving probiotics presented reduction of *Salmonella* in gastrointestinal tract (crop and cecum) of the birds and a better performance.

La Ragione & Woodward (2003) verified that the administration of viable spores of *Bacillus subtilis* to birds free from specific pathogens challenged with *C. perfringens* reduced the number of pathogens in the spleen, duodenum, colon and cecum, reporting similar results with a probiotic based on *Lactobacillus johnsonii* (La Ragione et al., 2004).

Haghighi et al. (2006) shown that a commercial probiotic containing *Lactobacillus acidophilus, Bifidobacterium bifidum,* and *Streptococcus faecalis* stimulated the production of antitoxin α IgA from *C. perfringens* in the intestine of non-vaccinated chicks.

In meat quails, Otutumi et al. (2010) evaluated the effect of probiotics based on *Lactobacillus spp* administered in the period of one to seven days of age on the counting of *Lactobacillus spp*, enterobacteria and *Escherichia coli* in the small intestine (at 7 and 14 days of age) and have not observed changes in the counting with the use of probiotic. However, it is worth mentioning that when evaluating the microbial population in the intestine, there is a very large standard deviation, which many times makes it difficult to identify differences by the use of inappropriate statistical models. And despite having used appropriate statistical analysis, the results were not significant.

Siriken et al. (2003) investigated the effect of two probiotics, alone and in combination with an antibiotic on the caecal flora of Japanese quail (*Coturnix coturnix japonica*) and no significant differences were detected among treatments for pH values and total count of aerobic bacteria, lactobacilli, enterobacteriaceae, coliforms, enteroccoci, salmonellae, except for sulphite-reducing anaerobic bacteria (P<0.001).

Unfortunately, more than 80% of gut bacteria cannot be cultured under current laboratory conditions, limiting assessment of the effects of probiotics on the gut microbiota. This drawback, however, has been overcome today to a large extent by employing molecular techniques (Ajithdoss et al., 2012).

The suggested mechanism by which probiotics might exert their protective or therapeutic effect against enteric pathogens include non immune mechanisms, such as the stabilization of the gut mucosal barrier, increasing the secretion of mucus, improving gut motility, and therefore interfering with their ability to colonize and infect the mucosa; competing for nutrients; secreting specific low molecular weight antimicrobial substances (bacteriocins) (Delgado et al., 2007; Liu et al., 2011), and influencing the composition and activity of the gut microbiota (regulation of intestinal microbial homeostasis) (Castilho et al., 2012).

5.3. Carcass quality and blood parameters

The quality of broiler meat as well as the reduction of fat levels in the carcass have been a constant concern of researchers. Thus, research directed to the improvement of meat quality has been made including the use of probiotics.

Santoso et al. (1995) demonstrated that the supplementation of *Bacillus subtilis* at the dose of 20g/Kg feed increased the level of phospholipids in blood serum, but reduced the concentration of phospholipids in carcass and triacylglycerol in liver, carcass and blood serum, as well as decreasing the percentage of abdominal fat. This parameter was also evaluated by Denli et al. (2003), who proved that the supplementation of *Saccharomyces cerevisiae* on the diet has decreased the weight and percentage of abdominal fat in broilers.

Equally, Pietras (2001) demonstrated that *L. acidophilus* and *Streptococcus faecium* decreased the plasmatic protein concentrations and the total cholesterol and high density lipoprotein (HDL) cholesterol levels, and that the meat from supplemented broilers presented a significant increase in protein content.

Other works with supplementation of probiotics based on *Lactobacillus spp.* demonstrated similar results, with reduction in the total cholesterol and low density lipoprotein (LDL) cholesterol levels (Kalavathy et al., 2003; Taherpour et al., 2009) and triglycerides (Kalavathy et al. 2003) in blood serum of broilers.

In Japanese quails with 4 weeks of age, Homma e Shinohara (2004) studying the effect of a commercial probiotic based on *Bacillus cereus toyoi* on the accumulation of abdominal fat verified that at eight weeks (four weeks of probiotic supplementation period), birds fed the control diet with probiotic had significantly less abdominal fat than those fed without the probiotic.

Moreover, probiotic supplementation has been shown to reduce the cholesterol concentration in egg yolk (Abdulrahim et al., 1996; Haddadin et al., 1996) and serum in chicken (Mohan et al., 1996; Jin et al., 1998a).

According to Matur & Eraslan (2012), hypocholesterolemic effect of probiotics depends on the species of the bacteria, and can occur by the assimilation of cholesterol from either endogen or hexogen origin in the intestinal tract, or de-conjugating bile acids by lactic acid bacteria (Gilliland et al., 1990) or the cholesterol and free bile acids bind to the cell surface of micro-organisms or co-precipitate with the free bile acids by probiotics (Guo & Zhang,

2010). However, recent research has revealed that probiotics affect gene expression of carrier proteins responsible for cholesterol absorption (Matur & Eraslan, 2012).

Regarding the microbiological quality of meat, Bailey et al. (2000) proposed that competitive exclusion cultures for broilers can be used to reduce contamination by *Salmonella* Enteritidis in processed carcasses, reducing therefore the exposure of consumers to food-borne infections.

Likewise, Estrada et al. (2001) observed a tendency to reduce total aerobic bacteria, coliforms and clostridia in broilers receiving *Bifidobacterium bifidum*, and proven a reduction in the number of carcass condemnation by cellulites in animals supplemented, and recently, Lilly et al. (2011) observed 86% reduction in contamination by *Salmonella* before slaughtering in broilers receiving probiotic with combination of *Lactobacillus acidophilus, Enterococcus faecium, Lactobacillus plantarum* and *Pediococcus acidilactici.*

Regarding the organoleptic quality, Kabir (2009), studying the supplementation of a commercial probiotic (Protexin® Boost, Novartis) in the ratio of 2g probiotic for every 10 liters of drinking water until 36 days of age in broilers, observed that the probiotic supplementation improved the organoleptic quality of broiler meat right after slaughtering, as well as after 21 days storage in freezer.

5.4. Bone quality in broilers

The surveys aiming the reduction in growth time in poultry, together with the increase of its live weight, have led to the development of broilers known as conformation or yield type. However, the development of this new broiler came together with some undesirable aspects associated to the fast growth which have compromised the performance of the birds (Leeson & Summers, 1988).

Among these aspects, it is notable the increase in bone problems, once the genetic selection for a high growth rate has promoted higher breast muscle weight when compared to the muscles and bones in legs, and therefore, this unbalanced redistribution of weight has increased the leg problems in poultry (Yalcin et al., 2001).

From an economic point of view, there is a great concern by the companies with the losses regarding bone anomalies in broilers, since they have contributed for the reduction in productivity and increase in mortality, as well as condemnation of whole carcasses or during the processing of meat.

The most prevalent bone problems in broilers are tibial dyschondroplasia, chronic painful lameness in older or reproductive broilers, condrodistrophy or bone angular deformity, valgus-varus angular deformities, spondylolisthesis, rickets, epiphyseal separation, femoral necrosis, curled toes and rupture of gastrocnemius tendon (Julian, 1998; Angel, 2007).

The etiology of bone abnormalities is generally complex and apparently it is not related to a single factor, and sometimes there is an overlapping among etiology, pathology and clinical signs of these conditions. Factors affecting the intestinal epithelium, leading to the reduction of nutrient absorption, as well as anti-nutritional factors of the ingredients can induce leg disorders caused by nutritional imbalance. Thus, genetics, handling, nutrition, hygiene and diseases will influence the occurrence of leg problems under field or experimental conditions. Therefore, even if the content of diets seems to be adequate, bone abnormalities can appear (Waldenstedt, 2006).

Although studies demonstrate probable influence of probiotics, prebiotics and symbiotics on the bone characteristics of poultry, it is not well established the relation between probiotics and mineral absorption or bone growth (Mutus et al., 2006).

Plavnick & Scott (1980) observed lower incidence of tibial dyschondroplasia and greater bone resistance in broilers receiving yeast extract supplementation. Likewise, Mutus et al. (2006) observed that at 42 days of age, the thickness of medial and lateral wall, tibia-tarsal index, percentages of ashes and phosphorus and the diameter of the medullar channel of the tibia in broilers fed with diets containing probiotics were higher than those receiving the control diet without supplementation.

Although the bone abnormality score has not been influenced, Panda et al. (2006) described positive effects of diets supplemented with *Lactobacillus sporogenes* (100mg/kg) on bone resistance to breakage and ash content from broiler tibiae. According to the authors, the supplementation of diets with probiotics resulted in higher serum concentration of calcium, which might explain the better resistance and ash concentration of bones.

Positive results as to morphometric (weight, length, tibia-tarsi and tibia-tarsal indexes, lateral and medial wall thickness), mechanical (elasticity module and draining tension) and mineral composition parameters (ashes, calcium and phosphorus) in the tibia of broilers receiving probiotics (150mg/kg) in feed were observed by Ziaie et al. (2011). According to the authors, the supplementation of diet with antibiotic substitutes can increase digestibility and availability of nutrients (such as calcium and phosphorus) due to the development of a desirable microflora in the digestive tract, which in turn results in an increase in mineral retention and bone mineralization.

Nahashon et al. (1994) reported a positive correlation between the diets containing probiotics (*Lactobacilus*) and the retention of calcium and phosphorus in laying hens. On the other hand, in a study with broilers, Maiorka et al. (2001) have not observed changes in the plasmatic levels of calcium and phosphorus of the broilers at 40 days of age receiving probiotic supplementation (*Bacillus subtilis*).

Working with broilers, Angel et al. (2005) demonstrated that the addition of probiotics based on Lactobacillus (0.9kg/ton) in feed has improved the retention of calcium and phosphorus by birds receiving feed that supply to their nutritional demands. However, birds receiving moderate density (18% less calcium and phosphorus in relation to the recommendation of the National Research Council - NRC) and low density feed (25% less calcium and phosphorus in relation to the recommendation by NRC) supplemented with probiotics presented bone breaking resistance and ash concentration in tibia similar to those receiving the control feed, without addition of additive. Data revealed that probiotics based on lactobacillus can improve the retention of nutrients, allowing its usage in feeds with lower nutritional levels, reducing excretion and costs.

Guçlu et al. (2011) analyzed the effect of different probiotic inclusion levels on the productive performance and quality of breeder quail eggs and reported that the improvement in the thickness of the shell observed with the addition of probiotic would probably be related with the greater absorption of calcium in the birds' intestines.

According to Scholz-Ahrens et al. (2007), as well as the stimulation of calcium entering enterocytes, another probable action mechanism of probiotics on bone health is the degradation of the mineral-phytic acid complex.

Lan et al. (2002) evaluated the effect of supplementation of an active culture of *Mitsuokella jalaludinii* (a kind of bacteria present in the rumen of cattle) in broiler feeds with high and low concentrations of non-phytate phosphorus and observed improvement in the performance, in the values of apparent metabolizable energy, in protein and dry matter digestibility, in the usage of calcium, phosphorus and copper, and bone mineralization of broilers receiving feed with lower concentrations of non-phytate phosphorus.

6. Conclusion

As it can be seen, the results of research available in literature with the use of probiotics are very variable, once several factors can interfere, such as the type of probiotic, its action mode, its interaction with the host and breeding environment. However, evidences presented in relation to the benefit of its use justify the continuity of research with the objective of expanding the knowledge on its action mechanism, its immune-modulation effect and methodologies that aid the maintenance of its viability for use in animal feed. Currently, research has evaluated the genomes of various probiotic species and the term "probiogenomics" has been proposed to denote the sequencing and analysis of probiotic genomes, for further development of strains and assessment of the safety of probiotics in order to aid the propagation of using probiotics in human and animal feed.

Author details

Luciana Kazue Otutumi and Marcelo Biondaro Góis
Universidade Paranaense, Brazil

Elis Regina de Moraes Garcia
Universidade Estadual do Mato Grosso do Sul, Brazil

Maria Marta Loddi
Universidade Estadual de Ponta Grossa, Brazil

7. References

Abdulrahim, S.M.; Haddadinm, M.S.Y.; Hashlamoun, E.A.R & Robinson, R.K. (1996). The influence of *Lactobacillus acidophilus* and bacitracin on layer performance of chickens and cholesterol content of plasma and egg yolk. *British of Poultry Science*, Vol.37, No.2, pp. 341-346, ISSN 1466-1799

Ajithdoss, D.K.; Dowd, S.E. & Suchodolski, J.S. Genomics of probiotic - host interactions. (2012). In: *Direct Fed Microbials and Prebiotics for Animals: Science and Mechanisms of Action*. Callaway, T.R.; & Ricke, S.C. (Eds.), pp. 35-60, Springer Science, retrieved from <www.springerlink.com>

Angel, R. (2007). Metabolic disorders: limitations to growth of and mineral deposition into the broiler skeleton after hatch and potential implications for leg problems. *Journal Applied Poultry Research*, Vol.16, No.1, (January 2007), pp. 138-149, ISSN 1537-0437

Angel, R.; Dalloul, R.A. & Doerr, J. (2005). Performance of broilers chickens fed diets supplemented with a direct-fed microbial. *Poultry Science*, Vol.84, (August 2005), pp. 1222-1231, 2005, ISSN 1525-3171

Arvola, T.; Laiho, K.; Torkelli, S.; Mykkanen, H.; Salminen, S.; Maunula, L. & Isolauri, E. (1999). Prophylactic *Lactobacillus* GG reduces antibiotic-associated diarrhea in children with respiratory infections: a randomized study. *Pediatrics*, Vol.104, No.5, (November 1999), pp. 64, 1999, ISSN 1098-4275

Ayasan, T.; Yurtseven, S.; Baylan, M. & Canogullari, S. (2005). The effects of dietary Yucca Schidigera on egg yield parameters and egg shell quality of laying Japanese quails (Coturnix coturnix japonica). *International Journal of Poultry Science*, Vol.4, No.3, pp. 159-162 ISSN 1682-8356

Bailey, J. S., Stern N. J., & Cox, N. A. (2000) Commercial field trial evaluation of mucosal starter culture to reduce *Salmonella* incidence in processed broiler carcasses. *Journal Food Protection*, Vol.63, No.7, pp. 867–870. ISSN 0362-028X

Blankenship, L. C.; Bailey, J. S.; Cox, N. A.; Stern, N. J.; Brewer, R. & Williams, O. (1993). Two-step mucosal competitive exclusion flora treatment to diminish salmonellae in commercial broiler chickens. *Poultry. Science*, Vol.72, No.9, (September 1993) pp. 1667-1672, ISSN 1525-3171

Casadei, M. A., Ingram, R., Hitchings, E., Archer, J. & Gaze, J. E. (2001). Heat resistance of Bacillus cereus, Salmonella Typhimurium and Lactobacillus delbrueckii in relation to pH and ethanol. *International Journal of Food Microbiology*, Vol.63, (January 2001), pp. 125–134 ISSN 0168-1605

Castilho, N.A.; De Leblanc, A.M.; Galdeano, C.M. & Perdigón, G. (2012). Probiotics: an alternative strategy for combating salmonellosis immune mechanisms involved. *Food Research International*, Vol.45, No.2, (March 2012), pp. 831-841, ISSN 0963-9969

Cole, C.B., & Fuller, R. (1984). A note on the effect of host specific fermented milk on the coliform population of the neonatal rat gut. *Journal of Applied Bacteriology*, Vol.56, pp. 495-498, ISSN 0021-8847

Corcoran, B.M.; Stanton, C.; Fitzgerald, G. & Ross, R.P. (2008). Life under stress: the probiotic stress response and how it may be manipulated. *Pharmaceutical Design*, Vol.14, No.14, pp. 1382-1399, ISSN 1381-6128

Cotter, P.F (1994). Modulation of immune response: current perceptions and future prospects with an example from poultry. *Proceedings of 10 Alltech's Annual Symposium on Biotechnology in Feed Industry*, UK: Nottingham University Press, 1994. pp. 105-203

Cuevas, A.C.; Gonzales, E.A.; Huguenin, M.C.; & Domingues, S.C. (2000). El efecto del *Bacillus toyoii* sobre el comportamiento productivo en pollos de engorda. *Veterinária México*, Vol.31, No.4, 05.04.2012, Available from
http:// www.ejournal.unam.mx/vet_mex/vol31-04/RVM31405.pdf

Dalloul, R.A.; Lillehoj, H.S.; Shellem, T.A. & Doerr, J.A. (2003). Enhanced mucosal immunity against *Eimeria acervulina* in broilers fed a *Lactobacillus*-based probiotic. *Poultry Science*, Vol.82, No.1, (January 2003), pp.62-66, ISSN 1525-3171

Davis, G.S. & Anderson, K.E. (2002). The effects of feeding the direct-fed microbial, Primalac, on growth parameters and egg production in single comb white leghorn hens. *Poultry Science*, Vol.81, No.6, (June 2002), pp.755–759, ISSN 1525-3171

De Angelis, M. & Gobbetti, M. (2004). Environmental stress responses in *Lactobacillus*: a review. *Proteomics*, Vol.4, No.1, (January 2004), pp. 106-122, ISSN 1615-9861

Delgado, S., O'sullivan, E., Fitzgerald, G., & Mayo, B. (2007). Subtractive screening for probiotic properties of lactobacillus species from the human gastrointestinal tract in the search for new probiotics. *Journal of Food Science*, Vol. 72, No. 8, (September 2007), pp. 310–315, ISSN 1750-3841

Denli, M.; Çelik, K. & Okan, F. (2003). Comparative effects of feeding diets containing Flavomycin, Bioteksin-L and dry yeast (*Saccharomyces cerevisiae*) on broiler performance. *Journal of Applied Animal Research*, Vol.23, No.2, pp. 139-144, ISSN 0974-1844

Desmond, C.; Stanton, C.; Fitzgerald, G.F.; Collins, K. & Ross, R.P. (2001). Environmental adaptation of probiotic lactobacilli towards improvement of performance during spray drying. *International Dairy Journal*, Vol.11, No.10, pp. 801–808, ISSN 0958-6946

Dilworth, B.C. & Day, E.J. (1978). Lactobacillus cultures in broiler diets (S.A.A.S. Abstract). *Poultry Science*, Vol.57, No.4, (July 1978), pp. 1101, ISSN 1525-3171

Edens, F. W. (2003). An alternative for antibiotic use in poultry: probiotic. *Revista Brasileira de Ciência Avicola*, Vol.5, No.2, (May/Aug 2003), pp. 75-97, ISSN: 1516-635X

Erickson, K. L. & Hubbard, N. E. (2000). Probiotic immunomodulation in health and diseases. *The Journal of Nutrition*, Vol.130, No.2, (February 2000), pp. 403-409, ISSN 1541-6100

Estrada, A.; Wilkie, D.C.; & Drew, M. (2001). Administration of *Bifidobacterium bifidum* to chicken broilers reduces the number of carcass condemnations for cellulitis at the abattoir. *Journal of Applied Poultry Research*, Vol.10, No.4, (January 2001), pp. 329-334, ISSN: 1537-0437

Faria-Filho, D.E.; Torres, K.A.A.; Faria, D.E.; Campos, D.M.B. & Rosa, P.S. (2006). Probiotics for broiler chickens in Brazil: systematic review and meta-analysis. *Revista Brasileira de Ciência Avícola*, Vol.8, No.2, (Apr/June 2006), pp. 89-98, ISSN 1516-635X

Fritts, C.A.; Kersn, J.H.; Motl, M.A.; Kroger, E.C.; Yan, E.; Si, J.; Jiang, Q.; Campos, M.M.; Waldroup, A.L. & Waldroup, P.W (2000). *Bacillus subtilis* C-3102 (Calsporin) improves live performance and microbiological status of broiler chickens. *Journal of Applied Poultry Research*, Vol.9, No.2, (January 2000), pp. 149-155, ISSN 1537-0437

Fuller R. (1995). Probiotics, their development and use. In: *Old Herborn University Seminar Monograph 8*, Van der Waaji, D.; Heidt, P.J.; Rusch, V.C. (Eds.), pp. 1-8, *Herborn-Dill*, Institute for Microbiology and Biochemistry

Fuller, R. (1989). Probiotics in man and animals. *Journal of Applied Bacteriology*, Vol.66, pp. 365-378, ISSN 0021-8847

Fuller, R. (1986). Probiotics. *Journal of Applied Bacteriology*, Vol.60, No.1, (January, 1986), pp. 1-6, ISSN 0021-8847

Fuller, R. (1997). The importance of lactobacili in maintaining normal microbial balance in the crop. *British Poultry Science*, Vol.18, pp. 85-94, ISSN 1466-1799

Fuller, R. (1975). Nature of the determinant responsible for the adhesion of lactobacilli to chicken crop epithelial cells. *Journal of General Microbiology*, Vol.87, pp. 245-250, ISSN 0022-1287

Gil De Los Santos, J.R.; Storch, O.B. & Gil- Turnes, C. (2005). *Bacillus cereus* Var. *Toyoii* and *Saccharomyces boulardii* increased feed efficiency in broilers infected with *Salmonella* Enteritidis. *British Poultry Science*, Vol.46, No.4, pp. 494-497, ISSN 1466-1799

Gill, H. S. (2003). Probiotics to enhance anti-infective defences in the gastrointestinal tract. *Bailliere's Best Practice and Research in Clinical Gastroenterology*, Vol.17, No.5, (October 2003) pp. 755–773, ISSN 1521-6918

Gilliland, S.E. & Walker, D.K. (1990). Factors to consider when selecting a culture of Lactobacillus acidophilus as a dietary adjunct to produce a hypocholesterolemic effect in humans. *Journal of Dairy Science*, Vol.73, No.4, (April 1990), pp. 905–11, ISSN 1525-3198

Goldin, B.R. & Gorbach, S.L. (1984). The effect of milk and lactobacillus feeding on human intestinal bacterial enzyme activity. American Journal of Clinical Nutrition, Vol.39, (May 1984), pp. 756-761, ISSN 1938-3207

Güçlü, B. K. (2011). Effects of probiotic and prebiotic (mannanoligosaccharide) supplementation on performance, egg quality and hatchability in quail breeders. *Ankara Üniveritesi Veteriner Fakültesi Dergisi*, Vol.58, pp. 27-32, ISSN 1308-2817

Guerra, N.P.; Bern'ardez, P.F.; M'endes, J.; Cachaldora, P. & Castro, L.P. (2007). Production of four potentially probiotic lactic acid bacteria and their evaluation as feed additives for weaned piglets. *Animal Feed Science and Technology*, Vol.134, No.1-2, (March 2007), pp. 89-107, ISSN: 0377-8401

Guo, C. & Zhang, L. (2010). Cholesterol-lowering effects of probiotics--a review. *Wei Sheng Wu Xue Bao*, Vol.50, No.12, (December 2010), pp. 590-599, ISSN 0001-6209

Gupta, V. & Garg, R. (2009). Probiotics. *Indian Journal of Medical Microbiology*, Vol.27, No.3, (July-September 2009), pp. 202-209, ISSN 1998-3646

Haddadin, M.S.Y.; Abdulrahim, S.M.; Hashlamoun, E.A.R. & Robinson, R.K. (1996). The effect of *Lactobacillus acidophilus* on the production and chemical composition of hen's eggs. *Poultry Science*, Vol.75, No.4, (April 1996), pp. 491-494, ISSN 1525-3171

Haghighi, H.R.; Gong, J.; Gyles, C.L.; Hayes, M.A.; Zhou, H.; Sanei, B.; Chambers, J.R. & Sharif, S. (2006). Probiotics stimulate production of natural antibodies in chickens. *Clinical and Vaccine Immunology*, Vol.13, No.9, (September 2006), pp. 975-980, ISSN 1556-679X

Hakkinen, M. & Schneitz, C. (1999). Efficacy of a commercial competitive exclusion product against *Campylobacter jejuni. British Poultry Science*, Vol.40, No.5, pp. 619-621, ISSN 1466-1799

Hamann, L.; EL-Samalouti, V.; Ulmer, A.J.; Flad, H.D. & Rietschel, E.T. (1998). Components of gut bacteria as immunomodulators. *International Journal of Food Microbiology*, Vol.41, No.2, (May 1998), pp. 141-154, ISSN 0168-1605

Havenaar, R. & Spanhaak, S. (1994). Probiotics from an immunological point of view. Current Opinion in Biotechnology, Vol.5, No.3, (June 1994) pp. 320-325, 1994, ISSN 0168-1605

Higgins, J.P.; Higgins, S.E.; Vicente, J.L.; Wolfenden, A.D.; Tellez, G. & Hargis, B.M. (2007). Temporal effects of lactic acid bacteria probiotic culture on *Salmonella* in neonatal broilers. *Poultry Science*, Vol.86, No.8, (August 2007), pp. 1662-1666, ISSN 1525-3171

Higgins, J.P.; Higgins, S.E.; Wolfenden, A.D.; Henderson, S.N.; Torres-Rodrigues, A.; Vicente, J.L.; Hargis, B.M. & Tellez, G. (2010). Effect of lactic acid bacteria probiotic culture treatment timing on *Salmonella* Enteritidis in neonatal broilers. *Poultry Science,* Vol.89, No.2, (February 2010), pp. 243-247, ISSN 1525-3171

Hinton, M. & Mead, G.C. (1991). *Salmonella* control in poultry: the need for the satisfactory evaluation of probiotics for this purpose. *Letters in Applied Microbiology*, Vol.13, No.2, (August 1991), pp. 49–50, ISSN: 1472-765X

Homma, H. & Shinohara, T. (2004). Effects of probiotic *Bacillus cereus* toyoi on abdominal fat accumulation in the Japanese quail (*Coturnix japonica*). *Animal Science Journal*, Vol.75, No.1, (February 2004) pp. 37-41, ISSN 1740-0929

Hong, H.A.; Duc, L.H. & Cutting, S.M. (2005). The use of bacterial spore formers as probiotics. (2005). *FEMS Microbiology Reviews*, Vol.29, No.4, (September 2005), pp. 813-835, ISSN 1574-6976

Hooper, L.V.; Midtvedt, T. & Gordon, J. I. (2002). How host-microbial interactions shape the nutrient environment of the mammalian intestine. *Annual Review of Nutrition*, Vol.22, (July 2002), pp. 283–307, ISSN 0199-9885

Huang, M.K.; Choi, Y.J.; Houde, R.; Lee, J.W.; Lee, B. & Zhao, X. (2004). Effects of Lactobacilli and an acidophilic fungus on the production performance and immune responses in broiler chickens. *Poultry Science*, Vol.83, No.5, (May 2004), pp. 788-795, ISSN 1525-3171

Huyghebaert, G.; Ducatelle, R. & Van Immerseel, F. (2011). An update on alternatives to antimicrobial growth promoters for broilers. *The Veterinary Journal*, Vol.187, No.2, (February 2011), pp. 182-188, ISSN 1090-0233

Impey, C.S.; Mead, G.C. & George, S.M. (1984). Evaluation of treatment with defined and undefined mixtures of gut microorganisms for preventing *Salmonella* colonization in chicks and turkey poults. *Food Microbiology*, Vol.1, No.2, (April 1984), pp. 143-147, ISSN 0740-0020

Jin, L.Z.; Ho, Y.W.; Abdullah, N. & Jalaludin, S. (1997). Probiotics in poultry: modes of action. *World's Poultry Science Journal*, Vol.53, No.4, (December 1997), pp. 351-368 ISSN: 1743-4777

Jin, L.Z., Ho, Y.W.; Abdullah, N. & Jalaludin, S. (1998a). Growth performance, intestinal microbial populations, and serum cholesterol of broilers fed diets containing *Lactobacillus* cultures. *Poultry Science*, Vol.77, No.9, (September 1998), pp. 1259-1265, ISSN 1525-3171

Jin, L.Z.; Ho, Y.W.; Abdullah, N.; Ali, A.M. & Jalaludin, S. (1998b). Effects of adherent lactobacillus cultures on growth, weight of organs and intestinal microflora and volatile fatty acids in broilers. *Animal Feed Science and Technology*, Vol.70, No.3, (February 1998), pp. 197-209, ISSN 0377-8401

Jin, L.Z.; Ho, Y.W.; Abdullah, N. & Jalaludin, S. (1996). Influence of dried *Bacillus subtilis* and Lactobacilli cultures on intestinal microflora and performance in broiler. *Asian-Australasian Journal of Animal Science*, Vol.9, No.4, (August 1996), pp. 397-404, ISSN 1076-5517

Julian, R. J. (1998). Rapid growth problems: ascites and skeletal deformities in broilers. *Poultry Science*, Vol.77, No.12, (December 1998), pp. 1773-1780, ISSN 1525-3171

Kabir, S.M.L.; Rahman, M.M.; Rahman, M.B. & Ahmed S.U. (2004). The dynamic of probiotics on growth performance and immune response in broiler. *International Journal of Poultry Science*, Vol.3, No. 5, (May 2004), pp. 361-364, ISSN 1682-8356

Kabir, S.M.L. (2009). The Role of Probiotics in the Poultry Industry, *International Journal of Molecular Sciences*, Vol.10, No.8, (August 2009), pp. 3531-3546, ISSN 1422-0067

Kalavathy, R.; Abdullah, N.; Jalaludin, S. & Ho, Y.W. (2003). Effects of Lactobacillus cultures on growth performance, abdominal fat deposition, serum lipids and weight of organs of broiler chickens. *British Poultry Science*,Vol.44, N.1, pp. 139–144, ISSN 1466-1799

Kalbane, V.H.; Gaffar, M.A. & Deshmukh, S.V. (1992). Effect of probiotic and nitrofurin on performance of growing commercial pullets. *Indian Journal of Poultry Science*, 27, pp. 116–117, ISSN 0974-8180

Knap, I.; Kehlet, A.B.; Bennedsen, M.; Mathis, G.F.; Hofacre, C.L.; Lumpkins, B.S.; Jensen, M.M.; Raun, M. & Lay, A. (2011). *Bacillus subtilis* (DSM 17299) significantly reduces Salmonella in broilers. *Poultry Science*, Vol.90, No.8, (August 2011), pp. 1690-1694, ISSN 1525-3171

Korver, D.R. (2012). Implications of changing immune function through nutrition in poultry. *Animal Feed Science and Technology*, Vol.173, No.1-2, (April 2012), pp. 54-64, ISSN 0377-8401

Kos, K. & Wittner, V. (1982). Use of probiotics in the nutrition of the fattening chicks. *Praxis Veterinary*, Vol.30, pp. 283-286, 1982.

Kurtoglu, V.; Kurtoglu, F.; Seker, E.; Coskun, B.; Balevi, T. & Polat, E.S. (2004). Effect of probiotic supplementation on laying hen diets on yield performance and serum and egg yolk cholesterol. *Food Additives and Contaminants*, Vol.21, No.9, (September, 2004), pp. 817–823. ISSN 1944-0057

La Ragione, R.M. & Woodward, M.J. (2003). Competitive exclusion by *Bacillus subtilis* spores of *Salmonella enterica* serotype Enteritidis and *Clostridium perfringens* in young chickens. *Veterinary Microbiology*, Vol.94, No.3, (July, 2003), pp. 245-256. ISSN 0378-1135

La Ragione, R.M.; Narbad, A.; Gasson, M.J. & Woodward, M.J. (2004). In vivo characterization of *Lactobacillus johnsonii* FI9785 for use as a defined competitive exclusion agent against bacterial pathogens in poultry. *Letters in Applied Microbiology*, Vol.38, No.3 (March 2004), pp. 197-205, ISSN 1472-765X

Lan,G.Q.; Abdullah, N.; Jalaludin, S. & Ho., Y.W. (2002). Efficacy of supplementation of a phytase-producing bacterial culture on the performance and nutrient use of broiler chickens fed corn-soybean meal diets. *Poultry Science*, Vol.81, No.10, (October 2002), pp. 1773–1780. ISSN 1525-3171

Lata, J.; Juránkova, J.; Doubek, J.; Příbramská, V.; Frič, P.; Dítě, P.; Kolář, M.; Scheer, P. & Kosáková, D. (2006). Labelling and content evaluation of commercial veterinary probiotics. *Acta Vet. Brno*, Vol.75, No.1, (March 2006), pp. 139-144, ISSN 1801-7576

Leandro, N.S.M.; Oliveira, A.S.C.; Gonzáles, E.; Café, M.B.; Stringhini, L.H. & Andrade, M.A. (2010). Probiótico na ração ou inoculado em ovos embrionados. 1. Desempenho de pintos de corte desafiados com *Salmonella* Enteritidis. *Revista Brasileira de Zootecnia*, Vol.39, No.7, (July 2010), pp. 1509-1516 ISSN 1806-9290

Leeson, S. & Summers, J.D. (1988). Some nutritional implications of leg problems with poultry. *British Veterinary Journal*, Vol.144, No.1 (January/February 1988), pp. 81-92, ISSN 1090-0233

Lilly, K.G.S.; Shires, L.K.; West, B.N.;, Beaman, K.R.; Loop, S.A.; Turk, P.J.; Bissonnette, G.K. & Moritz, J.S. (2011). Strategies to improve performance and reduce preslaughter *Salmonella* in organic broilers *Journal of Applied Poultry Research*, Vol.20, No.3 (September 2011), pp. 313–321, ISSN 1537-0437

Lima, A.C.F.; Pizauro Júnior, J.M.; Macari, M. & Malheiros, E.B. (2003). Efeito do uso de probiótico sobre o desempenho e atividade de enzimas digestivas de frangos de corte. *Revista Brasileira de Zootecnia*, Vol. 32, No.1, (January/February 2003), pp. 200-207, ISSN 1806-9290

Liu, G.; Griffiths, M. W.; Wu, P.; Wang, H.; Zhang, X. & Li, P. (2011). *Enterococcus faecium* LM-2, a multi-bacteriocinogenic strain naturally occurring in "Byaslag", a traditional cheese of Inner Mongolia in China. *Food Control*, Vol.22, No.2, (February 2011), pp. 283–289, ISSN 0956-7135

Liu, J.R.; Lai, S.F. & Yu, B. (2007). Evaluation of an intestinal *Lactobacillus reuteri* strain expressing rumen fungal xylanase as a probiotic for broiler chickens fed on a wheat-based diet. *British Poultry Science*, Vol.48, No.4, pp. 507-514, ISSN 1466-1799

Loddi, M. M. (2003). *Probióticos, prebióticos e acidificantes orgânicos em dietas para frangos de corte*. 52f. Tese (Doutorado em Zootecnia) – Faculdade de Ciências Agrárias e Veterinárias, Universidade Estadual Paulista "Júlio de Mesquita Filho", Jaboticabal.

Loddi, M.M.; Gonzales, E.; Takita, T.S.; Mendes, A.A. & Roça, R.O. (2000). Uso de probiótico e antibiótico sobre o desempenho, o rendimento e a qualidade de carcaça de frangos de corte. *Revista Brasileira de Zootecnia*, Vol.29, No.4, (July/August 2000), pp. 1124-1131, ISSN 1806-9290

Maiorka, A.; Santin, E.; Sugeta, S.M.; Almeida, J.G. & Macari, M. (2001). Utilização de prebióticos, probióticos ou simbióticos em dietas para frangos. *Revista Brasileira de Ciência Avícola*, Vol.3, No.1, (January/April 2001), pp. 75-82, ISSN 1516-635X

Majarmaa, H. & Isolauri, E. (1997). Probiotics: a novel approach in the management of food allergy. *Journal of Allergy and Clinical Immunology*, Vol.99, No.2, (February 1997), pp. 179–185, ISSN 0091-6149

Mattar, A.; Daniel, H.; Drongawski, R.; Wongyi, F.; Harmon, C. & Coran, A. (2002). Probiotics up-regulate MUC-2 mucin gene expression in a Caco-2 cell-culture model. *Pediatric Surgery International*, Vol.18, No.7, (October 2002), pp. 586-590, ISSN 0179-0358

Matur, E. & Eraslan, E. (2012). The impact of probiotics on the gastrointestinal physiology. In: *New advances in the basic and clinical gastroenterology*. Brzozowski, T. (Ed.), pp. 51-74, ISBN 978-953-51-0521-3, InTech, 10.04.2012, Available from: http://www.intechopen.com/books/new-advances-in-the-basic-and-clinical-gastroenterology

Mazmanian, S.K.; Round, J.L. & Kasper, D.L. (2008). A microbial symbiosis factor prevents inflammatory disease. *Nature*, Vol.453, (May 2008), pp. 620–625, ISSN 0028-0836

Menconi, A.; Wolfenden, A.D.; Shivaramaiah, S.; Terraes, J.C.; Urbano, T.; Kuttel, J.; Kremer, C.; Hargis, B.M. & Tellez, G. (2011). Effect of lactic acid bacteria probiotic culture for the treatment of *Salmonella enterica* serovar Heidelberg in neonatal broiler chickens and turkey poults. *Poultry Science*, Vol.90, No.3, (March 2011), pp. 561-565, ISSN 1525-3171

Menten, J. F. M. & Loddi, M. M. (2003). Probióticos, Prebióticos e aditivos fitogênicos na nutrição de aves. *Proceedings of Simpósio de Nutrição de Aves e Suínos*, Campinas, São Paulo, pp. 107-138

Mikulec, Z.; Serman, V.; Mas, N. & Lukac, Z. (1999). Effect of probiotic on production results of fattened chickens fed different quantities of protein. *Veterinarski Arhiv*, Vol.69, No.4, pp. 199-209, ISSN 1331-8055

Miles, R.D., (1993). Manipulation of the microflora of the gastrointestinal tract: natural ways to prevent colonization by pathogens. Biotechnolgy in the Feed Industry. *Proceeding of Altechs Ninth Annual Symposium*, 1993, pp. 133–150

Mills, S.; Stanton, C.; Fitzgerald, G.F. & Ross, R.P. (2011). Enhancing the stress responses of probiotics for a lifestyle from gut to product and back again. *Microbial Cell Factories*, Vol. 10, No.1, (August 2011), pp. 1-15, ISSN 1475-2859

Mohan, N.; Kadirvel, R.; Natarajan, A. & Bhaskaran, M. (1996). Effect of probiotic supplementation on growth, nitrogen utilisation and serum colesterol broilers. *British Poultry Science*, Vol.37, No.2, pp. 395-401, ISSN 1466-1799

Montes, A.J. & Pugh, D.G., (1993). The use of probiotics in food-animal practice. *Veterinary Medicine*, (March 1993), pp. 282–288

Mountzouris, K.C.; Tsirtsikos, P.; Kalamara, E.; Nitsch, S.; Schatzmayr, G. & Fegeros, K. (2007). Evaluation of the efficacy of a probiotic containing *Lactobacillus*, *Bifidobacterium*, *Enterococcus*, and *Pediococcus* strains in promoting broiler performance and modulating caecal microflora composition and metabolic activities. *Poultry Science*, Vol.86, No.2, (February 2007), pp. 309-317, ISSN 1525-3171

Mountzouris, K.C.; Tsitrsikos, P.; Palamidi, I.; Arvaniti, A.; Mohnl, M.; Schatzmayr, G. & Fegeros, K. (2010). Effects of probiotic inclusion levels in broiler nutrition on growth performance, nutrient digestibility, plasma immunoglobulins, and cecal microflora composition. *Poultry Science*, Vol.89, No.1, (January 2010), pp. 58–67, ISSN 1525-3171

Murry, A.C.; Hinton, A.J. & Buhr, R.J. (2006). Effect of botanical probiotic containing Lactobacilli on growth performance and populations of bacteria in the ceca, cloaca, and carcass rinse of broiler chickens. *International Journal of Poultry Science*, Vol.5, No.4, pp. 344-350, ISSN 1682-8356

Mutus, R.; Kocabagli, N.; Alp, M.; Acar, N.; Eren, M. & Gezen, S.S. (2006). The effect of dietary probiotic supplementation on tibial bone characteristics and strength in broilers. *Poultry Science*, Vol.85, No.9, (September 2006), pp. 1621-1625, ISSN 1525-3171

Nahashon S.N., Nakaue H. S. & Mirosh L.W. (1996). Performance of Single Comb White Leghorn fed a diet supplemented with a live microbial during the growth and egg laying phases. *Animal Feed Science and Technology*, Vol.57, No.1-2, (January 1996), pp. 25–38, ISSN 0377-8401

Nahashon, S. N.; Nakaue, H.S. & Mirosh, L.W. (1994). Production variable and nutrient retention in Single Comb White Leghorn laying pullets fed diets supplemented with direct-fed microbials. *Poultry Science*, Vol.73, No.11, (November 1994), pp. 1699–1711, ISSN 1525-3171

Neurath, M.F. (2007). IL-23: a master regulator in Crohn disease. *Nature Medicine*, Vol.13, No.1, (January, 2007), pp. 26-28, ISSN 1546-170X

Ng, S.C.; Hart, A.L.; Kamm, M.A.; Stagg, A.J. & Knight, S.C. (2009). Mechanisms of Action of Probiotics: Recent Advances. *Inflammatory Bowel Diseases*, Vol.15, No.2, (February 2009), pp.300-310, ISSN 1536-4844

Nunes, A.D. (2008). *Influencia do uso de aditivos alternativos a antimicrobianos sobre o desempenho, morfologia intestinal e imunidade de frangos de corte.* 111f. Dissertação (Mestrado em Medicina Veterinária) – Faculdade de Medicina Veterinária e Zootecnia, Universidade de São Paulo, São Paulo, 2008

Nurmi, E. & Rantala, M. (1973). New aspects of Salmonella infection in broiler production. *Nature,* Vol.241, No.111, (February 1973), pp. 210-211, ISSN 0028-0836

Oliveira-Sequeira, T.C. G., Melo, C. & Gomes, M.I.T.V. (2008). Potencial bioterapêutico dos probióticos nas parasitoses intestinais. *Ciência Rural,* Vol. 38, No. 9, (December 2008), pp. 2670-2679, ISSN 0103-8478

Otutumi, L.K.; Furlan, A.C.; Martins, E.N.; Nakamura, C.V.; Garcia, E.R.M. & Loose, P.V. (2010). Diferentes vias de administração de probiótico sobre o desempenho, o rendimento de carcaça e a população microbiana do intestino delgado de codornas de corte. *Revista Brasileira de Zootecnia,* Vol.39, No.1, (January 2010), pp. 158-164, ISSN 1806-9290

Oumer, A.; Garde, S.; Gaya, P.; Medina, M.; Nunez, M. (2001). The effects of cultivating lactic starter cultures with bacteriocin producing lactic acid bacteria. Journal of Food Protection Vol.64 No.1 (January 2001) pp. 81–86, ISSN 0162-7278

Panda, A.K., Rama RAO, S.S., Raju, M.V.L.N. & Sharma, S.S., (2008). Effect of probiotic (*Lactobacillus sporogenes*) feeding on egg production and quality, yolk cholesterol and humoral immune response of white leghorn layer breeders. *Journal of the Science of Food and Agriculture,* Vol.88, No.2 (January 2008), pp.43–47, ISSN 1097-0010

Panda, A.K.; Saravam, V.R.R.; Mantena, V.L.N.R. & Sita, R.S. (2006). Dietary supplementation of Lactobacillus Sporogenes on performance and serum biochemico-lipid profile of broiler chickens. *The Journal of Poultry Science,* Vol.43, No.3 (August 2006), pp.235-240 ISSN 1349-0486

Patterson, J. A. & Burkholder, K.M. (2003). Application of prebiotics and probiotics in poultry production. *Poultry Science,* Vol.82, No.4, (April 2003), pp. 627-631, ISSN 1525-3171

Pelicano, E.R.L.; Souza, P.A.; Souza, H.B.A; Leonel, F.R.; Zeola, N.M.B.L. & Bonago, M.M. (2004). Productive Traits of Broiler Chickens Fed Diets Containing Different Growth Promoters. *Brazilian Journal of Poultry Science,* Vol.6, No.3, (September 2004), pp.177-182 ISSN 1516-635x

Perić, L.; Žikić, D. & Lukić, M. (2009). Aplication of alternative growth promoters in broiler production. *Biotechnology in Animal Husbandry,* Vol.25, No.5-6, pp. 387-397, ISSN 1450-9556

Pietras, M. (2001). The effect of probiotics on selected blood and meat parameters of broiler chickens. *Journal of Animal and Feed Sciences,* Vol.10, No.2, pp. 297-302, ISSN 1230-1388

Plavnik, I. & Scott, M.L. (1980). Effects of additional vitamins, minerals or brewers yeast upon leg weaknesses in broiler chickens. *Poultry Science,* Vol.59, No.2, (February 1980), pp. 459–464, ISSN 1525-3171

Rantala, M. & Nurmi, E. (1974). Hazards involved in the use of furazolidone for the prevention of salmonellosis in broiler chickens. *Journal of Hygiene*, Vol.72 No.3 (June 1974), pp.349–354, ISSN 0950-2688

Revolledo, L.; Ferreira, A.J.P. & Mead, G. C. (2006). Prospects in *Salmonella* Control: Competitive Exclusion, Probiotics, and Enhancement of Avian Intestinal Immunity *The Journal Applied Poultry Research*, Vol.15, No.2, pp. 341–351, ISSN 1537-0437

Rigobelo, E.C.; Maluta, R.P. & Ávila, F.A. (2011). Desempenho de frangos de corte suplementados com probiótico. *Ars Veterinaria*, Jaboticabal, Vol.27, No.2, pp. 111-115, ISSN 2175-0106

Sahin, T.; Kaya, I.; Unal, Y.; Elmali, D.A. (2008). Dietary supplementation of probiotic and prebiotic combination (combiotics) on performance, carcass quality and blood parameters in growing quails. *Journal of Animal and Veterinary Advances*, Vol.7, No.11, pp. 1370-1373 ISSN 1993-601x

Salminen, S. Isolauri, E. (1996). Clinical uses of probiotics for stabilizing the gut mucosal barrier: successful strains and future challenges. Antonie van Leeuwenhoek , Vol. 70, No.2-4, pp.347–358, ISSN 1572-9699

Salzman, N.H.; Ghosh, D.; Huttner, K.M.; Paterson, Y. & Benvis, C.L. (2003). Protection against enteric salmonellosis in transgenic mice expressing a human intestinal defensin. *Nature*, Vol. 422, No.3 (April 2003), pp. 522–526, ISSN 0028-0836

Santoso U.; Tanaka, K. & Ohtani, S. (1995). Effect of dried *Bacillus subtilis* culture on growth, body composition and hepatic lipogenic enzyme activity in female broiler chicks. *British Journal of Nutrition*, Vol.74, No.4, (October 1995), pp.523-529, ISSN 0007-1145

Scanlan, C.M. (1997). Current concepts of competitive exclusion cultures for the control of *Salmonellae* in domestic poulty. *Advances in Experimental medical Biology*, Vol.421, pp. 421-426, ISSN 0065-2598

Schneitz, C. & Nuotio, L. (1992). Efficacy of different microbial preparations for controlling Salmonella colonization in chicks and turkey poults by competitive exclusion. *British Poultry Science*, Vol.33, No.1, pp. 207-211, ISSN 1466-1799

Schneitz, C.; Nuotio, L.; Kiiskinen, T. & Nurmi, E. (1991). Pilot-scale testing fo the competitive exclusion method in chickens. *British Poultry Science*, Vol.32, N.04, pp. 877-880, ISSN 1466-1799

Schocken-Iturrino, R.P.; Urbano, T.; Trovó, K.V.P.; Tremiliosi, N.G.; Medeiros, A.A.; Ishi, M.; Paulillo, A.C. & Carneiro, A.P.M. (2004). The use of probiotics for poultry: evaluation of the productive performance in chicken challenged with *Clostridium perfringes*. *Ars Veterinaria*, Vol.20, pp. 249-255, ISSN 0102-6380

Scholz-Ahrens, K.E.; Ade, P.; Marten, B.; Weber, P.; Timm, W.; Asil, Y.; Gluer, C. & Schrezenmeir, J. (2007). Prebiotics, probiotics, and synbiotics affect mineral absorption, bone mineral content and bone structure. *The Journal of Nutrition*,Vol. 137, No.3, (March, 2007), pp. 839S-846S (Suplement), ISSN 1541-6100

Seuna, E.; Raevuori, M. & Nurmi, E. (1978). An epizootic of *Salmonella* typhimurium var. copenhagen in broilers and the use of cultured chicken intestinal flora its control. *British Poultry Science*, Vol.19, No.3, pp. 309-314, 1978, ISSN 1466-1799

Shane, S. M. (2001). Mananoligossacarídeos em nutrição de aves: mecanismos e benefícios. Proceedings 17º Simpósio Anual da Alltech, Lexington, 2001, pp. 65-77

Simon, O.; Jadamus, A. & Vahjen, W. (2001). Probiotic feed additives, effectiveness and expected modes of action. *Journal of Animal and Feed Sciences*, Vol.10, Suppl. 1, pp. 51-67, ISSN 1230-1388

Siriken, B.; Bayram, I. & Önol, A.G. (2003). Effects of probiotics: alone and in a mixture of Biosacc plus Zinc Bacitracin on the caecal microflora of Japanese quail. *Research in Veterinary Science*, Vol.75, No.1, (August 2003), pp. 9-14, ISSN 0034-5288

Soerjadi, A.S.; Rufner, R.; Snoeyenbos, G.H. & Weinack, O.M. (1982). Adherence of salmonellae and native gut microflora to the gastrointestinal mucosa of chicks. *Avian Diseases*, Vol.26, No.3, (July –September, 1982), pp. 520–524, ISSN 1938-4351

Stavric, S. (1992). Defined cultures and prospects. *International Journal of Food Microbiology*, Vol.15, No.3-4. (March –April 1992), pp. 245–263, ISSN 0168-1605

Stavric, S.T.M.; Gleeson, R. & Blanchfield, B. (1991). Efficacy of undefined and defined bacterial treatment in competitive exclusion of Salmonella from chicks. In: *Colonization control of human bacterial enteropathogens in poultry*, Blankenship, L.C. (Ed.), pp. 323–330, *Academic Press*, San Diego, Calif

Szajewska, H.; Kotowska, M.; Mrukowicz, J.Z.; Armanska, M. & Mikolajczyk, W. (2001). Efficacy of *Lactobacillus* GG in prevention of nosocomial diarrhea in infants. *The Journal of Pediatrics*, Vol.138, No.3, (March 2001), pp.361–365, ISSN 0022-3476

Taherpour, K.; Moravej, H.; Shivazad, M.; Adibmoradi, M. & Yakhchali, B. (2009). Effects of dietary probiotic, prebiotic and butyric acid glycerides on performance and serum composition in broiler chickens. *African Journal of Biotechnology*, Vol.8, No.10, (May 2009), pp. 2329-2334, ISSN 1684-3646

Timmerman, H.M.; Mulder, L.; Everts, H.; Van Espen, D.C.; Van Der Wal, E.; Klaassen, G.; Rouwers, S.M.; Hartemink, R.; Rombouts, F.M. & Beynen, A.C. (2005). Health and growth of veal calves fed milk replacers with or without probiotics. *Journal of Dairy Science*, Vol.88, No.6, (June 2005), pp. 2154–2165, ISSN 1525-3198

Timmerman, H.M.; Veldman, A.; Van Den Elsen, E.; Rombouts, F.M. & Beynen, A.C. (2006). Mortality and growth performance of broilers given drinking water supplemented with chicken specific probiotics. *Poultry Science*, Vol.85, No.8, (August 2006), pp. 1383-1388, ISSN 1525-3171

Tournut, J.R. Probiotics. (1998). Proceedings of 35ª Reunião Anual da Sociedade Brasileira de Zootecnia, Botucatu, 1998, pp. 179-199

Waldenstedt, L. (2006). Nutritional factors of importance for optimal leg health in broilers: a review. *Animal Feed Science and Technology*, Vol.126, No.3-4, (March 2006), pp. 291-307, ISSN 0377-8401

Wang, Y. & Gu, Q. (2010). Effect of probiotic on growth performance and digestive enzyme activity of Arbor Acres broilers. *Research in Veterinary Science*, Vol.89, No. 2, (October 2010), pp. 163-167, ISSN 0034-5288

Weese, J.S. (2002). Microbiologic evaluation of commercial probiotics. *Journal of the American Veterinary Medical Association*, Vol.220, No.6, (March 2002), pp. 794-797, ISSN 0003-1488

Weinack, O.M.; Snoeyenbos, G.H.; Soerjadi-Liem, A.S. & Smyser, C.F. (1985). Influence of temperature, social and dietary stress on development and stability of protective microflora in chickens against S. typhimurium. *Avian Diseases*, Vol.29, No.4, (October-December 1985), pp.1177-1183, ISSN 1938-4351

Willis, W.L. & Reid, L. (2008). Investigating the effects of dietary probiotic feeding regimens on broiler chicken production and *Campylobacter jejuni* presence. *Poultry Science*, Vol.87, No.4, (April 2008), pp. 606-611, ISSN: 1525-3171

Yalcin, S.; Özkan, S.; Coskuner, E.; Bilgen, G.; Delen, Y.; Kurtulmus, Y. & Tanyalçin, T. (2001). Effects of strain, maternal age and sex on morphological characteristics and composition of tibial bone in broilers. *British Poultry Science*, Vol.42, No.2, pp.184-190, ISSN 1466-1799

Yang,Y., Iji, P.A. & Choct, M. (2009) Dietary modulation of gut microflora in broiler chickens: a review of the role of six kinds of alternatives to in-feed antibiotics. *World's Poultry Science Journal*, Vol.65, No.1, (March 2009), pp. 97-114, ISSN 1743-4777

Yeo, J. & Kim, K. (1997). Effect of feeding diets containing an antibiotic, a probiotic, or yucca extract on growth and intestinal urease activity in broiler chicks. *Poultry Science*, Vol.76, No.2, (February 1997), pp. 381-385, ISSN 1525-3171

Yörük, M.A.; Gül, M.; Hayirli, A. & Macit, M. (2004). The effects of supplementation of humate and probiotic on egg production and quality parameters during the late laying period in hens. *Poultry Science*, Vol.83, No.1, (January 2004), pp. 84-88, ISSN 1525-3171

Yurong, Y.; Ruiping, S.; Shimin, Z. & Yibao J. (2005). Effect of probiotics on intestinal mucosal immunity and ultrastructure of cecal tonsils of chickens. *Archives of Animal Nutrition*, Vol.59, No.4, pp. 237–246, ISSN 1477-2817

Zhang, Z.; Hinrichs, D.J.; Lu, H.; Chen, H.; Zhong, W. & Kolls, J.K. After interleukin-12p40, are interleukin-23 and interleukin-17 the next therapeutic targets for inflamematorybowel disease? *Int Immunopharmacol*, 200 Vol.7, No.4, (April, 2007), pp. 409–416, ISSN 1567-5769

Ziaie, H.; Bashtani, M.; Torshizi, M.A.; Naeeimipour, H.; Farhangfar, H. & Zeinali, A. (2011). Effect of antibiotic and its alternatives on morphometric characteristics, mineral content and bone strength of tibia in Ross broiler chickens. *Global Veterinaria*, Vol.7, No.4, pp. 315-322, ISSN 1992-6197

Ziprin, R.L.; Corrier, D.E. & Deloach, J.R. (1993). Control of established *Salmonella typhimurium* intestinal colonization with in vivo-passaged anaerobes. *Avian Diseases*, Vol.37, No.1, (January – March 1993), pp.183–188, ISSN 1938-4351

Zulkifli, I., Abdullah, N., Azrin, N.M. & Ho, Y.W. (2000). Growth performance and immune response of two commercial broiler strains fed diets containing Lactobacillus cultures and oxytetracycline under heat stress conditions. *British Poultry Science*, Vol.41, No.5, pp. 593-597, ISSN 1466-1799

Chapter 9

Dairy Propionibacteria:
Less Conventional Probiotics to
Improve the Human and Animal Health

Gabriela Zárate

Additional information is available at the end of the chapter

1. Introduction

Probiotics are live microorganisms that confer health benefits to the host when administered in adequate amounts. In the last decades there has been a great interest from food and pharmaceutical industries to develop products containing probiotics due to the great demands of healthy foods and alternatives to conventional chemotherapy.

Although the great bulk of evidence concerns lactobacilli and bifidobacteria, since they are members of the resident microbiota in the gastrointestinal tract, other less conventional genera like *Saccharomyces, Streptococcus, Enterococcus, Pediococcus, Leuconostoc* and *Propionibacterium* have also been considered.

The genus *Propionibacterium* has been historically divided, based on habitat of origin, into "dairy" and "cutaneous" microorganisms which mainly inhabit dairy/silage environments and the skin/intestine of human and animals, respectively. Dairy propionibacteria are generally recognized as safe microorganisms whereas members of the cutaneous group have shown to be opportunistic pathogens in compromised hosts. In consequence, the economic relevance of propionibacteria derives mainly from the industrial application of dairy species as cheese starters and as biological producers of propionic acid and other metabolites like exopolysaccharides and bacteriocins to be used as thickeners and foods preservers, respectively.

However, the ability of dairy propionibacteria to improve the health of humans and animals by being used as dietary microbial adjuncts has been extensively investigated. In this sense, our research group has been studying for the last two decades the probiotic properties of dairy propionibacteria isolated from different ecological niches. In the present article the current evidences supporting the potential of dairy propionibacteria to be used as probiotics are reviewed focusing in a less studied mechanism such as the protection of the intestinal mucosa by the binding of dietary toxic compounds.

Nowadays there are clear evidences that propionibacteria used alone or combined with other microorganisms can exert beneficial effects in the host. Dairy propionibacteria have proven to posses many promising properties such as the production of nutraceuticals like vitamin B_2, B_{12}, K and conjugated linoleic acid, and their health promoting effects could be attributed to one or more of the following modes of action: *i)* influence on gut microbial composition and exclusion of pathogens; *ii)* modulation of the metabolic activities of the microbiota and host, and *iii)* immunomodulation. The most documented probiotic effects for propionibacteria within these categories include: bifidogenic effect in the human gut, improvement of nutrients utilization, hypocholesterolemic effect and anticarcinogenic potential immune system stimulation.

Different studies have also described the ability of dairy propionibacteria to bind and remove toxic compounds from different environments such as the gut and food. Some of them have focused in the removal of mycotoxins, like Aflatoxin B and Fusarium sp. toxins by *in vitro*, *ex vivo* and *in vivo* assays whereas others have reported the binding of cyanotoxins and some heavy metals like cadmium and lead. It has been proposed that probiotic microorganisms may reduce by binding, the availability of free toxic compounds within the intestinal tract which reduces in turn, their negative effects. In this respect, in recent years we have been investigating the potential of dairy propionibacteria to protect the intestinal mucosa from the toxic and antinutritional effects of some common dietary substances like the plant lectins from the *Leguminosae* family. By *in vitro* and *in vivo* studies we have determined that certain strains are able to bind and remove different dietary lectins from media, preventing their cytotoxic effects on intestinal epithelial cells. Daily ingestion of *P. acidipropionici* CRL 1198, a dairy strain studied in our laboratory, at the same time than concanavalin A prevented the deleterious effects caused by this lectin on some morphological and physiological parameters related to intestinal functionality in mice. Propionibacteria reduced the incidence of colonic lesions, the enlargement of organs, the disruption of brush border membranes and the decrease of their disaccharidase activities. Since consumption of suitable propionibacteria may be an effective tool to avoid lectin-epithelia interactions, further investigations on their potential as probiotic detoxifying agents are actually ongoing

With regard to animals' health it has been reported that dairy propionibacteria directly fed to farm animals increased weight gain, food efficiency and health of many animals like chickens, laying hens, piglets and cows. With a wider insight, propionibacteria may be assayed as probiotics for other ruminants like goats and sheep since their milk-derived products are highly appreciated by consumers.

It should be emphasized that much of the health benefits described above could be related to the ability of propionibacteria to remain in high numbers in the gastrointestinal tract by surviving the adverse environmental conditions and adhering to the intestinal mucosa.

On the basis of the GRAS status of dairy propionibacteria and the positive results obtained by us and other authors, further studies are encouraged in order to select the appropriate strains for developing new functional foods that include these bacteria for human and animal nutrition.

2. The genus propionibacterium

2.1. General features and taxonomy

Propionibacteria are Gram positive, catalase positive, high G+C%, non spore forming and non motile pleomorphic bacteria [1, 2]. In general, microorganisms of the genus *Propionibacterium* are anaerobic to slightly aerotolerant and morphologically heterogeneous including rod-shaped and filamentous branched cells that may occur singly, in pairs forming a V or a Y shape, or arranged in "Chinese characters". They have a peculiar metabolism leading to the formation of propionic acid as main end-product of fermentation.

Although in 1861, Louis Pasteur demonstrated that propionic fermentation was due to the biochemical activity of microorganisms, the first studies about the morphology and physiology of propionibacteria were carried out by Albert Fitz (1879) [3], who observed that organisms from cheeses with "eyes" ferment lactate to propionic and acetic acids and liberate carbon dioxide.

By the beginning of the XXth century, E. Von Freudenreich and Sigurd Orla-Jensen (1906) [4] isolated the bacteria responsible for the "eyes" formation in Emmental cheese and some years later, the name *Propionibacterium* was suggested by Orla-Jensen [5] for referring to bacteria that produced large amounts of propionic acid. Although several strains were isolated during the following years these microorganisms were not included in the Bergey's Manual of Determinative Bacteriology till the third edition published in 1930. Since then, new species were described on the basis of their morphological and biochemical characteristics such as their typical pattern of Chinese characters, propionic acid production, and carbohydrate fermentation profile.

In 1972, Johnson and Cummins [6], classified strains with several common features into eight homology groups based on DNA-DNA hybridization and peptidoglycan characteristics. This study was the basis for the classification of propionibacteria into "dairy or classical" and "cutaneous" groups included in the 8th edition of Bergey's Manual of Determinative Bacteriology (1974). Four dairy species were recognized in this edition: *P. freudenreichii* and their three subspecies (*freudenreichii, shermanii* y *globosum*), *P. thoenii, P. jensenii* and *P.acidipropionici* whereas other four species that inhabit the human skin were ascribed to the cutaneous propionibacteria: *P. acnes, P. avidum, P.*

lymphophylum and *P.granulosum*. The same scheme was followed in the first edition of Bergey's Manual of Systematic Bacteriology [1]. In 1988, on the basis of 16S rRNA sequences, the species *Arachnia propionica* was reclassified as *Propionibacterium propionicus* [7]. Then, in Bergey's Manual 9th edition (1994), the classification of previous edition was maintained but the subspecies *P. freudenreichii* subsp. *globosum* was removed without justification. Other species like *P. inoccuum* and *P lymphophilum* were then also reclassified as *Propioniferax innocua* [8] and *Propionimicrobium lymphophilum* [9], respectively.

In the last two decades six new species were isolated: *P. cyclohexanicum* was obtained from spoiled orange juice [10]; *P. microaerophilum* was isolated from olive mill wastewater [11]; *P. australiense* came from granulomatous bovine lesions [12] and *P. acidifaciens* from human carious dentine [13]. Recently, a new species isolated from human humerus, *P. humerusii*, has been proposed [14].

At present, the genus *Propionibacterium* is classified as Actinobacteria with a high G+C content, that make them more related to corynebacteria and mycobacteria than lactic acid bacteria. The current taxonomic position of propionibacteria is the following [2]: **Phylum** *Actinobacteria*; **Class** *Actinobacteria*; **Subclass** *Actinobacteridae*; **Order** *Actinomycetales*; **Suborder** *Propionibacterineae*; **Family** *Propionibacteriaceae*; **Genus** *Propionibacterium*.

In the more conventional and general way, propionibacteria are divided based on habitat of origin, in two main groups:

- *"Dairy* or *classical propionibacteria"* that inhabit dairy environments and silages, and
- *"Cutaneous propionibacteria"* that inhabit the skin and the intestine of humans and animals.

Classical propionibacteria include among their main habitats: raw milk and cheese [1, 2] but have been obtained also from silages and vegetables for human consumption [15], and from ruminal content and feces of cows and calves [16]. Furthermore, they are not limited to the gastrointestinal tract of ruminants being also isolated from the intestine of pigs and laying hens [17].

On the other side, cutaneous species are found mainly in the human skin, but have been isolated also from the intestine of humans, chicken and pigs [1, 2, 18], being best represented by the acne bacillus, *Propionibacterium acnes*.

The 13 species known up to now are listed in Table 1.

From a safety point of view, classical species have a long history of safe application on industrial processes whereas members of the cutaneous group are commonly considered opportunistic pathogens in compromised hosts. In consequence, the economic relevance of propionibacteria derives mainly from the industrial application of dairy species as cheese starters and as biological producers of propionic acid and other metabolites with a more recent interest on their usage as health promoters.

"Dairy or classical" propionibacteria	"Cutaneous" propionibacteria
P. acidicpropionici	*P. acidifaciens*
P. cyclohexanicum	*P. acnes*
P. freudenreichii	*P. australiense*
P. jensenii	*P. avidum*
P. microaerophilum	*P. granulosum*
P. thoenii	*P. humerusii*
	P. propionicus

Table 1. Current species of the genus *Propionibacterium*

Isolation and enumeration of propionibacteria can be made by microbial culture and molecular methods [19]. Various agarized media with different degrees of selectivity have been used for detection and enumeration of classical propionibacteria in dairy environments, animal and human fecal samples. Among them it could be mentioned YELA [20], Pal Propiobac® medium, which contains glycerol, lithium lactate and antibiotics [21] or others including lithium chloride and sodium lactate in concentrations high enough to limit the growth of accompanying bacteria [22]. In all cases, incubations are made in anaerobiosis with an atmosphere of 10–20% CO_2. Although these media may be successful for the isolation of classical and cutaneous strains of *Propionibacterium*, they have limitations for selective enumeration of bacteria in very complex ecosystems like intestinal microbiota. Furthermore, plate count methods for propionibacteria are time consuming since long incubation periods for at least 6 days are needed to obtain typical colonies and enumerations may be underestimated due to aggregation of bacteria in the diluents used, and/or growth inhibition by the selective agents used.

Molecular methods are a valuable alternative to plating assays, being far more specific, and unhindered by the presence of non-target microorganisms. Different fingerprinting methods such as SDS-PAGE of whole cell proteins [23], 16s rDNA targeted PCR-RFLP [24], ribotyping [25], 16S-23S ribosomal spacer amplification and restriction [26], Pulsed-Field Gel Electrophoresis [27], Conventional Gel Electrophoresis Restriction Endonuclease Analysis (CGE-REA) and Randomly Amplified Polymorphic DNA-PCR [28] have been used for detection and accurate identification of dairy propionibacteria from various environments like milk, cheese, whey and flour. Genus and species-specific primers targeted to the genes encoding 16S rRNA for PCR-based assays were also designed for detection of dairy propionibacteria [29].

Recently, a multicolor fluorescent *in situ* hybridization (FISH) assay targeting the 16S rRNA [30] or 23S rRNA [31] of *P.acnes* was developed and used to detect this bacterium in blood samples and tissues of patients with prostate cancer, respectively. A FISH protocol and oligonucleotide probes targeting the 16S rRNA of dairy propionibacteria were developed in our laboratory [32] and successfully used for enumeration of *P. acidipropionici* in cecal samples of mice fed with a strain of this species [33].

Finally, a real-time PCR method, based on the transcription of the enzyme transcarboxylase involved in propionic fermentation, was successfully used to detect a strain of *P. freudenreichii* in the intestinal ecosystem [34] and would be a valuable tool for monitoring survival and metabolic activity of propionibacteria in different environments.

2.2. Genotypic characteristic of *Propionibacterium*

The members of the genus *Propionibacterium* possess a circular-shaped chromosome like most bacteria that varies in size between 2.3 and 3.2 Mb depending on the different species [35]. The G+C content in their DNA is in the range of 53-68 mol% and although they generally do not possess plasmids their existence has been reported in strains of *P. acidipropionici*, *P. freudenreichii* and *P. jensenii* [36]. In fact, it has been informed that between 10 and 30% of *P. freudenreichii* strains possess one or two cryptic plasmids [37]. The presence of two types of bacteriophages has also been described for propionibacteria. One of them, the bacteriophage B22, belongs to the Group B1 of Bradley classification, whereas the other, bacteriophage B5, would be the first infectious filamentous virus described in a Gram positive bacterium [38].

Up to few years ago, the only completely sequenced and publicly available genome within the genus *Propionibacterium* was that of the commensal cutaneous species *P. acnes* [39]. However, in the year 2010, the complete genome of a species that belongs to the taxonomic group of dairy propionibacteria was described for the first time.

The genome of the type strain, *P. freudenreichii subsp. shermanii* strain CIRM-BIAI_T, was sequenced with an 11-fold coverage [40]. It consists of a circular chromosome of 2,616,384 base pairs (bp) with 67% GC content, 2 rRNA operons and 45 tRNAs. The chromosome is predicted to contain 2439 protein-coding genes and also contains 22 different insertion sequences that represent 3.47% (in base pairs) of the genome. Insertion sequences and transposable elements may promote genome plasticity and induce phenotypic changes that contribute to bacterial adaptation to different environments; being particular for propionibacteria the synthesis of capsular EPS and the ability to ferment lactose [40].

P. freudenreichii subsp. *shermanii* CIRM-BIAI_T is able to metabolize lactose, although this trait is strain-dependent, since the Lac genes may have been acquired through a horizontal transfer event mediated by phage infection. In this sense it should be emphasized that the presence of the enzyme β-galactosidase should be the only feature that allows these bacteria to adapt to dairy niches like cheeses.

The genome sequence also showed that *P. freudenreichii* possesses a complete enzymatic machinery for de novo biosynthesis of aminoacids and vitamins (except panthotenate and biotin) and genes involved in the metabolism of carbon sources, immunity against phages, chaperones for stress resistance, and storage of inorganic polyphosphate, glycogen and compatible solutes such as trehalose that confer these bacteria a long survival in stationary phase [40]. Although propionibacteria are usually described as anaerobes, all the genes encoding enzymes required for aerobic respiration such as NADH dehydrogenase, succinate dehydrogenase, cytochrome bd complex, ATPase and the complete pathway for heme synthesis have been identified in the genome of *P. freudenreichii* [40].

With respect to technological application in dairy industries, various pathways for formation of cheese flavor compounds were identified in the genome of this strain such as the enzymes involved in the production of propionic acid, volatile branched chain fatty acids from amino acid degradation, and free fatty acids and esters from lipids catabolism.

In relation to probiotic functionality, it has been identified the complete biosynthesis pathway for a bifidogenic compound (DHNA) as well as the sequences corresponding to a high number of surface proteins involved in the interactions with the host (like adhesion and immunomodulation). By comparative genomics with *P. acnes*, no pathogenicity factors were identified in *P. freudenreichii*, which is consistent with the Generally Recognized As Safe and Qualified Presumption of Safety status of this species.

2.3. Main physiological characteristics of *Propionibacterium*

Propionibacteria are heterotrophic microorganisms that mean they need an organic carbon source to grow and posses a fermentative metabolism [41-43]. They degrade carbohydrates like glucose, galactose, lactose, fructose and other sugars; poliols like glycerol; erythritol and others; and organic acids such as lactic and gluconic acids producing propionic, acetic and CO_2 as the main fermentation end-products [1].

The production of propionic acid by these bacteria involves a complex metabolic cycle with several reactions in which substrates are metabolized to pyruvate via glycolysis, pentose phosphate or the Entner-Doudoroff pathways, generating ATP and reduced co-enzymes. Pyruvate is then oxidised to acetate and CO_2 or reduced to propionate. The latter transformation occurs via the Wood-Werkman cycle or transcarboxilase cycle which represents the key component of the central carbon metabolic pathway in propionibacteria [41].

The most important reaction of this cycle is transcarboxylation that transfers a carboxyl group from methyllmalonyl-CoA to pyruvate to form oxaloacetate and propionyl-CoA, without ATP consumption. The enzyme catalyzing this reaction is a methylmalonyl-CoA carboxytransferase that has been fully characterized and its structure resolved [34; 40].

Then, oxaloacetate is reduced to succinate, via malate and fumarate in two NADH requiring reactions. Succinate is then converted to propionate via methylmalonyl-CoA intermediates (succinyl-CoA and propionyl-CoA); the carboxyl group removed from methylmalonyl-CoA is transferred to pyruvate to yield oxaloacetate, thus completing one cycle. Methylmalonyl-CoA is also regenerated from succinyl-CoA during propionate production, thus creating the second of the two transcarboxylase cycles, and can react with a new molecule of pyruvate. All the reactions of this cycle are reversible. It must be emphasized that the Wood Werkman cycle used by propionibacteria to produce propionate is coupled to oxidative phosphorylation and yields more ATP than in the other bacteria producing propionic acid [42, 43].

Depending on the strains, the substrate used, and the environmental conditions, propionibacteria modulate the proportions of pyruvate either reduced to propionate, or oxidised to acetate and CO_2, to maintain the redox balance [43]. In this way the oxidation of glucose and lactic acid leads to a molar ratio of propionate:acetate of 2:1 whereas the oxidation of glycerol leads to the formation of propionate only. The co-metabolism of aspartate/asparagine and lactate has also been reported [44]. During lactate fermentation, aspartate is deaminated to fumarate by an aspartate ammonia lyase; fumarate is then converted to succinate, with a concomitant production of NAD and ATP. Cells using this pathway convert less pyruvate to propionate and oxidised more pyruvate to acetate+CO_2.

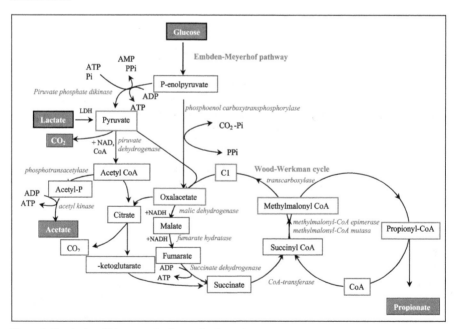

Figure 1. Propionic acid fermentation in propionibacteria

Propionibacteria are also mesophilic microorganisms, with optimal growth conditions at 30 ℃ and pH 6.8. However, they grow in a temperature range between 15 a 40 ℃ and tolerate pH variations between 5.1 and 8.5 [1, 2]. Their nutritional requirements are low and almost the same for all the species. Dairy propionibacteria like *P. freudenreichii* are able to synthesize all amino acids [40]. They can grow in a minimal medium containing ammonium as the sole nitrogen source, but a higher growth is observed in media containing amino acids [45].

Although *P. freudenreichii* subspecies *shermanii* is able to ferment lactose, dairy propionibacteria show poor growth in milk, as they do not possess proteases capable of hydrolyzing milk caseins [46]. Some proteinases have been described for *Propionibacterium*, one cell wall associated and one intracellular or membrane bound but their activities are weak. By contrast, different peptidases such as aminopeptidases, proline iminopeptidase, proline imidopeptidase, X-prolyl-dipeptidyl-amino-peptidase, endopeptidases and carboxypeptidase, have been described. and characterized. Amino acids, especially aspartic acid, alanine, serine and glycine, are degraded by *Propionibacterium*, with variations among species and strain [47]. On the other side, cutaneous propionibacteria, have the ability to hydrolyze different proteins, like gelatin and fibronectin, and to promote damages and inflammation of the host tissues.

Regarding vitamins, all propionibacteria strains require pantothenate (vitamin B5) and biotin (vitamin H). In addition, some strains require thiamine (B1) and p-aminobenzoic acid [40, 41].

2.4. Long term and stress survival of Propionibacteria

It is known that propionibacteria are able to adapt and survive to different stresses like industrial processes and the gastrointestinal transit, as well as to remain active for long periods of time in such adverse environments [43].

In this sense, the manufacture of a swiss type cheese represents for microbial starters successive stresses like acidification of the curd, heating during cooking, osmotic stress due to brining, and low temperature (4 to 12 °C) during cheese ripening. The transit through the digestive tract also suppose stressful conditions for bacteria such as gastric acidity and the presence of other aggressive intestinal fluids like bile and pancreatic enzymes.

Interestingly, the cell machinery involved in general stress adaptation in *P. freudenreichii* was shown to be encoded by multicopy stress-induced genes [40]. The redundancy and inducibility of this chaperone and protease machinery is in agreement with the ability of *P. freudenreichii* to adapt rapidly and efficiently to various unfavorable conditions [48-50].

The stress adaptation proteins were particularly investigated in *P. freudenreichii* and its genome, finding out that they are differentially expressed depending on the strain and the stress [40, 48-50]. Acid and bile stresses, induce the synthesis of the following proteins: pyruvate-flavodoxin oxidoreductase and succinate dehydrogenase which are involved in electron transport and ATP synthesis, as well as glutamate decarboxylase and aspartate ammonia-lyase, which are involved in intracellular pH homeostasis. Bile also induces oxidative stress so that survival and activity within the gut depend on remediation of oxidative damages. *P. freudenreichii* possesses an arsenal of genes for disulfide-reduction and elimination of reactive oxygen species. Moreover, in response to bile salts, *P. freudenreichii* overexpresses the iron/manganese superoxide dismutase, Glutathione-S-transferase, two cysteine synthases and S-adenosylmethionine synthetase [40]. The occurrence of a sodium/bile acid symporter (PFREUD_14830) reflects adaptation to the gut environment. Other inducible proteins involved in protection and repair of DNA damages include Ssb protein which is involved in DNA recombination and repair, as well as Dps which protects DNA against oxidative stress are stress-induced in *P. freudenreichii* [49].

With respect to thermotolerance, the over-expression of constitutive stress-related molecular chaperones and ATP-dependent proteases as well as the induction of the dihydroxyacetone kinase locus (dhaKL, PFREUD_07980 and PFREUD_07990) by stress and starvation seems to be related to survival to thermal stress by difference to thermosensitive strains [40, 50].

Stress tolerance and cross-protection in strains of *Propionibacterium freudenreichii* were examined after exposure to heat, acid, bile and osmotic stresses. Cross-protection between bile salts and heat adaptation was demonstrated. By contrast, some other heterologous pretreatments (hypothermic and hyperosmotic) had no effect on tolerance to bile salts. Furthermore, acid pretreatment sensitized cells to bile salts challenge and vice versa. Heat and acid responses did not present significant cross-protection and no cross-protection of salt-adapted cells against heat stress was observed for these propionibacteria [48-50].

In addition, long term survival of propionibacteria on adverse environments could be due to the accumulation of storage compounds, compatible solutes, and the induction of a multi-tolerance response under carbon starvation [40]. In contrast to other bacteria that use ATP, *P. freudenreichii* accumulates inorganic polyphosphate (polyP) as energy reserve. Short chains of PolyP are synthesized when bacteria grow on glucose whereas long chains are accumulated when the main carbon source is lactate. The synthesis of PolyP is catalysed by polyphosphate kinase (PPK) that transfers the terminal phosphate of ATP to polyP. It is proposed that PolyPs enable microorganisms to tolerate adverse conditions since ppk mutants are unable to survive during stationary phase [51]. The genes encoding for polyP or pyrophosphate (instead of ATP) using enzymes were found in the genome of *P.freudenreichii* CIRM-BIA1T [40].

Propionibacteria is also able to synthesize glycogen and all the genes related to glycogen metabolism were identified in the genome of the strain *P.freudenreichii* CIRM-BIA1T [40]. Some of these genes were also found in *P. acnes*. These enzymes seem to be involved in intracellular accumulation and hydrolysis of glycogen as neither *P. freudenreichii* nor *P. acnes* are able to ferment extracellular glycogen

It has been reported that propionibacteria are able to withstand osmotic stress by accumulation of compatible solutes like glycine betaine and trehalose [52]. Trehalose is a non-reducing disaccharide that can be used by bacteria as a carbon and energy source and also can be accumulated as a compatible solute. All dairy propionibacteria are able, in a strain dependent manner, to synthesize and accumulate trehalose from glucose and pyruvate [53]. Both processes are enhanced at stationary phase and under oxidative, osmotic, and acid stress conditions [54]. Trehalose is commonly synthesised via the trehalose-6-phosphate synthase/phosphatase (OtsA–OtsB) pathway and catabolised by trehalose synthase (TreS). The genes otsA, otsB, and treS were identified in *P. freudenreichii* by Cardoso et al., 2007 [55] and Falentin et al 2010 [40].

It is also known that dairy propionibacteria survive for many months at room temperature even under conditions of carbon starvation, being the majority of the strains non-lytic [2]. This long-term survival in stationary phase or dormant phase could be the consequence of a multi-tolerance response that involves the synthesis and accumulation of polyP, glycogen, trehalose and the over-expression of molecular protein chaperones. Besides, a gene encoding an Rpf (resuscitation promoting factor) protein which is essential for the growth of dormant cells from actinobacteria has been described in the genome of *P freudenreichii* and is probably involved in long-term survival of propionibacteria [40].

3. Technological importance of dairy propionibacteria

3.1. Dairy starters for Swiss-type cheeses and other products

The main industrial application of the genus *Propionibacterium* is the usage of "classical propionibacteria" as dairy starters for the manufacture or Swiss type cheeses. This denomination refers to cheese varieties, such as Sbrinz, Emmental, Gruyère, Compté, Appenzeller and others riddled with holes and made with raw or pasteurized milk (depending on the variety).

In these products propionibacteria are responsible for the typical sweet, nutty taste by production of acetic and propionic acids; aminoacids like proline and leucine but mainly for the characteristic "eyes" formation by releasing of CO_2 [56-57]. However, propionibacteria can also be used in the manufacture of various cheeses without eyes just to enhance flavour formation [58].

In swiss type cheeses, propionibacteria may be present either as contaminants of raw milk or as components of starter cultures. The typical starter for this variety includes *Streptococcus thermophilus*, *Lactobacillus helveticus*, *Lactobacillus delbrueckii* subsps. *lactis* or *bulgaricus* and *Propionibacterium freudenreichii*. During manufacture and early stages of ripening, the thermophilic bacteria develop at expense of lactose of milk being responsible for lactic acid production, and also contributing to casein hydrolysis during pressing of the cheese.

Interactions between microbiota and milk throughout ripening lead to biochemical changes that result in the development of the typical texture and flavor. During maturation in the cold room (15 °C) most of lactic starter lyse and release peptidases that produce free amino acids, which are precursors of many flavor compounds. The subsequent period of warm room ripening is characterized by a marked growth of propionibacteria that metabolize the lactate produced by the lactic acid bacteria into propionate, acetate and CO_2. At the end of maturation that ranges from 6 weeks to 12 - 18 months in the hardest varieties, the number of propionibacteria reaches 10^8 - 10^9 cfu/g of cheese [41, 57].

P. freudenreichii greatly contributes to Swiss-type cheese flavour by producing compounds from three main pathways: lactate and aspartate fermentation, amino acid catabolism, and fat hydrolysis [59]. As described above, the end-products of propionic fermentation are considered as flavour compounds in cheese whereas the co-metabolism of aspartate leads to additional CO_2 production. However, strains with a high ability to metabolise aspartate can be associated with undesirable slits and cracks [60].

Propionibacteria degrade branched-chain amino acids to branched-chain volatile compounds mainly 2-methylbutanoic acid and 3-methylbutanoic acid, which derive from isoleucine and leucine degradation, respectively [61]. These important flavour compounds are almost entirely produced in cheese by propionibacteria that synthesize them in closely related manner to that of cell membrane fatty acids [62].

P. freudenreichii also contributes in a great manner to cheese lipolysis by releasing free fatty acids from fat during cheese ripening. Two esterases, one extracellular and other surface-exposed seem to be involved in lipolysis of milk glycerides [63, 64]. Furthermore, ten intracellular esterases were found in the *P. freudenreichii* genome that could be involved in the synthesis of the volatile esters associated with the fruity flavor of cheese [65].

In contrast, although it possesses diverse intracellular peptidases, *P. freudenreichii* has a limited role in secondary proteolysis, compared to starter and non-starter lactic acid bacteria (NSLAB), because it does not lyse in cheese [66].

It is important to emphasize that propionibacteria maintain metabolic activity up to the end of ripening, as shown by molecular methods [68] producing flavour compounds during growth in cheeses at 24 °C, and further cold storage [60].

Other dairy products such as yogurt and fermented milks seem to be less appropriated for delivery of propionibacteria due to their weak proteolitic activity, the presence of inhibitory substances and the low pH attained by lactic acid fermentation that do not allow their development. Currently, yogurt is used to deliver probiotic propionibacteria to the host's intestine or to produce nutraceuticals, but in both cases inoculums higher than those used for cheese manufacturing are necessary.

3.2. Antimicrobials production: Propionic acid and bacteriocins

Propionic acid and its salts, as well as *Propionibacterium* spp strains, are widely used as food and grain preservatives due to their antimicrobial activity at low pH. They are commonly incorporated in the food industry to prolong the shelf-life of many products by suppressing the growth of mold and spoilage microorganisms in bread and cakes, on the surface of cheeses, meats, fruits, vegetables, and tobacco.

Most commercial propionic acid is produced by petrochemical processes since biosynthesis by microbial fermentation is limited by low productivity, low conversion efficiency, by-product formation (acetic acid and succinic acid) and end-product inhibition. However, different attempts have been made to improve biological production of propionic acid for industrial applications [68]. In this sense, it has been determined that the most appropriated species for bioproduction of propionic acid from carbohydrate-based feedstock, including glucose and whey lactose, is *P.acidipropionici* [69, 70]. Since the use of glycerol as the principal carbon source enables the production of propionic acid without acetic acid, recent investigations have focused on the optimization of this particular homopropionic fermentation by propionibacteria [71, 72].

Two commercial products that include propionibacteria or their metabolites aimed for controlling spoilage microorganisms are currently available at market. Microgard™ is a food grade biopreservative obtained by fermentation of skim milk with *Propionibacterium shermanii* that is active against some fungi and Gram negative bacteria, but not against Gram positive ones [73]. The other product named BioProfit, contains viable cells of *P. freudenreichii* subsp *shermanii* strain JS and is effective for inhibiting yeasts growth in dairy products, *Bacillus* spp. in sourdough bread [74]; and also used to preserve grain and produce good quality silages [75].

Propionic acid, produced *in vivo* in the gut by viable bacteria, is also a desired healthy metabolite, as it is related to many probiotic properties of propionibacteria (as will be described below). In this respect, it has been demonstrated that SCFA favours the colonic recovery of water and electrolytes counteracting the osmotic diarrhea induced by lactose and/or other unabsorbed carbohydrates [76]. Besides, they exert anticarcinogenic effects by inducing apoptosis of neoplastic cells but not of healthy mucosa [77]. Finally, SCFA may exert hypocholesterolemic effects, since propionate lowers blood glucose and alters lipid metabolism by suppressing cholesterol synthesis in the liver and intestine [78].

Bacteriocins are antimicrobial peptides or proteins encoded by plasmid or chromosomal DNA of a wide range of Gram positive and negative bacteria. They have an antagonistic activity against species genetically related to the producer strain, but many of them exhibit a rather wide spectrum of activity and inhibit the growth of spoilage and pathogenic bacteria belonging to other genera [79].

Both starters and naturally occurring bacteria on food have the ability to produce bacteriocins. Hence, they may have potentially important applications as food biopreservatives or bacteriocin-producer probiotics to inhibit intestinal pathogens [80].

However, only nisin, a bacteriocin produced by *Lactococcus lactis subsp. lactis*, has attained the GRAS status of the FDA for use in certain foods.

Different bacteriocins produced by both dairy and cutaneous propionibacteria have been reported and characterized. Among them it could be mentioned: Propionicin PLG-1 and GBZ-1 produced by *P. thoenii* 127 [81]; Jenseniin G isolated from *P. thoenii* P126 [82]; Propionicins SM1 and SM2 produced by *P. jensenii* DF1 [83]; Propionicin T1 synthesized by *P. thoenii* 419 and LMG2792 [84]; Thoenicin 447 isolated from *P. thoenii* 447 [85]; Acnecin produced by a strain of *P. acnes* [86] and several other propionicins [87-89].

These bacteriocins are active against other propionibacteria, lactic acid bacteria (*Lactobacillus, Lactococcus* and *Streptococcus*), other Gram positive bacteria (*Clostridium botulinum* types A, B and E), Gram negative bacteria (*Campylobacter jejuni, E. coli, Ps. fluorescens, Ps. aeruginosa, Vibrio parahaemolyticus Salmonella typhimurium, Yersinia enterocolitica*); yeasts (*Saccharomyces, Candida* y *Scopularopsis sp*) and molds (*Aspergillus ventii, Apiotrichum curvatum, Fusarium tricinctum, Phialophora gregata*).

Although the ability of dairy propionibacteria to produce bacteriocins *in situ* in food products or inside the intestine has not been demonstrated yet, they have a potential application as safe biopreservatives. In this respect, some efforts have been made to improve the production processes [90] since the slow growth, late bacteriocin synthesis and low production represent limitations for the practical application of bacteriocin-producer propionibacteria.

Propionibacteria also produce other peptides and organic acids (2-pyrrolidone-5-carboxylic acid, 3-phenyllactic acid, hydroxyphenyl lactic acid 3-phenyllactic acid) with antiviral, antiyeasts and antifungal activities [91-93].

3.3. Nutraceuticals production: CLA, vitamins, EPS and trehalose

Propionibacteria are able to produce many biological compounds that enhance the human health so they can be used as "nutraceuticals cell factories" for food enrichment. In this regard, propionibacteria have already been considered as rich sources of conjugated linoleic acid, vitamins, exopolysaccharides and trehalose.

Many health benefits have been attributed to consumption of CLA-containing foods such as anticarcinogenic, antiatherogenic, antidiabetogenic and antioxidative properties, immune system modulation and reduction of body fat gain [94]. CLA-isomers are formed by biohydrogenation of LA in the rumen and through conversion of vaccenic acid by $\Delta 9$-destaurase in the mammary gland so that ruminant meats and milk-derived products are main dietary sources of CLA. However, some microorganisms like *Bifidobacterium, Lactobacillus, Enterococcus* and *Propionibacterium* posses a linoleic acid isomerase that allow them to form CLA as a detoxification mechanism [95]. In consequence, they have been intended, either as starter or adjunct cultures, to increase the CLA level and nutritional value of some fermented products like yoghurt and cheese.

In this regard, several studies have shown the potential of propionibacteria for producing CLA enriched products. Both growing and resting cells of dairy (*P. freudenreichii*) [96, 97] and cutaneous propionibacteria (*P. acnes*) [98] produce cis-9, trans-11 and trans-10, cis-12, the major isomers with biological activity, on different growth media: culture broths [97], lipid containing plant materials [99], milk and ripening cheese [100].

By varying the source of LA for conjugation and the fermentation conditions it has been observed that *P. freudenreichii* convert free LA to mainly extracellular CLA with a high efficiency (50-90%), being the optimal conditions that favor the accumulation of CLA also determined [97, 101]. Besides, it has been observed that CLA formation and growth of dairy propionibacteria in fermented milks were enhanced in the presence of yogurt microorganisms whereas organoleptic attributes obtained with yogurt starter cultures were not affected by co-cultures with the propionibacteria [100].

Vitamin B12 also called cobalamin, is an essential nutrient for the human body that plays a key role in the normal functioning of the brain and nervous system, the formation of blood and also the metabolism of every cell, especially affecting DNA synthesis and regulation, fatty acid synthesis and energy production. Its deficiency leads to a serious physiological disorder called pernicious anemia.

The pathway of vitamin B12 synthesis in *Propionibacterium freudenreichii* has been completely elucidated [40, 102]. This microorganism synthesizes cobalamin as a cofactor for propionic acid fermentation [41] and is the only bacteria, among B12 producers that possess the GRAS status of the United States Food and Drug Administration.

In consequence dairy propionibacteria are the preferred microorganisms for the industrial production of this vitamin and many efforts have been made to improve the production process by using genetic engineering [102, 103] and other biotechnological strategies like fermentation manipulations [104, 105].

Vitamin B2, also known as riboflavin, is the central component of the cofactors FAD and FMN, and is therefore required by all flavoproteins. As such, vitamin B2 is required for a wide variety of cellular reactions and is involved in vital metabolic processes in the body. It has been reported that *P. freudenreichii* NIZO2336, a mutant strain that produces larger amounts of riboflavin than the parental strain, improved riboflavin content of yogurt and riboflavin status of rats fed with this product [106].

Different studies have shown the possibility to obtain genetically modified strains of *P. freudenreichii* that overproduce B12 vitamin [102, 107], porphyrin [108], and riboflavin (vitamin B2) [107].

Propionibacteria also produce Vitamin B7 (biotin) and Vitamin B9 (folic acid), so that propionibacteria-containing products could be expected to be good sources of B-group vitamins.

Vitamin K (a group of 2-methyl-1,4-naphthoquinone derivatives), is an essential cofactor for the formation of γ-carboxyglutamic acid-containing proteins that bind calcium ions and are involved in blood coagulation and tissue calcification. Its deficiency has been associated with low bone density and increased risk of fractures from osteoporosis and intracranial hemorrhage in newborns [109]. Vitamin K1 or phylloquinone is present in plants, and vitamin K2, also called menaquinone, is produced in animals and bacteria that live in the intestine.

It has been reported that *Propionibacterium freudenreichii* produces large amounts of tetrahydromenaquinone-9 (MK-9 (4H)) and the precursor 1,4-dyhidroxy-2-naphtoicacid (DHNA) which is a known bifidogenic factor [110-112]. In order to improve the production of these metabolites, different laboratory culture protocols that could be applied to an industrial scale have been assayed finding out that DHNA production is markedly influenced by carbon source limitation and the oxygen supply. An improvement in DHNA production could be obtained by a cultivation method that combines anaerobic fed-batch and aerobic batch cultures [112, 113].

In another study, Hojo et al. [114] assessed the concentration of MK-9 (4H) in commercial propionibacteria-fermented cheeses finding out a positive correlation between the increase in propionibacteria and the generation of MK-9 (4H) in cheese. Due to their high MK-9 (4H) concentrations (200 to 650 ng/g), Emmental and Jarlsberg cheeses should be a meaningful source of vitamin K and potential protectors against osteoporosis.

Exopolysaccharides-producing bacteria and their secreted EPS are important biological thickeners for food industry. Besides, some health promoting properties such as immunomodulation and cholesterol lowering activities have been ascribed to EPS [115].

In dairy propionibacteria *(P.freudenreichii* subsp. *shermanii)*, the single gene *gtf* encoding for a β-d-glucan synthase that is responsible for the synthesis of surface polysaccharide has been identified [40, 116] and the EPS produced was also characterized. Both homopolysaccharide [116, 117] and heteropolymers [118] were described and it has been reported that production of EPS by propionibacteria is a strain-dependent property (due to an IS element in the gtf promoting sequence) that is influenced by the medium composition and the fermentation conditions [119, 120]. Further studies are needed to elucidate the role of these polymers and their potential applications.

Trehalose has been proposed as a healthy sugar substitute in foods because of its anticariogenic and dietetic properties. As described in paragraphs above, propionibacteria synthesize trehalose as a reserve compound and as a stress-response metabolite [52-55]. With respect to the production of this sugar in situ in food products, it has been observed that *P. freudenreichii* ssp. shermanii NIZO B365 produces high levels of trehalose in skim milk [54].

Technological property	General comments	References
Dairy starter	*Propionibacterium freudenreichii* is included in the starter of Swiss type cheeses. It contributes to the typical flavor and the development of characteristic "eyes"	[56, 57], [59].
Antimicrobials	*P. acidipropionici* could be considered for biological production or propionic acid to be used as food preservative. Microgard™ and BioProfit are commercial products that include propionibacteria aimed for controlling spoilage microorganisms. Different bacteriocins are produced by both dairy and cutaneous propionibacteria that are active against gram positive and gram negative bacteria. They have a potential application as safe biopreservatives	[68-71]. [73-75]. [81-89].
CLA	Propionibacteria produce cis-9, trans-11 and trans-10, cis-12, CLA isomers on culture broths; lipid containing plant materials; milk and ripening cheese. They have potential for producing CLA enriched products.	[96-101].
Vitamins	*Propionibacterium freudenreichii* is the only GRAS status producer of Group B vitamins: B2, B7 (biotin), B9 (folic acid) and B12. Genetically modified overproducer strains have been experimentally obtained. Propionibacteria produces vitamin K (MK-9 (4H) and its precursor DHNA with bifidogenic activity.	[103-108]. [110, 114].
EPS	Propionibacteria produce homo and heteropolysaccharides that could be used as food thickeners.	[117, 121].
Trehalose	*P. freudenreichii* synthesizes trehalose that coud be used as sugar substitute in foods	[54].

Table 2. Technological relevance of the genus *Propionibacterium*

4. Probiotic application of dairy propionibacteria

Since the last decades, there has been an increasing interest from food and pharmaceutical industries to develop healthy foods and therapeutic alternatives to conventional antibiotic treatments in response to consumers' demands of natural products. Probiotics are "live microorganisms that confer health benefits to the host when administered in adequate amounts" [121]. In this respect, the great bulk of evidence concerning the beneficial effects of microorganisms both in human and animal health refers to lactic acid bacteria and bifidobacteria as they are common inhabitants of the gastrointestinal tract. However, in recent years several potential probiotic properties of propionibacteria have been reported and many studies on this subject have been published. In the following sections, safety aspects and the major health benefits ascribed to dairy propionibacteria are reviewed.

4.1. Safety and persistence in the gut

Strains selected on the basis of their potential beneficial effects by *in vitro* tests, must demonstrate their safety both in humans and animals, before they could be incorporated as probiotics, either in food or pharmaceutical products.

In this sense, dairy propionibacteria have a long history of safe use in human diet and animal feed. *P. freudenreichii* is widespread consumed in Swiss type cheeses in which they are present in concentrations close to 10^9 bacteria/g. Besides, classical propionibacteria have been isolated from soil, silage, vegetables, raw milk, secondary flora of cheese and other naturally fermented food. Therefore, it could be considered that they would arrive to the gut of different organisms, including the man, at least once in their lives.

At present, no cases of sickness or toxicity after the ingestion of dairy propionibacteria have been reported [122] neither for humans (for a review of human trials see [123]) nor for animals [124-126]. In fact, it has been reported that propionibacteria did not translocate to blood, liver or spleen and no adverse effects on body weight gain and general health status was observed after short [124, 127] and long terms [125] administration of strains of *Propionibacterium acidipropionici, P. freudenreichii and P. jensenii,* respectively.

Most studies have been performed with strains of *P. freudenreichii* since it is the traditional component of cheese starters being this species granted the Generally Recognized As Safe (GRAS) status from the US Food and Drug Administration. Furthermore, *P. freudenreichii* belongs with *P. acidipropionici,* to the list of agents recommended for Qualified Presumption of Safety (QPS) by the European Food Safety Authority [122, 128].

On the other side, most strains isolated from humans and animals belong to the "cutaneous group" [18, 129] and their use as probiotics is discouraged since they are potential pathogens. However, propionibacteria isolated from the intestine of animals and identified by molecular tools as dairy species, were not associated to pathogenesis.

Besides safety, other criteria to take into account in the selection of strains for dietary adjuncts are the absence of antibiotic resistances (due to the risk of spreading any resistance to intestinal microbiota) and virulence factors. Dairy propionibacteria have natural resistance to some antibiotics and this resistance does not appear to be encoded by plasmids or other mobile genetic elements [36, 122, 130]. By comparative genomics, no virulence factors found in *P. acnes* or in other pathogenic species were identified in *P. freudenreichii*, although some *P. thoenii* and *P. jensenii* strains have β-haemolytic activity [40, 122].

In order to exert their beneficial effects in the host, it is generally accepted that ingested microorganisms must survive the hostile environmental conditions of the gastrointestinal tract represented by the low pH of the stomach and intestinal fluids such as bile and pancreatic enzymes. Many studies have demonstrated by *in vitro* assays the ability of dairy propionibacteria to survive and tolerate the gastrointestinal conditions [130-134]. This tolerance could be improved by a pre-adaptation of the microorganisms to the adverse conditions of the gut by a brief exposure to the stressful conditions at a non-lethal level [48, 135].

Both acid and bile tolerance have shown to be strain-dependent properties. In previous studies [131, 132] we observed that dairy propionibacteira developed in a medium containing bile (0 – 0.5%) behaved as "bile-tolerant" and "non bile-tolerant" strains and that there were differences among *P. freudenreichii* and *P. acidipropionici* strains in their tolerance to pancreatic enzymes when subjected to sequential digestion with artificial gastric and intestinal fluids.

It has also been demonstrated that the vehicle used for delivery of probiotics is important for digestive stress tolerance since cells included in food matrices like milk or cheese had better tolerance to acid challenge than free cultures [132]. Similar results were obtained by Huang and Adams [134], by protecting propionibacteria from acid and bile stresses with a soymilk and cereal beverage, and Leverrier et al. [136], who used yoghurt-type fermented milk.

Survival of propionibacteria during gastrointestinal transit has also been reported *in vivo* in rats [125, 126]; mice [124, 137] and humans [127, 130, 133]. Furthermore, Herve et al. [34], demonstrated that propionibacteria remain metabolically active since the *P. freudenreichii*-specific transcarboxylase mRNA was detected in human faeces. In most studies, a high level of propionibacteria was detected in intestinal contents and feces during the feeding period but this concentration gradually declined and returned to the initial levels a few weeks after consumption ceased.

Besides surviving the gastrointestinal digestion, intended probiotics must remain in high levels in the intestine avoiding normal washout by peristaltic contractions of the gut. Therefore, microorganisms with a short generation time and/or the ability to adhere to the mucosa would have an extended survival in the body of the host. Bacterial adhesion to intestinal cells and mucus is generally considered as the initial step in the colonization of the gut and has been related to many of the health effects of probiotics, as it prolongs the time that beneficial bacteria can influence the gastrointestinal microbiota and immune system [138]. Since propionibacteria grow slowly in natural environments and culture media, adhesion ability becomes an important property in the selection of strains for probiotic purposes.

Dairy propionibacteria have demonstrated to adhere to immobilized mucus [139]; to isolated mouse intestinal epithelial cells [140,141], to human intestinal cell lines [142-144] and in vivo to intestinal cells as was assessed by counting the adhering propionibacteria on the mucosa by a plate count method [124, 125, 137, 145].

In previous studies, we have correlated the *in vitro* and *in vivo* abilities of dairy *Propionibacterium* strains to adhere to intestinal epithelial cells and observed by scanning electron microscopy, that *P.acidipropionici* CRL 1198 adheres well to IEC or the mucus layer covering them [141]. Microscopic examination revealed two adhesion patterns in propionibacteria: autoaggregating strains adhere in clusters, with adhesion being mediated by only a few bacteria, whereas nonautoaggregating propionibacteria adhere individually making contact with each epithelial cell with the entire bacterial surface [140].

Besides, the adhesion of propionibacrteria of different dairy species such as *P. freudenreichii* subsp. *shermanii* JS, *P. jensenii* 702 and *P. acidipropionici* Q4 to Caco-2, C2BBe1 and HT29 cells respectively, was clearly stated [142-144].

Interactions with the host gut mucosa are also suggested by the analysis of the genome of *P. freudenreichii* that revealed the presence of genes encoding for a high number of surface proteins involved in adhesion and present in other probiotic bacteria [40].

To date, the ability of dairy propionibacteria (used alone or combined with other microorganisms) to improve the health of humans and animals by being used as dietary microbial adjuncts has been extensively investigated. Their health promoting effects could be attributed to one or more of the following modes of action: *i)* immunomodulation; *ii)* influence on gut microbial composition and exclusion of pathogens; and *iii)* modulation of the metabolic activities of the microbiota and host. Main evidences obtained by *in vitro* and *in vivo* studies supporting the potential of dairy propionibacteria to be used as probiotics are summarized below.

4.2. Propionibacteria for improving animal health

Nowadays, the usage of probiotics as an alternative to antibiotics to enhance the growth and health of domestic animals is a growing practice. With this aim, different bacterial genera have been isolated from the intestine of farm animals and pets and employed as probiotics, such as *Lactobacillus*, *Bifidobacterium* and *Enterococcus* [146].

To date, most animal studies have been performed with ruminants (cows, calves, steers), chicken, pigs, and to a lesser extent with horses and pets. In this sense, it has been reported that dairy propionibacteria administered alone or combined with other microorganisms increase the weight gain, feed efficiency and health of different animals such as laying hens and broilers [147], pigs [148] and calves [149, 150].

Propionibacteria are natural inhabitants of the rumen microbiota. In consequence, they have been used as direct-fed microbial (DFM) feed additives in ruminant nutrition with strain-dependant results on animal performances.

One desired effect for ruminant probiotics is an improvement in propionate production as it is considered the major precursor for hepatic gluconeogenesis that provides substrate for lactose synthesis in lactating dairy cows. Various strains of *Propionibacterium* have increased the molar proportion of ruminal propionate when fed to ruminants [151, 152]. In this respect, many researches have been done with the dairy strain *Propionibacterium acidipropionici* P169. It has been reported that, when administered to beef cattle, this microorganism was able to increase hepatic glucose production via enhanced ruminal propionate production and absorption, whereas directly fed to early lactating dairy cows, it tended to improve milk proteins content and energetic efficiency during early lactation, without affecting the reproductive function [152-154]. In general, these authors concluded that strain P169 might have potential as an effective direct-fed microorganism to increase milk production in dairy cows.

In other studies, the supplementation of lactating dairy cows with a DFM product containing a mixture of *L. acidophilus* and *P. freudenreichii* improved milk and protein yield, and apparent digestibility of crude protein, neutral detergent fiber, and acid detergent fiber, so that it could be used to enhance the performance of cows subject to heat stress during hot weather [155].

With respect to calves, a preparation called Proma, which is a blended culture of lactic acid bacteria plus *P. freudenreichii* and a DFM product containing *P. jensenii* 702 showed to be effective to improve weight gain during pre-weaning and weaning periods [149, 150].

Propionibacteria have also been assayed as health and growth promoters in monogastric animals like pigs, with positive results. Mantere-Alhonen [148] was the first to achieve growth promotion in piglets fed with different species of propionibacteria being *P freudenreichii* ssp *shermanii* the most effective probiotic among the species tested. When propionibacteria were fed to piglets in a daily concentration of 2×10^9 cfu/g, the weight gain was 9.2-14.5% higher, the fodder demand was 7.2-46.1% lower than the control group and the animals had less diarrhoea. In bigger swine, the effects were even more evident.

Cutaneous propionibacteria have also been used to improve the health of swine. *Propionibacterium* avidum KP-40 showed to be a potent immunomodulator that stimulated granulopoiesis as well as a faster body weight gain in pregnant swine and their offspring [156]. The usefulness of the prophylactic application of this strain, against porcine microbial infections was tested in swine finding out that propionibacteria application caused positive immunoregulation of porcine innate immune system effectors, non-specific activation of lymphocytes and antibody production that resulted in milder clinical symptoms, faster recovery and a larger body weight gain [157, 158].

In chicken, both undefined and defined "Nurmi Cultures" have been used to establish an intestinal flora that will prevent colonization by pathogenic bacteria in young animals. These formulas have shown to be effective for the protection against species of *Salmonella* and other avian pathogens; for immune system stimulation in newborn chicks, and also had growth promoting effects [159, 160]. The most frequently assayed bacteria as avian probiotics were several species of lactic acid bacteria [146, 159, 160]. Propionibacteria have not been widely studied in this ecological niche. However, some authors demonstrated the presence of this bacterial group in the ileum and cecum of chickens [161], and cecal Nurmi cultures characterized by microbiological and PCR-DGGE techniques, evidenced the presence of *Propionibacterium propionicus* [147].

In recent studies, the occurrence of *Propionibacterium* in different segments of the gastrointestinal tract of laying hens was demonstrated. Bacteria from this genus were evidenced in 27% of the animals sampled. Half of these isolates were identified by genus and species specific PCR as *P. acidipropionici,* belonging the others to the propionibacteria cutaneus group. This report represents the first evidence of dairy propionibacteria as inhabitants of the gastrointestinal tract of chickens. Some preliminary studies on the probiotic properties of these strains, suggest their potential application as probiotic to prevent intestinal infections in poultry [17].

4.3. Probiotic properties for human application

Inmunomodulation: One of the most promoted properties of probiotics is their ability to regulate in a positive manner the innate and adaptive responses of the human immune system. It is well-documented that cutaneous propionibacteria are potent immunomodulators, since they have been tested in several assays both in humans and rodents used as animal models [162]. Administration of cutaneous propionibacteria (*P. avidum, P. granulosum, P. acnes*) have shown to be beneficial in the treatment of neoplastic and infectious diseases [163-165]. Besides, dead *Propionibacterium acnes* or a polysaccharide extracted from its cell wall have proven to be effective in the induction of macrophages with an antitumor effect [166] and in modulating an experimental immunization against *Trypanosoma cruzi* [167].

With respect to the immunomodulatory properties of dairy propionibacteria, many researches have been done in *vitro* and *in vivo* with the strain *P. freudenreichii subsp. shermanii* JS. It has been reported that this microorganism stimulated the proliferative activity of B and T lymphocytes depending on doses administration and treatment duration in mice [168]. Regarding to cytokine production, *P. freudenreichii* JS was able to induce TNF-α and IL-10 production in human PBMCs [169] and inhibited the H. pylori-induced IL-8 and PGE2 release in human intestinal epithelial cells [170].

Other dairy *P. freudenreichii* strains also showed promising immunomodulatory properties by strongly inducing the synthesis of anti-inflammatory IL-10 by human PBMCs and could be helpful in the treatment of inflammatory conditions or diseases [171].

Further beneficial results with *P. freudenreichii* JS were obtained with different randomised, placebo-controlled, double-blind trials in humans such as: reduction in the serum level of C-reactive protein (an inflammation marker) [172];   induction of IL-4 and IFN-gamma production in PBMCs of infants with cow's milk allergy [173]; prevention of IgE-associated allergy in caesarean-delivered children [174] and increase in the resistance to respiratory infections during the first two years of life [175].

With respect to other dairy species, an increase in the phagocytic activity of peritoneal macrophages and the phagocytic function of the reticuloendothelial system was observed in mice fed with *Propionibacterium acidipropionici* CRL 1198 [124]. In addition, administration of this strain prior to infection of mice with *Salmonella* Typhimurium led to an increase of the anti-*Salmonella* IgA level and the number of IgA producing cells [176].

Dairy propionibacteria may also act as safe adjuvant for development of oral vaccines. Adams et al [177] found that *Propionibacterium jensenii* 702 co-administered orally with soluble *Mycobacterium tuberculosis* antigens to mice stimulate T-cell proliferation of splenic lymphocytes in a significant manner so that the strain PJ702 could act as a potential living vaccine vector to be used against mucosal transmitted diseases.

4.4. Gut microbial modulation

Stimulation of bifidobacteria: It is well-documented that propionibacteria can modulate gut microbiota in a positive manner by enhancing bifidobacterial growth. This property has been demonstrated both *in vitro* [110, 111, 178, 179], and *in vivo* [127, 180-182] and the bifidogenic growth stimulators (BGS) involved in this effect were identified. The active compounds that were present in supernatants of *P. freudenreichii*, *P. jensenii* and *P. acidipropionici* were purified and identified as 2-amino-3-carboxy-1,4-naphtoquinone (ACNQ) [110, 178] and 1,4-dihydroxy-2-naphtoic acid (DHNA) a precursor of menaquinone (vitamin K2) biosynthesis [111]. It has been proposed that these compounds serve as electron transfer mediators for NADP regeneration in bifidobacteria [183], thus favoring growth.

The bifidogenic effect of selected strains of *P. freudenreichii* [127, 180-182] or purified BGS [184] was assessed in independent studies performed on human volunteers. As a general result, increased fecal bifidobacterial populations were observed even after some days after stopping the consumption of propionibacteria. Besides a reduced colonic transit time and a reduction in the numbers of clostridia were evidenced in some studies.

Inhibition of pathogens: There are several reports on the ability of dairy propionibacteria to inhibit exogenous and opportunistic pathogens. *In vitro* studies have demonstrated that *P. freudenreichii* strain JS was able to inhibit, alone or combined with other probiotics the adhesion of different pathogens including *H .pylori* to intestinal mucus and Caco2 cell line also improving the epithelial barrier function [170, 185]. Other dairy species like *P. acidipropionici* strain Q4 was able to prevent the adhesion of *Salmonella enteritidis* and *Escherichia coli* to HT29 cells [144] whereas *P. acidipropionici* CRL 1198 regulates *in vitro* the growth of *Bacteroides* and *Clostridium* in cecal homogenates of mice supplemented with propionibacteria and/or inulin [33]. Mice consuming this strain delivered in water, milk or cheese showed a decrease in the number of anaerobes and coliforms in the caecal content one week after feeding [124, 137, 145]. *P. acidipropionici* CRL 1198 also prevented tissue colonization by *Salmonella* Typhimurium in mice [176].

In humans, propionibacteria have been used in combination with *Lactobacillus spp.* and *Bifidobacterium spp.* in the treatment of intestinal disorders and regulation of gut flora and motility. It has been demonstrated that the consumption of probiotic mixtures containing *Propionibacterium freudenreichii* JS reduced oral *Candida* in elderly [186] and gastric inflammation of the mucosa caused by *H.pylori* in the host. [187]. Besides, infants and children fed with Propiono-Acido-Bifido (PAB) milk [188] or milk containing *P. freudenreichii* subsp. *shermanii* and *L. acidophilus* [189], showed a reduction in coliforms with an increase in lactobacilli and bifidobacteria population.

Alleviation of IBD: It has been demonstrated that consumption of either isolated BGS or *P. freudenreichii* strains ameliorate experimental colitis in mice and human ulcerative colitis [171, 189-192]. The mechanism proposed for this effect was restoring of microbiota intestinal balance and suppressing inflammatory lymphocyte infiltration. In this respect, it has been proposed that some surface compounds should be involved in immunomodulatory effects of propionibacteria since removal of surface layer proteins decreased the in vitro induction of anti-inflammatory cytokines [171]. By their side, Michel et al. [193] demonstrated that colonic infusion with *P. acidipropionici* reduced the severity of TNBS induced colitis in rats whereas Kajander et al [194] reported that the multispecies probiotic mixture containing *Propionibacterium freudenreichii* JS was effective in alleviating irritable bowel syndrome symptoms.

4.5. Modulation of the host and resident microbiota metabolism

Lactose malabsorption: The ability of probiotics to alleviate lactose intolerance by supplying β-galactosidase for the intraintestinal hydrolysis of lactose has been widely reported for LAB and bifidobacteria [196]. However there are no clinical reports on this property for dairy propionibacteria. Several evidences suggest the potential of *Propionibacterium acidipropionici* strains on this subject: they have high β-galactosidase activity that remain unaltered in the conditions of the human's intestine, and cells are permeabilized by bile, which in turn may favour the hydrolysis of lactose within the intestine [131, 132]. Besides, the manufacture conditions of Swiss-type cheese did not decrease the synthesis and activity of the β-galactosidase of these propionibacteria [197]. When mice were fed with *P.acidipropionici* CRL 1198 included in milk or cheese, the β-galactosidase levels in the small bowel and the propionic acid concentration in the caecum were significantly increased. High SCFA concentration in the colon could counteract diarrhea induced by non-digested carbohydrates [137].

Hypocholesterolemic properties: The reduction of cholesterol has been assessed for many probiotics with conflicting results. Somkuti and Johnson [198] evidenced the ability of *P. freudenreichii* cells to remove by surface adsorption up to 70% of the cholesterol from the medium, whereas Perez Chaia et al [124] demonstrated, in an animal study, that *P. acidipropionici* CRL 1198 was able to reverse the hyperlipemic effect of a diet with a high lipid content. However, the mechanisms underlying this beneficial effect were not determined in this investigation.

Antimutagenic properties: Vorobjeva [199] demonstrated the antimutagenic activity (AM) of *Propionibacterium freudenreichii* against the mutations induced by 4-nitro-quinoline and N-nitro-N-nitrosoguanidine (transition mutations), and by 9-aminoacridine and 2-nitrofluorene (frame-shift mutations). This AM activity was exerted by live and dead cells and by the cultured media. The active compound responsible for this activity was identified as a cysteine synthase which is induced by some stress factors.

Anticarcinogenic properties: Several *in vitro* and *in vivo* studies (mainly in animal models) have suggested the potential of probiotics to prevent have suggested the potential of probiotics to prevent colon cancer as evidenced by colon cancer as evidenced by a decrease in the incidence and magnitude of tumours and preneoplastic lesions [200]. Among the mechanisms involved it could be mentioned: inhibition of enzyme activities that convert procarcinogens into carcinogens, control of harmful bacteria, antigenotoxicity, production of active metabolites and immunomodulation.

Regarding propionibacteria, it has been demonstrated that *P.acidipropionici* CRL1198 fed to mice was able to modulate the metabolism of the resident microbiota as it prevented the induction of azoreductase, nitroreductase and β-glucuronidase activities caused by a cooked red-meat supplemented diet. Furthermore, feeding with propionibacteria resulted in a remarkable reduction of β-glucuronidase activity and slight reductions of azo and nitroreductase activities [201]. In humans, independent researches have shown that consumption of *P. freudenreichii* subsp. *shermanii* JS decreased to different extents fecal azoreductase activity in elderly subjects, β-glucosidase and urease in healthy young men and β-glucuronidase activity of irritable bowel syndrome patients [202, 203].

Other studies have reported that dairy propionibacteria kill human colorectal adenocarcinoma cells *in vitro* through apoptosis via their metabolites, propionate and acetate [204, 205]. In addition, consumption of *P. freudenreichii* TL133 by human microbiota associated rats significantly increased the number of apoptotic cells in the colon of 1,2-dimethylhydrazine treated rats but have no effect on healthy colonic mucosa [77]. The authors suggest that dairy PAB may help in the elimination of damaged cells by apoptosis within the colon epithelium after genotoxic insult. Long term studies assessing the protective role of PAB against colon cancer are still missing.

4.6. A less studied mechanism: *Binding of toxic compounds*

Foods daily ingested by humans and animals may possess besides nutrients, many toxins and antinutrititive factors that could be endogenous (i.e., compounds naturally occurring because of the inherent genetic characteristics of the plant or animal used as food) or produced by the action of microorganisms, under the influence of physical factors, or by chemical reactions between food constituents. Among these deleterious compounds it could be mentioned: trypsin inhibitors, lectins, biogenic amines, mycotoxins, etc. In this respect, several studies have focused, in recent years, on the ability of safe bacteria to bind and remove toxic compounds from different environments such as the gut and food.

Numerous findings have shown that intestinal microorganisms and lactic acid bacteria ingested with food, including probiotics, play a role in detoxification of various classes of DNA-reactive carcinogens such as heterocyclic aromatic amines (HAs), pyrolysis products of amino acids contained in meat and fish products [206-209].

Most studies have ascribed this effect to the physical binding of the mutagenic compounds to the bacteria rather than their metabolism. The binding of the HAs (Trp-P-2, PhIP, IQ and MeIQx) to bacteria is generally measured by HPLC and/or the decrease in mutagenicity in bacterial assays (mainly in *Salmonella* frameshift tester strains) and genotoxicity by comet assay. In attempts to elucidate the mechanisms involved in the binding of Tryptophan pyrolysates it was found that the structure of the cell wall plays a role in the inactivation and that the effect may involve cation exchange processes. Although gram-positive strains were more effective than gram-negative to remove HAs, these compounds bound both to peptidoglycan and outer membrane. Sreekumar and Hosono [209] studied the binding of Trp-P-1 to *Lactobacillus gasseri*, and postulated that the binding receptors of the HAs are the carbohydrate moieties of the cell walls and that glucose molecules play a key role in the binding reaction. By comparing, the effects of heat inactivated cells with those of living cells, it was suggested that living bacteria may also produce metabolites or catalyze reactions which lead to the detoxification of the amines [208]. However there are no reports on the ability of propionibacteria to detoxify HAs.

Another detoxification property proposed for probiotics is their ability to remove mycotoxins. These fungal metabolites are carcinogens that unavoidable contaminate cereals and grains destined for human consumption. Mycotoxins are also forage contaminants, which impair animal performances and health. Several probiotic bacteria, commonly used in food products, have been shown to bind Aflatoxin B1 and the toxins produced by *Fusarium* sp such as zearalenone, fumonisins B1 and B2 and trichothecenes, like deoxynivalenol (DON), nivalenol (NIV) and T-2 toxin (T-2) preventing their absorption in the gastrointestinal tracts of animals and humans [210-214].

The capacity of *Propionibacterium freudenreichii* strain JS used alone and combined with lactobacilli (*L. rhamnosus* GG or LC705) to remove mycotoxins has been studied by *in vitro* [210-212], *ex vivo* [211] and *in vivo* assays [213-214]. It has been determined that both viable and heat-killed forms of propionibacteria are able to remove efficiently aflatoxin B1, fumonisins and trichotecenes from liquid media. Binding, not biodegradation appeared to be the mode of action, as no toxin derivatives were observed and removal was not impaired in nonviable bacteria. Kinetics of adsorption and desorption of Aflatoxin B1 by viable and no viable bacteria have also been determined [215]. Tested ex vivo in the intestinal lumen of chicks, there was a 63% reduction in the uptake of AFB1 by the intestinal tissue in the presence of *P.freudenreichii* JS and its binding ability seems to be even better than in vitro results [211]. When combined with *L. rhamnosus* LC-705, 57-66% of AFB1 was removed by the probiotic mixture *in vitro* whereas 25% of AFB1 was bound by bacteria in *ex vivo* experiments being tissue uptake of AFB1 also reduced when probiotic bacteria were present in the duodenal loop [211]

Intestinal mucus significantly reduced AFB1 binding by the probiotic mixture and vice-versa (preincubation with AFB1 reduced mucus binding) [216]. However, similar binding sites are unlikely to be involved, since heat-treated bacteria lost their ability to bind intestinal mucus, whereas AFB1 binding was found to be enhanced by heat treatment. It has been proposed that proteins must be involved in the binding of mucus, whereas carbohydrates must bind AFB1 [217, 218]. Other mechanisms, such as steric hindrance, may cause interference in AFB1 and mucus binding by bacteria. These findings have relevance, since probiotics adhering to the intestinal wall are less likely to bind and consequently accumulate AFB1 in the host. On the other hand, probiotics with AFB1 bound to their surfaces are less likely to adhere to the intestinal wall and prolong exposure to dietary AFB1. Specific probiotics may be significant and safe means to reduce absorption and increase excretion of dietary AFB1 from the body.

On clinical trials it has been observed that the consumption of a probiotic preparation containing both *P. freudenreichii* JS and *L. rhamnosus* LC-705 reduced in a significant manner the levels AFB1 in fecal samples [213] and the concentration of urinary AFB-N7-guanine [214] of healthy volunteers during treatment and even after several days after probiotic consumption ceased. These results suggest that the probiotic bacteria used in these trials could block the intestinal absorption of aflatoxin B1

Dietary exposure to heavy metals and cyanotoxins may have detrimental effects on human and animal health, even at low concentrations. Specific probiotic bacteria may have properties that enable them to bind these toxins from food and water. In this respect, it has been reported that *P. freudenreichii* spp. *shermanii* JS alone and combined with other probiotics have the ability to remove microcystin-LR [219] and also cadmium and lead from aqueous solution [219, 220] and could be considered a promising microorganism for decontamination in food and intestinal models.

Lectins are proteins which interact selectively and reversibly with specific residues of carbohydrates present in glycoconjugates [221]. Although their biological relevance as recognition molecules is well-known their physiological role and impact on health is controversial since both beneficial and deleterious effects have been ascribed to different lectins [222, 223]. Plant lectins are widespread in the human diet, in food items such as vegetables, fruits, cereals, legumes, etc, so their ingestion could be significant [224]. They are also present in other members of the *Leguminosae* and *Gramineae* Families that are used as farm feeds.

Most plant lectins are highly resistant to degradation by cooking and by digestive processes, so after consumption, they reach the intestinal lumen in a bioactive state and bind specifically to carbohydrate moieties expressed on the glycocalix of enterocytes affecting cellular physiology [221]. In general, lectins from the *Leguminosae* Family are considered as antinutritive or toxic substances since they lead to deleterious morphological and physiological changes after binding to the intestinal mucosa. Those changes include the thinning of the mucus lining, reduction of the absorptive function and nutrient utilization, genotoxic effects like single strand breaks in the DNA and stimulation of cellular proliferation and turnover that could lead to tumors development [225-229]. Some of these alterations could be initially unnoticed but lead to important nutritional deficiencies in the long term, being their impact on health of significant relevance.

Different alternatives have been proposed in order to prevent or counteract the deleterious effects of toxic or antinutritional dietary compounds on the GIT (Figure 2), being of particular interest those that focus on a suitable complementary diet. Regarding lectins, it has been proposed that a high dietary intake of carbohydrate-containing foods, complementary to most toxic lectin expected in the diet, would offer protection by binding free lectin in the colonic lumen (Figure 2a). In this sense, it has been reported that the consumption of sucrose may reduce the toxic effects of legume lectins such as red kidney beans by protecting barrier function, bacterial overgrowth and bacterial translocation [230]. In the same way, it has been proposed, that a high consumption of galactose-containing carbohydrates, such as galactose-containing vegetable fiber, would offer protection against binding and proliferative effects of galactose-N-acetylgalactosamine-binding dietary lectins (such as PNA) on colonic neoplastic epithelium [229, 231].

The same role could be played by bacteria with suitable sugar residues on their surface, that would reduce the interaction between dietary lectins and cells by competing for the sites where these molecules bind (Figure 2b), by capturing and removing free lectins (Figure 2c) or by binding to different receptors and blocking lectin access to their receptors (Figure 2d). .

With this concept in mind, it could be proposed that probiotic microorganisms with the appropriate surface glycosidic moieties could be consumed as a part of human or animal diets to interfere with the cell-lectin recognition process preventing some toxic effects. In consequence, in recent years we have initiated a research line aimed to assess the capacity of dairy propionibacteria to protect the intestinal mucosa from the deleterious effects of dietary lectins.

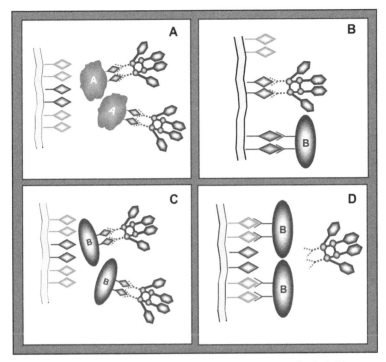

Figure 2. Mechanisms proposed to counteract the interaction lectin-intestinal cell. A) Dietary carbohydrates complimentary to free lectin in the intestinal lumen; B) Bacterial binding analogous to lectin binding; C) Microorganisms that bind free lectins; D) Microorganisms that adhere to the epithelium blocking the binding of lectins to intestinal receptors.

In a recent study [232], we have assessed *in vitro* the citotoxic effects of three plant lectins: concanavalin A (Con A), peanut agglutinin (PNA) and jacalin (AIL) on intestinal epithelial cells (IEC) of mice finding out that the three lectins used in the study induced cells death in a different extent. The effect was remarkable only with Con A and AIL since they reduced the percentage of viable cells from 88 ± 12% to 63 ± 10% and 64 ± 12% respectively after 120 min of contact as determined by Trypan Blue dye exclusion.

Then we evaluated the ability of different dairy propionibacteria to bind those lectins decreasing their citotoxic effects and the relation between bacterial adhesion to epithelial cells and protection against lectins. Two bacterial strains, with and without the property of adhesion to IEC, were studied for their ability to remove lectins from the reaction mixture. Both *Propionibacterium acidipropionici* (adh+) and *P. freudenreichii* (adh-) were able to remove 60–70% of Con A and AIL as determined by the free protein detected in the interaction supernatants. Removal was due to binding with specific sugar moieties on the bacterial surfaces, as was evidenced by inhibition in the presence of sugars specific for each lectin. It is known that dairy propionibacteria possess residues of glucose, mannose and galactose in their cell walls depending on the species [233] that would allow their interactions with ConA and AIL. Besides, no growth or production of SCFA was observed in a synthetic medium supplemented with ConA or AIL as sole carbon and energy sources confirming the binding hypothesis.

When the supernatants of the interactions bacteria-lectin reaction mixtures were assayed for their toxic effect against IEC a great reduction on the percentages of necrotic cells was observed for both lectins (Table 3)

Conditions	Percentage of cells		
	Viable	Necrotic	Apoptotic
Control	85 ± 6	10 ± 7	5 ± 2
Con A	58 ± 3	35 ± 5	7 ± 5
P. acidipropionici + Con A	82 ± 4	9 ± 1	11 ± 4
P.freudenreichii+ Con A	89 ± 2	5 ± 4	6 ± 2
AIL	62 ± 13	36 ± 5	2 ± 3
P. acidipropionici + AIL	78± 9	8 ± 2	13 ± 5
P.freudenreichii+ AIL	75 ± 5	15 ± 2	10 ± 1

Table 3. Cytotoxic effects of lectins, and protection of colonic cells by lectin removal by propionibacteria. *Control*: Cells exposed to PBS. *Con A* and *AIL*: Cells exposed to 100 μg/mL of lectins; *Propionibacteria+lectins*: Supernatant of interactions bacteria-lectins after removal of bacteria. Viability was assessed by counting cells under the fluorescence microscope after propidium iodide/fluorescein diacetate/Hoescht staining. Adapted from Zárate and Pérez Chaia, J. Appl. Microbiol (2009)106: 1050-1058 [232].

Since the cellular damage was almost completely abolished when lectin solutions were preincubated with bacteria it is evident that microorganisms remove these compounds from the media avoiding their deleterious effects on cells.

Both strains were subjected to chemical and enzymatic treatments used to remove surface structures previous to their interaction with Con-A, and then were assayed for their ability to bind this lectin and to adhere to IEC. As shown in the Figure 3 different components are involved in the Con A-bacteria interaction depending on the strain studied.

In adherent *P. acidipropionici* both carbohydrates and proteins seemed to be involved in Con A removal since high cytotoxic effects of interaction supernatants was observed when these surface structures were removed. In contrast, the lectin removal by a nonadherent strain of *P. freudenreichii* only depended on cell wall carbohydrates as periodate treatment of bacterial cells was the only responsible for the loss of protective effect on IEC of this strain (Figure 3a, right). Besides, in adherent *P. acidipropionici* the lectin receptors on the bacterial surface and the adhesion determinants seem to be related, since both the abilities to adhere to IEC and to remove Con A were lost after treatments with periodate and pronase E (Fig. 3a left and 3b). Con A bound to *P. acidipropionici*, reduced but not abolished adhesion of *P. acidipropionici* to IEC suggesting that carbohydrates other than glucose and mannose on the bacterial surface are also involved in the bacteria-IEC interaction (Fig. 3b)

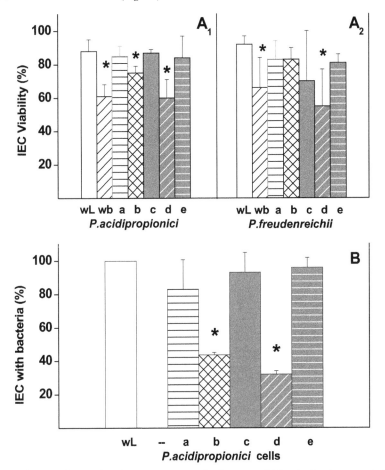

Figure 3. Influence of bacterial surface components on lectins removal (a) and adhesion property (b). (a) Viability of IEC exposed to the interaction supernatants of Con A and propionibacteria treated with chemical agents in order to remove cell surface structures. (b) Adhesion ability (%) of treated propionibacteria after incubation with Con A. **wL:** propionibacteria without lectin interaction, **wb:** lectin without bacteria; **a:** Non-treated bacteria; **b:** protease treatment (cell wall proteins remotion); **c:** LiCl treatment (S-layer); **d:** periodate treatment (polysaccharides); **e:** phenylmethylsulfonylfluoride treatment (lectin-like adhesins). Reproduced from: Zárate and Perez Chaia, Journal of Applied Microbiology (2009) 106: 1050–1057 [232].

Although Con A is not a regular component of human diets, it is a good model to study the behaviour of members of the mannose binding lectins family, which include, among others, lectins found in lentils and kidney beans. However, Con-A and other lectins like WGA (from wheat) and SBA (from soy) could be found in feed formulations for broilers leading to epithelial damages and growth depression of BB chicks. In consequence, probiotic bacteria could be considered also by avian industry to avoid the undesirable effects of lectins on animal's health by capturing them or by blocking their ligands in the mucosa. In this respect, it has been observed that some LAB and *P. acidipropionici* isolated from the chicken gut were able to bind Con A and WGA (Babot et al 2012 unpublished results) so that further studies are actually ongoing in order to develop a lectin-protector probiotic for broilers.

Since the removal *in vitro* of Con A and AIL by dairy propionibacteria was an effective way to avoid the toxic effects against intestinal cells, we assessed *in vivo* the effects of Con A on some morphological and physiological parameters related to intestinal functionality such as small bowel architecture, main microflora components and disaccharidase activities of Balb/c mice after long term feeding with this lectin alone (8 mg/kg/day of Con A for 3 weeks) or with the simultaneous consumption of *Propionibacterium acidipropionici* CRL 1198 (5 x 10^8 CFU/mice/day) [145].

Long-term inoculation of adult Balb/c mice with Concanavalin A resulted in a less food efficiency since food consumption was not affected but animals gained less weights during this treatment, suggesting an alteration of the digestion/absorption function of the intestine in the presence of lectin. Other deleterious effects observed during Con A feeding include a significant increase of the stomach size and transient enlargement of other organs such as liver, small bowel and cecum; and histomorphological and physiological alterations. In fact, an increased intestinal epithelial cell proliferation, evidenced by the higher cellularity of the epithelium lining the villus and the disarrangement and stratification of nuclei was observed at the optical microscopic level. At the ultrastructural level, a marked shortening and shedding of microvilli were evidenced in the lectin treated group as could be seen in Fig. 4(a) and (b). Similar results were reported previously by Lorenzsonn and Olsen [225] who observed in the jejunum of normal rats, an increased shedding of brush border membranes, acceleration of cell loss and shortening of villi as acute effects after an intraluminal injection of Con A. or WGA.

The histomorphological modifications induced by Con A were greatly prevented by consumption of propionibacteria at the same time than Con A (Fig. 4c and 4d). By their side, mice that consumed *P. acidipropionici* CRL 1198 showed no remarkable differences with respect to the control animals.

Intestinal microbial populations were also modified by lectin feeding. Mice fed Con A showed increased enterobacteria and enterococci populations whereas lactobacilli, bifidobacteria and propionibacteria were not affected. Inclusion of *P. acidipropionici* CRL 1198 in the diet prevented these microbial modifications induced by Con A.

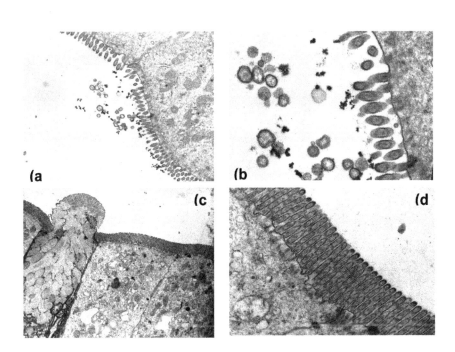

Figure 4. Transmission electron microscopy photomicrographs of the microvillous surface of the small bowel of mice fed with Con A (Group 2) (panels a-b) and those that consumed lectin plus propionibacteria (Group 4) (Panels c-d). Reproduced from Zárate and Perez Chaia, Food Research International (2012), 47(1): 13-22 [145].

With respect to physiological effects, since lectins interact in the intestine with the mucosa membrane; it could be expected that the processes that take place at this level, such as hydrolysis of dietary components and nutrients transport may be affected leading to a low nutritional status. Besides, structural alterations could also contribute to physiological changes. The four dissacharidases assessed in this study were affected by Con A to some extent. Daily Con-A feeding led to a significant decrease of lactase, sucrase, and trehalase activities whereas maltase seemed to be less affected. One week after treatments were finished sucrase and trehalase were still below control values. In general, consumption of propionibacteria with Con A resulted in activities similar to those of untreated animals and those fed propionibacteria alone (Figure 5).

From the results obtained up to now it could be suggested that consumption of foods containing these propionibacteria would be a valuable tool for protecting the intestinal mucosa of humans and animals from the undesirable interactions with antinutritional lectins.

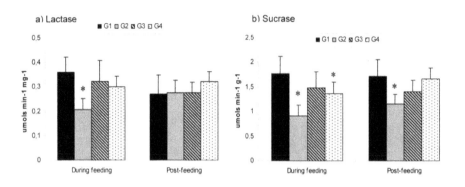

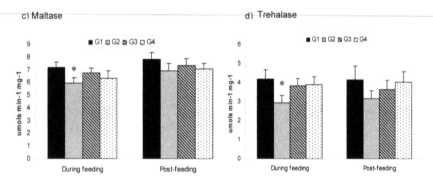

Figure 5. Effect of Concanavalin A, *P.acidipropionici* CRL 1198 and lectin plus propionibacteria feeding on the disaccharidase activities of intestinal mucosa homogenates of Balb/c mice. G1: Control; G2: Con A, G3: *P. acidipropionici* CRL 1198, G4: Con A+ CRL 1198. Values are means ± SD. The asterisk indicates significant differences with the control group (G1) (P<0.05). Reproduced from Zárate and Perez Chaia, Food Research International (2012), 47(1): 13-22 [145].

Although probiotic microorganisms are considered a promising alternative to physico-chemical methods to be used as biological sequestering agents of toxins, further in vivo studies are needed in order to confirm that the inclusion of such microorganisms in the diet may reduce the absorption of deleterious compounds in the gastrointestinal tract.

5. Concluding remarks

From the extensive data reviewed in the present article it can be concluded that dairy propionibacteria are valuable microorganisms for both technological applications and health promotion. Although many studies have been made and the current knowledge of the genus has increased in different and well-defined fields further studies are needed in order to select the best strains and their most appropriate delivery vehicles. In this sense the unique nature of the genus *Propionibacterium* (such as the resistance to stress and particular technological and probiotic properties) turns it, and particularly dairy species, as promising microorganisms to be incorporated in new types of food products. However, randomized, placebo-controlled, double blind human trials that confirm the properties of individual propionibacteria are still lacking. It could be expected that in the near future this void will be filled and new possible applications for propionibacteria will be discovered on the basis of newly available genome sequence and the recent development of molecular tools.

Author details

Gabriela Zárate
Centro de Referencias para Lactobacilos (CERELA)-CONICET, San Miguel de Tucumán, Argentina

Acknowledgement

This review was supported by grants of Consejo Nacional de Investigaciones Científicas y Técnicas (CONICET - PIP 0043), and Consejo de Investigaciones de la Universidad Nacional de Tucumán (CIUNT 26/D429).

6. References

[1] Cummins C.S., Johnson J.L. Propionibacterium. In: Holt JG. (ed.) Bergey's Manual of Systematic Bacteriology. Baltimore, MD, USA: The Williams & Wilkins Co. 1986. p1346-1353.

[2] Stackebrandt E., Cummins C.S., Johnson J.L. Family Propionibacteriacea: The genus *Propionibacterium*. In: Dworkin M, Falkow, S., Rosemberg, E., Schleifer, K. H., and Stackebrandt, E. (ed.). The Prokaryotes: A handbook on the Biology of Bacteria. Singapur: Springer. 2006. p400-418.

[3] Fitz A. Ueber Spaltpilzgährungen. Ber. Dtsch. Chem. Ges 1879; 12: 474–481. doi: 10.1002/cber.187901201136.

[4] Von freudenreich E., Orla-Jensen S. Über die im Emmentalerkase staffindene Propionsauregarung. Zbl Bakteriol 1906; 2: 529-546.

[5] Orla-Jensen S. Die hauptlien des natürlichen bakteriensystems. Centrlbl Bakteriol Hyg II Abt. 1909; 22: 305-346.

[6] Johnson J.L., Cummins C.S. Cell wall composition and deoxyribonucleic acid similarities among the anaerobic coryneforms, classical propionibacteria, and strains of *Arachnia propionica*. J Bacteriol 1972; 109: 1047-1066.

[7] Charfreitag O, Collins, M.D., Stackebrandt E. Reclassification of *Arachnia propionica* as *Propionibacterium propionicus* comb. Nov. Int J Syst Bacteriol 1988; 38: 354-357.

[8] Yokota A., Tamura T., Takeuchi M., Weiss N., Stackebrandt E., Transfer of *Propionibacterium innocuum* Pitcher and Collins 1991 to Propioniferax gen. nov., as *Propioniferax innocua* comb. nov. Int J Syst Bacteriol 44; 1994: 579–582.

[9] Stackebrandt E., Schumann P., Schaal K.P., Weiss N. Propionimicrobium gen. nov., a new genus to accommodate *Propionibacterium lymphophilum* (Torrey 1916) Johnson and

Cummins 1972, 1057(AL) as *Propionimicrobium lymphophilum* comb. nov., Int J Syst Evol Microbio. 2002, 52: 1925–1927.

[10] Kusano K, Yamada, H., Niwa, M., Yamasato K. *Propionibacterium cyclohexanicum* sp. nov., a new acid-tolerant omega-cyclohexyl fatty acid-containing *Propionibacterium* isolated from spoiled orange juice. Int J Syst Bacteriol 1997; 47: 825-831.

[11] Koussemon M., Combet-Blanc Y., Patel B.K., Cayol J.L., Thomas P., et al. *Propionibacterium microaerophilum* sp. nov., a microaerophilic bacterium isolated from olive mill wastewater. Int J Syst Evol Microbiol 2001; 51: 1373-1382.

[12] Bernard K.S.L, Munroa C., Forbes-Faulknerb J.C., Pittb D., Nortonb J.H., Thomas A.D. *Propionibacterium australiense* sp. nov. Derived from Granulomatous Bovine Lesions. Taxonomy/Systematics 2002; 8: 41-47.

[13] Downes J., Wade, W.G. *Propionibacterium acidifaciens* sp. nov., isolated from the human mouth. Int J Syst Evol Microbiol 2009; 59: 2778-2781.

[14] Butler-Wu S.M., Sengupta D.J., Kittichotirat W., Matsen III F. A., Bumgarner R.E. Genome Sequence of a Novel Species, *Propionibacterium humerusii*. J Bacteriol 2011; 193(14): 3678.

[15] Mantere-Alhonen S., Ryhänen E.L. Lactobacilli and Propionibacteria in living food. M.A.N. 1994; 12: 399 -405.

[16] Rinta-Koski M., Montoten L., Mantere-Alhonen S. Propionibacteria isolated from rumen used as possible probiotics together with bifidobacteria. Milchwissenschaft 2001; 56(1): 11-13.

[17] Argañaraz Martínez E., Babot J.D., Zárate G., Apella M.C., Perez Chaia, A. Presencia de propionibacterias clásicas de potencial efecto probiótico en intestino de aves de consumo humano. Revista Chilena de Nutrición 2009; 36 (Suppl 1): 677.

[18] Macfarlane G.T., Allison C., Gibson S.A., Cummings J.H. Contribution of the microflora to proteolysis in the human large intestine. J Appl Bacteriol 1988; 64: 37-46.

[19] Zárate G., Lorenzo-Pisarello M.J., Babot J., Argañaraz-Martinez E., Pérez Chaia A. Dairy Propionibacteria: Technological importance and Probiotic Potential for Application on Human and Animal Nutrition. In: Rosana Filip (ed.). Multidisciplinary Approaches on Food Science and Nutrition for the XXI Century. Research Signpost, India; 2011. Chapter 10 p75-213.

[20] Malik A.C., Reinbold G.W., Vedamuthu E.R. An evaluation of the taxonomy of *Propionibacterium*. Can J Microbiol 1968; 14: 1185-1191.

[21] Thierry A., Madec M. N. Enumeration of propionibacteria in raw milk using a new selective medium. Lait 1995; 75: 315-323.

[22] Bujazha M., Perez Chaia A., Oliver G. Desarrollo de un medio de cultivo para el recuento de propionibacterias en contenido intestinal. Proc. of COMBHAL 98 VI Simp. Bras. Microbiol. Aliment. Sao Paulo, Brasil.1998; p. 45, B 4.3.

[23] Baer A. Identification and differentiation of propionibacteria by electrophoresis of their proteins. Milchwissenschaft 1987; 42: 431-433.

[24] Riedel K.H.J., Wingfield B.D., Britz T.J. Justification of the 'classical' *Propionibacterium* species concept by restriction analysis of the 16s ribosomal RNA genes. Syst Appl Microbiol 1994; 17: 536-542.

[25] Riedel K.H.J., Britz T.J. Justification of the 'classical' *Propionibacterium* species concept by ribotyping. Syst Appl Microbiol 1996; 19: 370-380.

[26] Rossi F., Sammartino M., Torriani S. 16S-23S Ribosomal spacer polymorphism in dairy propionibacteria. Biotechnol Tech 1997; 11:159–161.

[27] Gautier M., de Carvalho, A.F., Rouault A. DNA fingerprinting of dairy propionibacteria strains by pulsed-field gel electrophoresis. Curr Microbiol 1996; 32: 17-24.

[28] Rossi F., Torriani S., Dellaglio F. Identification and clustering of dairy propionibacteria by RAPD-PCR and CGE-REA methods. J Appl Microbiol 1998; 85: 956-964.

[29] Rossi F., Torriani S., Dellaglio F. Genus- and species-specific PCR-based detection of dairy propionibacteria in environmental samples by using primers targeted to the genes encoding 16S rRNA. Appl Environ Microbiol 1999; 65: 4241-4244.

[30] Poppert S., Riecker M., Essig A. Rapid identification of *Propionibacterium acnes* from blood cultures by fluorescence in situ hybridization. Diagn Microbiol Infect Dis 2010; 66: 214-216.

[31] Alexeyev O.A., Marklund I., Shannon B., Golovleva I., Olsson J., et al. Direct visualization of *Propionibacterium acnes* in prostate tissue by multicolor fluorescent in situ hybridization assay. J Clin Microbiol 2007; 45: 3721-3728.

[32] Babot J.D., Hidalgo M., Argañaraz-Martínez E., Apella M.C., Perez Chaia A. Fluorescence *in situ* hybridization for detection of classical propionibacteria with specific 16S rRNA-targeted probes and its application to enumeration in Gruyère cheese. Int J Food Microbiol 2011; 145 (1): 221-228.

[33] Lorenzo-Pisarello M.J., Gultemirian M.L., Nieto-Peñalver C., Perez Chaia A. *Propionibacterium acidipropionici* CRL 1198 influences the production of acids and the growth of bacterial genera stimulated by inulin in a murine model of cecal slurries. Anaerobe 2010; 16: 345-354.

[34] Hervé C., Fondrevez M., Cheron A., Barloy-Hubler F., Jan G. Transcarboxylase mRNA: a marker which evidences P. freudenreichii survival and metabolic activity during its transit in the human gut. Int J Food Microbiol 2007; 113: 303-314.

[35] Gautier M., Mouchel N., Rouault A., Sanseau P. Determination of genome size of four *Propionibacterium* species by pulsed-field gel electrophoresis. Lait 1992; 72: 421-446.

[36] Rehberger T.G., Glatz B.A. Characterization of *Propionibacterium* plasmids. Appl Environ Microbiol 1990; 56: 864-871.

[37] van Luijk N., Stierli M.P., Miescher Schwenninger S., Hervé C., et al. Review: Genetics and molecular biology of propionibacteria. Lait 2002; 82: 45-57.

[38] Gautier M., Rouault A., Hervé C., Sommer P., Leret V., et al. Bacteriophage of dairy propionibacteria. Lait 1999; 79: 93-104.

[39] Bruggemann H., Henne A., Hoster F., Liesegang H., Wiezer A., et al. The complete genome sequence of *Propionibacterium acnes*, a commensal of human skin. Science 2004; 305: 671–673.

[40] Falentin H., Deutsch S.M., Jan G., Loux V., Thierry A., et al. The complete genome of *Propionibacterium freudenreichii* CIRM-BIA1, a hardy actinobacterium with food and probiotic applications. PloS One 2010; 5, e11748.

[41] Hettinga D.H., Reinbold G.W. The propionic acid bacteria - a review. II. Metabolism. J Milk Food Technol 1972; 35: 358-372.

[42] Piveteau P. Metabolism of lactate and sugars by dairy propionibacteria: a review.Le Lait 1999; 79: 23–41.

[43] Thierry A. Deutsch S-M., Falentin H., Dalmasso M., Cousin F.J., Jan G. New insights into physiology and metabolism of *Propionibacterium freudenreichii*. Int J Food Microbiol 2011;149: 19-27.

[44] Crow V. Utilization of lactate isomers by *Propionibacterium freudenreichii subsp. shermanii*: regulatory role for intracellular pyruvate. Appl Environ Microbiol 1986; 52: 352-358.

[45] Peberdy M.F., Fryer T.F. Improved selective media for the enumeration of propionibacteria from cheese. N Z J Dairy Sci Technol 1976; 11: 10-15.

[46] Dupuis C., Corre C., Boyaval P. Proteinase activity of dairy *Propionibacterium*. Appl Microbiol Biotechnol 1995; 40: 750-755.

[47] Langsrud T., Serhauq T., Vegarud G.E. Protein degradation and amine acid metabolism by propionibacteria. Lait 1995; 75: 325-330.

[48] Leverrier P., Dimova D., Pichereau V., Auffray Y., Boyaval P., Jan G.L. Susceptibility and adaptive response to bile salts in *Propionibacterium freudenreichii*: physiological and proteomic analysis, Appl Environ Microbiol 2003; 69: 3809–3818.

[49] Leverrier P., Vissers J.P.C., Rouault A., Boyaval P., Jan G. Mass spectrometry proteomic analysis of stress adaptation reveals both common and distinct response pathways in *Propionibacterium freudenreichii*. Arch Microbiol 2004; 181: 215–230.

[50] Anastasiou R., Leverrier P., Krestas I., Rouault A., Kalantzopoulos G., et al. Changes in protein synthesis during thermal adaptation of *Propionibacterium freudenreichii subsp. shermanii*. Int J Food Microbiol 2006; 108: 301–314.

[51] Clark J.E., Beegen H., Wood H.G. Isolation of intact chains of polyphosphate from *Propionibacterium shermanii* grown on glucose or lactate. J Bacteriol 1986; 168: 1212–1219.

[52] Boyaval P., Deborde C., Corre C., Blanco C., Begue E. Stress and osmoprotection in propionibacteria. Lait 1999; 79: 59-69.

[53] Deborde C., Corre C., Rolin D.B., Nadal L., De Certaines J.D., et al. Trehalose biosynthesis in dairy *Propionibacterium*. J Magn Reson Analysis 1996; 2: 297–304

[54] Cardoso F.S., Gaspar P., Hugenholtz J., Ramos A., Santos H. Enhancement of trehalose production in dairy propionibacteria through manipulation of environmental conditions. Int J Food Microbiol 2004; 91: 195-204.

[55] Cardoso F.S., Castro R.F., Borges N., Santos H. Biochemical and genetic characterization of the pathways for trehalose metabolism in *Propionibacterium freudenreichii*, and their role in stress response. Microbiology 2007;153: 270–280.

[56] Langsrud T., Reinbold G.W. Flavour development and microbiology of Swiss cheese. A review. II Starters, manufacturing process and procedure. J Milk Food Technol 1973; 36: 531-542.

[57] Langsrud T., Reinbold G.W. Flavor development and microbiology of Swiss cheese. A review. III Ripening and flavor production. J Milk Food Technol 1973; 36: 593-609.

[58] Thierry A., Maillard M.B., Bonnarme P., Roussel E. The addition of *Propionibacterium freudenreichii* to Raclette cheese induces biochemical changes and enhances flavour development. J Agric Food Chem 2005 ; 53: 4157–4165.

[59] Thierry A., Maillard M.B., Richoux R., Kerjean J.R., Lortal S. *Propionibacterium freudenreichii* strains quantitatively affect production of volatile compounds in Swiss cheese. Lait 2005; 85: 57–74.

[60] Wyder M.T., Bosset J.O., Casey M.G., Isolini D., Sollberger H. Influence of two different propionibacterial cultures on the characteristics of Swiss-type cheese with regard to aspartate metabolism. Milchwissenschaft 2001; 56: 78–81.

[61] Thierry A., Maillard M.B. Production of cheese flavour compounds derived from amino acid catabolism by *Propionibacterium freudenreichii*. Lait 2002; 82: 17–32.

[62] Dherbécourt J., Maillard M.B., Catheline D., Thierry A. Production of branched chain aroma compounds by *Propionibacterium freudenreichii*: links with the biosynthesis of membrane fatty acids. J Appl Microbiol 2008; 105: 977–985.

[63] Dupuis C., Corre C., Boyaval P. Lipase and esterase of *Propionibacterium freudenreichii* subsp. *freudenreichii*. Appl Environ Microbiol 1993; 59: 4004-4009.

[64] Dherbécourt J., Falentin H., Jardin J., Maillard M.B., Baglinière F., et al. Identification of a secreted lipolytic esterase in *Propionibacterium freudenreichii*, a ripening process bacterium involved in Emmental cheese lipolysis. Appl Environ Microbiol 2010; 76: 1181–1188.

[65] Dherbécourt J., Falentin H., Canaan S., Thierry A. A genomic search approach to identify esterases in *Propionibacterium freudenreichii* involved in the formation of flavour in Emmental cheese. Microb Cell Fact 2008; 7: 16. doi: 10.1186/1475-2859-7-16

[66] Gagnaire V., Thierry A., Léonil J. Propionibacteria and facultatively heterofermentative lactobacilli weakly contribute to secondary proteolysis of Emmental cheese. Lait 2001; 81: 339–353.

[67] Falentin H., Postollec F., Parayre S., Henaff N., Le B.P., et al. Specific Metabolic Activity of Ripening Bacteria Quantified by Real-time Reverse Transcription PCR throughout Emmental Cheese Manufacture. Int J Food Microbiol 2010; 144: 10–19.

[68] Boyaval P., Corre C. Production of propionic acid. Lait 1995; 75: 453-461.

[69] Himmi E.H., Bories A., Boussaid A., Hassani L. Propionic acid fermentation of glycerol and glucose by *Propionibacterium acidipropionici* and *Propionibacterium freudenreichii* ssp. *shermanii*. Appl Microbiol Biotechnol 2000; 53: 435-440.

[70] Coral J., Karp S.G., Porto de Souza Vandenberghe L., Parada J.L., Pandey A., et al. Batch fermentation model of propionic acid production by *Propionibacterium acidipropionici* in different carbon sources. Appl Biochem Biotechnol 2008; 151: 333-341.

[71] Zhang A., Yang, S. Propionic acid production from glycerol by metabolically engineered *Propionibacterium acidipropionici*. Proc Biochem 2009; 44: 1346-1351.

[72] Liu L., Zhu Y., Li J., Wang M., Lee, P., et al. Microbial production of propionic acid from propionibacteria: Current state, challenges and perspectives Critical Reviews in Biotechnology 2012; 1 DOI: 10.3109/07388551.2011.651428.

[73] Al-Zoreky N., Ayres J.W., Sandine W.E. Antimicrobial activity of Microgard against food spoilage and pathogenic microorganisms. J Dairy Sci 1991; 74: 758-763.

[74] Suomalainen T.H., Mäyrä-Makinen A.M. Propionic acid bacteria as protective cultures in fermented milks and breads. Lait 1999; 79: 165-174.

[75] Florez-Galarza R.A., Glatz B., Bern C.J., Van Fossen L.D. Preservation of high-moisture corn by microbial fermentation. J Food Prot 1985; 48: 407-411.

[76] Holtug K., Clausen M.R., Hove N., Christiansen J., Mortensen P.B. The colon in carbohydrate malabsorption: Short Chain Fatty Acids, pH, and osmotic diarrhea. Scand J Gastroenterol 1992; 27: 545-552.

[77] Lan A., Bruneau A., Bensaada M., Philippe C., Bellaud P., et al. Increased induction of apoptosis by *Propionibacterium freudenreichii* TL133 in colonic mucosal crypts of human microbiota-associated rats treated with 1,2-dimethylhydrazine. Br J Nutr 2008; 100: 1251-1259.

[78] Hara H., Haga S., Aoyama Y., Kiriyama S. Short-chain fatty acids suppress cholesterol synthesis in rat liver and intestine. J Nutr 1999; 129: 942-948.

[79] Tagg J.R., Dajani A.S., Wannamaker L.W. Bacteriocins of gram-positive bacteria. Bacteriol Rev 1976; 40: 722-756.

[80] Gillor O., Etzion A., Riley M.A. The dual role of bacteriocins as anti- and probiotics. Appl Microbiol Biotechnol 2008; 81: 591-606.

[81] Lyon W.J., Sethi J.K., Glatz B.A. Inhibition of psychrotrophic organisms by propionicin PLG-1, a bacteriocin produced by *Propionibacterium thoenii*. J Dairy Sci 1993; 76: 1506-1513.

[82] Grinstead D.A., Barefoot S.F. Jenseniin G, a heat-stable bacteriocin produced by *Propionibacterium jensenii* P126. Appl Environ Microbiol 1992; 58: 215-220.

[83] Miescher S., Stierli M.P., Teuber M., Meile L. Propionicin SM1, a bacteriocin from *Propionibacterium jensenii* DF1: isolation and characterization of the protein and its gene. Syst Appl Microbiol 2000; 23: 174-184.

[84] Faye T., Langsrud T., Nes I.F., Holo H. Biochemical and genetic characterization of propionicin T1, a new bacteriocin from *Propionibacterium thoenii*. Appl Environ Microbiol 2000; 66: 4230-4236.

[85] Van der Merwe I.R., Bauer R., Britz T.J., Dicks L.M. Characterization of thoeniicin 447, a bacteriocin isolated from *Propionibacterium thoenii* strain 447. Int J Food Microbiol 2004; 92: 153-160.

[86] Paul G.E., Booth S.J. Properties and characteristics of a bacteriocin-like substance produced by *Propionibacterium acnes* isolated from dental plaque. Can J Microbiol 1988; 34: 1344-1347.

[87] Ratnam P., Barefoot S.F., Prince I.U., Bodine A.B. McCaskill L.H. Partial purification of the bacteriocin produced by *Propionibacterium jensenii* B1264. Lait 1999; 79: 125-136.

[88] Brede D.A., Faye T., Johnsborg O., Odegard I., Nes I.F., et al. Molecular and genetic characterization of propionicin F, a bacteriocin from *Propionibacterium freudenreichii*. Appl Environ Microbiol 2004; 70: 7303-7310.

[89] Gwiazdowska D., Trojanowska K. Antimicrobial activity and stability of partially purified bacteriocins produced by *Propionibacterium freudenreichii* ssp. *freudenreichii* and ssp. *shermanii*. Lait 2006; 86: 141-154.

[90] Ekinci F.Y., Barefoot S.F. Fed-batch enhancement of jenseniin G, a bacteriocin produced by *Propionibacterium thoenii* (jensenii) P126. Food Microbiol 2006; 23: 325-330.

[91] Ramanathan S., Wolynec C., Cutting W. Antiviral principles of Propionibacteria-isolation and activity of propionins B and C. Proc Soc Exp Biol Med 1968; 129: 73-77.

[92] Faye T., Brede D.A., Langsrud T., Nes I.F., Holo H. An antimicrobial peptide is produced by extracellular processing of a protein from *Propionibacterium jensenii*. J Bacteriol 2002; 184: 3649-3656.

[93] Lind H., Sjogren J., Gohil S., Kenne L., Schnurer J., Broberg A. Antifungal compounds from cultures of dairy propionibacteria type strains. FEMS Microbiol Lett 2007; 271: 310–315.

[94] Benjamin S., Spener F. Conjugated linoleic acids as functional food: an insight into their health benefits. Nutr Metab 2009; 6: 36.
http://www.nutritionandmetabolism.com/content/6/1/36

[95] Sieber R., Collomb M., Aeschlimann A., Jelen P., Eyer H. Impact of microbial cultures on conjugated linoleic acid in dairy products. Int Dairy J 2004; 14: 1-15.

[96] Rainio A., Vahvaselkä M., Suomalainen T., Laakso S. Production of conjugated linoleic acid by *Propionibacterium*. Lait 8 2002; 2: 91-101.

[97] Wang L.M. Lv J.P., Chu Z.Q., Cui Y.Y., Ren X.H. Production of conjugated linoleic acid by *Propionibacterium freudenreichii*. Food Chem 2007; 103: 313-318.

[98] McIntosh F.M., Shingfield K.J., Devillard E., Russell W.R., Wallace R.J. Mechanism of conjugated linoleic acid and vaccenic acid formation in human faecal suspensions and pure cultures of intestinal bacteria. Microbiology 2009; 155: 285-294.

[99] Vahvaselka M., Laakso S. Production of cis-9,trans-11-conjugated linoleic acid in camelina meal and okara by an oat-assisted microbial process. J Agric Food Chem 2010; 58: 2479-2482.

[100] Xu S., Boylston T.D., Glatz B.A. Conjugated linoleic acid content and organoleptic attributes of fermented milk products produced with probiotic bacteria. J Agric Food Chem 2005; 53: 9064-9072.

[101] Xu S., Boylston T.D., Glatz B.A. Effect of lipid source on probiotic bacteria and conjugated linoleic acid formation in milk model systems. J Am Oil Chem 2004; 81: 589-595.

[102] Murooka Y., Piao Y., Kiatpapan P., Yamashita M. Production of tetrapyrrole compounds and vitamin B12 using genetically engineering of *Propionibacterium freudenreichii* An overview. Le Lait 2005; 85: 9–22.

[103] Piao Y., Yamashita M., Kawaraichi N., Asegawa R., Ono H., Murooka Y. Production of vitamin B12 in genetically engineered *Propionibacterium freudenreichii*. J Biosci Bioeng 2004;.98: 167–173.

[104] Ye K., Shijo M., Jin S., Shimizu K. Efficient production of vitamin B12 from propionic acid bacteria under periodic variation of dissolved oxygen concentration J Ferment Bioeng 1996; 82: 484-491.

[105] Hunik J.H Improved process for the production of vitamin B12. 2000; Patent WO00/37669.

[106] LeBlanc J.G., Rutten G., Bruinenberg P., Sesma F., de Giori G.S., et al. A novel dairy product fermented with *Propionibacterium freudenreichii* improves the riboflavin status of deficient rats. Nutrition 2006; 22: 645-651.

[107] Burgess C.M., Smid E.J., Van Sinderen D. Bacterial vitamin B2, B11 and B12 overproduction: an overview. Int J Food Microbiol 2009; 133: 1–7.

[108] Piao Y., Kiatpapan P., Yamashita M., Murooka Y. Effects of expression of hemA and hemB genes on production of porphyrin in *Propionibacterium freudenreichii*. Appl Microbiol Biotechnol 2004; 70: 7561–7566.

[109] Shearer M.J. Vitamin K and vitamin K-dependent proteins. Br J Haematol 1990; 75: 156-162.

[110] Mori H., Sato Y., Taketomo N., Kamiyama T., Yoshiyama Y., et al. Isolation and structural identification of bifidogenic growth stimulator produced by *Propionibacterium freudenreichii*. J Dairy Sci 1997; 80: 1959-1964.

[111] Isawa K., Hojo K., Yoda N., Kamiyama T., Makino S., et al. Isolation and identification of a new bifidogenic growth stimulator produced by *Propionibacterium freudenreichii* ET-3. Biosci Biotechnol Biochem 2002; 66: 679-681.

[112] Furuichi K., Hojo K., Katakura Y., Ninomiya K., Shioya S. Aerobic culture of *Propionibacterium freudenreichii* ET-3 can increase production ratio of 1,4-dihydroxy-2-naphthoic acid to menaquinone. J Biosci Bioeng 2006; 101: 464-470.

[113] Furuichi K., Katakura Y., Ninomiya K., Shioya S. Enhancement of 1,4-dihydroxy-2-naphthoic acid production by *Propionibacterium freudenreichii* ET-3 fed-batch culture. Appl Environ Microbiol 2007; 73: 3137-3143.

[114] Hojo K., Watanabe R., Mori T., Taketomo N. Quantitative measurement of tetrahydromenaquinone-9 in cheese fermented by propionibacteria. J Dairy Sci 2007; 90: 4078-4083.

[115] Badel S., Bernardi T., Michaud P. New perspectives for Lactobacilli exopolysaccharides. Biotechnol Adv 2011; 29(1): 54-66.

[116] Deutsch S.M., Le Bivic P., Herve C., Madec M.N., LaPointe G., Jan G., Le Loir Y., Falentin H. Correlation of the capsular phenotype in *Propionibacterium freudenreichii* with the level of expression of gtf, a unique polysaccharide synthase encoding gene. Appl Environ Microbiol 2010 ;76: 2740–2746.

[117] Nordmark E.L., Yang Z., Huttunen E., Widmalm G. Structural studies of the exopolysaccharide produced by *Propionibacterium freudenreichii* ssp. *shermanii* JS. Biomacromolecules 2005; 6: 521-523.

[118] Dobruchowskaa J.M., Gerwig G.J., Babuchowski A., Kamerling J.P. Structural studies on exopolysaccharides produced by three different propionibacteria strains. Carbohydrate Research 2007; 343: 726-745.

[119] Racine M., Dumont J., Champagne C.P., Morin A. Production and characterization of the exopolysaccharide from *Propionibacterium acidipropionici* on whey-based media. J Appl Bacteriol 1991; 71:233-238

[120] Gorret N., Maubois J.L., Engasser J.M., Ghoul M. Study of the effects of temperature, pH and yeast extract on growth and exopolysaccharides production by *Propionibacterium acidipropionici* on milk microfiltrate using a response surface methodology. J Appl Microbiol 2001; 90: 788-796.

[121] FAO/WHO (2002) Guidelines for the Evaluation of Probiotics in Food. Food and Agriculture Organization of the United Nations - World Health Organization. London, Ontario.

[122] Meile L., Le Blay G., Thierry A. Safety assessment of dairy microorganisms: *Propionibacterium* and *Bifidobacterium*. Int J Food Microbiol 2008; 126: 316-320.

[123] Cousin F., Mater D.D.G., Foligné B., Jan G. Dairy propionibacteria as human probiotics: a review of recent evidence. Dairy Sci Technol 2010. doi:10.1051/dst/2010032.

[124] Perez Chaia A., Nader de Macias M.E., Oliver G. Propionibacteria in the gut: effect on some metabolic activities of the host. Lait 1995; 75: 435-445.

[125] Huang Y., Kotula L., Adams M.C. The in vivo assessment of safety and gastrointestinal survival of an orally administered novel probiotic, *Propionibacterium jensenii* 702, in a male Wistar rat model. Food Chem Toxicol 2003; 41: 1781-1787.

[126] Lan A., Bruneau A., Philippe C., Rochet V., Rouault A., et al. Survival and metabolic activity of selected strains of *Propionibacterium freudenreichii* in the gastrointestinal tract of human microbiota-associated rats. Br J Nutr 2007; 97: 714-724.

[127] Bougle D., Roland N., Lebeurrier F., Arhan P. Effect of propionibacteria supplementation on fecal bifidobacteria and segmental colonic transit time in healthy human subjects. Scand J Gastroenterol 1999; 34: 144-148.

[128] EFSA, 2009. Scientific opinion of the panel on biological hazards on the maintenance of the list of QPS microorganisms intentionally added to food or feed. The EFSA Journal 2009; 7: 1–93.

[129] Funke G., von Graevenitz A., Clarridge J.E.3rd., Bernard K.A. Clinical microbiology of coryneform bacteria. Clin Microbiol Rev 1997; 10: 125-159.

[130] Suomalainen T., Sigvart-Mattila P., Matto J., Tynkkynen S. In vitro and in vivo gastrointestinal survival, antibiotic susceptibility and genetic identification of *Propionibacterium freudenreichii* ssp. shermanii JS. Int Dairy J 2008; 18: 271–278.

[131] Zárate G., González S., Pérez-Chaia A., Oliver G. Effect of bile on the β-galactosidase activity of dairy propionibacteria. Lait 2000; 80: 267-276.

[132] Zarate G., Chaia A.P., Gonzalez S., Oliver G. Viability and beta-galactosidase activity of dairy propionibacteria subjected to digestion by artificial gastric and intestinal fluids. J Food Prot 2000; 63: 1214-1221.

[133] Jan G., Leverrier P., Proudy I. Survival and beneficial effects of propionibacteria in the human gut: in vivo and in vitro investigations. Lait 2002; 82: 131-144.

[134] Huang Y., Adams M.C. In vitro assessment of the upper gastrointestinal tolerance of potential probiotic dairy propionibacteria. Int J Food Microbiol 2004; 91: 253-260.

[135] Jan G., Leverrier P., Pichereau V., Boyaval P. Changes in protein synthesis and morphology during acid adaptation of *Propionibacterium freudenreichii*, Appl. Environ. Microbiol. 67 (2001) 2029–2036.

[136] Leverrier P., Fremont Y., Rouault A., Boyaval P., Jan G. In vitro tolerance to digestive stresses of propionibacteria: influence of food matrices. Food Microbiol 2005; 22: 11-18.

[137] Perez Chaia A., Zárate G. Dairy propionibacteria from milk or cheese diets remain viable and enhance propionic acid production in the mouse cecum. Lait 2005; 85: 85-98.

[138] Havenaar R., Ten-Brink B., Huis in't Velt J.H. Selection of strains for probiotic use. In: Fuller R. (ed.). Probiotics: The Scientific Basis. London: Chapman & Hall. 1992.

[139] Thiel A., Eikmanns B., Salminen S., Ouwehand A.C. In vitro adhesion of propionibacteria to human intestinal mucus. Ital J Food Sci 2004; 16: 245-254.

[140] Zarate G., Morata de Ambrosini V.I., Pérez Chaia A., Gonzalez S.N. Adhesion of dairy propionibacteria to intestinal epithelial tissue in vitro and in vivo. J Food Prot 2002; 65: 534-539.

[141] Zarate G., Morata De Ambrosini V., Perez Chaia A., Gonzalez S. Some factors affecting the adherence of probiotic *Propionibacterium acidipropionici* CRL 1198 to intestinal epithelial cells. Can J Microbiol 2002; 48: 449-457.

[142] Lehto E.M., Salminen S. Adhesion of two *Lactobacillus* strains, one *Lactococcus* and one *Propionibacterium* strain to cultured human intestinal Caco-2 cell line. Biosci Microflora 1997; 16: 13-17.

[143] Huang Y., Adams M.C. An in vitro model for investigating intestinal adhesion of potential dairy propionibacteria probiotic strains using cell line C2BBe1. Lett Appl Microbiol 2003; 36: 213-216.

[144] Zárate G.; Villena J.; Zúñiga-Hansen M. E., Pérez-Chaia A. Inhibition of adhesion of enteropathogens to human enterocyte-like HT29 cell line by a dairy strain of *Propionibacterium acidipropionici*. 3rd International Symposium on Propionibacteria and Bifidobacteria: Dairy and Probiotic Applications, Oviedo, España. 2010.

[145] Zárate G., Perez Chaia A. Feeding with dairy *Propionibacterium acidipropionici* CRL 1198 reduces the incidence of Concanavalin-A induced alterations in mouse small intestinal epithelium. Food Res Int 2012; 47(1): 3-22.

[146] Mountzouris K.C., Tsirtsikos P., Kalamara E., Nitsch S., Schatzmayr G., et al. Evaluation of the efficacy of a probiotic containing *Lactobacillus*, *Bifidobacterium*, *Enterococcus*, and *Pediococcus* strains in promoting broiler performance and modulating cecal microflora composition and metabolic activities. Poult Sci 2007; 86: 309-317.

[147] Waters S.M., Murphy R.A., Power R.F. Characterisation of prototype Nurmi cultures using culture-based microbiological techniques and PCR-DGGE. Int J Food Microbiol 2006; 110: 268-277.

[148] Mantere Alhonen S. Propionibacteria used as probiotics. A review. Lait 1995; 75: 447 - 452.

[149] Cerna B., Cerny M., Betkova H., Patricny P., Soch M., Opatrna I. Effect of the Proma probiotics on calves. From Dairy Sci Abstr 1991; 55: 1735.

[150] Adams M., Luo J., Rayward D., King S., Gibson R., et al. Selection of a novel direct-fed microbial to enhance weight gain in intensively reared calves. Anim Feed SciTechnol 2007; 145: 41-52.

[151] Kim S.W., Standorf D.G., Roman-Rosario H., Yokoyama M.T., Rust S. R. Potential use of *Propionibacterium acidipropionici*, strain DH42 as a direct-fed microbial for cattle. J. Dairy Sci. 2000; 83(Suppl. 1):292 (Abstr.).

[152] Stein D.R., Allen D.T., Perry E.B., Bruner J.C., Gates K.W., et al. Effects of feeding propionibacteria to dairy cows on milk yield, milk components, and reproduction. J Dairy Sci 2006; 89: 111-125.

[153] Francisco C.C., Chamberlain C.S., Waldner D.N., Wettemann R.P., Spicer L.J. Propionibacteria fed to dairy cows: effects on energy balance, plasma metabolites and hormones, and reproduction. J Dairy Sci 2002; 85: 1738-1751.

[154] Weiss W. P., Wyatt D.J.,. McKelvey T.R. Effect of Feeding Propionibacteria on Milk Production by Early Lactation Dairy Cows. J Dairy Sci 2008; 91: 646–652. doi:10.3168/jds.2007-0693.

[155] Boyd J., West J.W., Bernard J.K. Effects of the addition of direct-fed microbials and glycerol to the diet of lactating dairy cows on milk yield and apparent efficiency of yield.J Dairy Sci 2011; 94(9):4616-4622.

[156] Markowska-Daniel I., Pejsak Z., Szmigielski S., Jeljaszewicz J., Pulverer G. Stimulation of granulopoiesis in pregnant swine and their offspring by *Propionibacterium avidum* KP-40. Br Vet J 1992; 148(2):133-145.

[157] Markowska-Daniel I., Pejsak Z., Szmigielski S., Jeljaszewicz J., Pulverer G. Prophylactic application of *Propionibacterium avidum* KP-40 in swine with acute experimental infections. II. Bacterial infections: pleuropneumonia and swine erysipelas. Dtsch Tierarztl Wochenschr 1993;100(5):185-188.

[158] Lo D.Y., Hung C.N., Lee W.C., Liao J.W., Blacklaws B.A., et al. Effect of immunostimulation by detoxified *E. coli* lipopolysaccharide combined with inactivated *Propionibacterium granulosum* cells on porcine immunity. J Vet Med Sci 2009; 71(7):897-903.

[159] Khan M, Raoult D, Richet H, Lepidi H, La Scola B Growth-promoting effects of single-dose intragastrically administered probiotics in chickens. Br Poult Sci 2007; 48: 732-735.

[160] Higgins S.E., Higgins J.P., Wolfenden A.D., Henderson S.N., Torres-Rodriguez A., et al. Evaluation of a *Lactobacillus*-based probiotic culture for the reduction of *Salmonella enteritidis* in neonatal broiler chicks. Poult Sci 2008; 87: 27-31.

[161] Salanitro J.P., Blake I.G., Muirehead P.A., Maglio M., Goodman J.R. Bacteria isolated from the duodenum, ileum, and cecum of young chicks. Appl Environ Microbiol 1978; 35: 782-790.

[162] Roszkowski W., Roszkowski K., Ko H.L., Beuth J., Jeljaszewicz J. Immunomodulation by propionibacteria. Zentralbl Bakteriol 1990; 274: 289-298.

[163] Mara M., Julak J., Bednar M., Ocenaskova J., Mikova Z., et al. The influence of *Propionibacterium acnes* (*Corynebacterium parvum*) fractions on immune response in vivo. Zentralbl Bakteriol 1994; 281: 549-555.

[164] Isenberg J., Ko H., Pulverer G., Grundmann R., Stutzer H., et al. Preoperative immunostimulation by *Propionibacterium granulosum* KP-45 in colorectal cancer. Anticancer Res 1994; 14: 1399-1404

[165] Isenberg J., Stoffel B., Wolters U., Beuth J., Stutzer H., et al. Immunostimulation by propionibacteria--effects on immune status and antineoplastic treatment. Anticancer Res 1995; 15: 2363-2368.

[166] Ananias R.Z., Rodrigues E.G., Braga E.G., Squaiella C.C., Mussalem J.S., et al. Modulatory effect of killed *Propionibacterium acnes* and its purified soluble polysaccharide on peritoneal exudate cells from C57Bl/6 mice: major NKT cell recruitment and increased cytotoxicity. Scand J Immunol 2007; 65: 538-548.

[167] Mussalem J.S., Vasconcelos J.R., Squaiella C.C., Ananias R.Z., Braga E.G, et al. Adjuvant effect of the *Propionibacterium acnes* and its purified soluble polysaccharide

on the immunization with plasmidial DNA containing a *Trypanosoma cruzi* gene. Microbiol Immunol 2006; 50: 253-263.

[168] Kirjavainen P.V., El Nezami H.S., Salminen S.J., Ahokas J.T., Wright P.F. Effects of orally administered viable *Lactobacillus rhamnosus* GG and *Propionibacterium freudenreichii* subsp. shermanii JS on mouse lymphocyte proliferation. Clin Diagn Lab Immunol 1999; 6: 799-802.

[169] Kekkonen R.A., Kajasto E., Miettinen M., Veckman V., Korpela R., et al. Probiotic *Leuconostoc mesenteroides* ssp. cremoris and *Streptococcus thermophilus* induce IL-12 and IFN-gamma production. World J Gastroenterol 2008; 14: 1192-1203.

[170] Myllyluoma E., Ahonen A.M., Korpela R., Vapaatalo H., Kankuri E. Effects of multispecies probiotic combination on *helicobacter pylori* infection in vitro. Clin Vaccine Immunol 2008; 15: 1472-1482.

[171] Foligné B., Deutsch S.M., Breton J., Cousin F., Dewulf J., et al. Promising immunomodulatory effects of selected strains of dairy propionibacteria evidenced *in vitro* and *in vivo*. Appl Environ Microbiol 2010; 76(24): 8259-8264.

[172] Kekkonen R.A., Lummela N., Karjalainen H., Latvala S., Tynkkynen S., et al. Probiotic intervention has strain-specific anti-inflammatory effects in healthy adults, World J Gastroenterol 2008; 14: 2029–2036.

[173] Pohjavuori E., Viljanen M., Korpela R., Kuitunen M., Tiittanen M., et al. *Lactobacillus* GG effect in increasing IFN-gamma production in infants with cow's milk allergy. J Allergy Clin Immunol 2004; 114:131–136.

[174] Kukkonen K., Savilahti E., Haahtela T., Juntunen-Backman K., Korpela R., et al. Probiotics and prebiotic galacto-oligosaccharides in the prevention of allergic diseases: a randomized, double-blind, placebo-controlled trial, J Allergy Clin Immunol 2007; 119: 192–198.

[175] Kukkonen K., Savilahti E., Haahtela T., Juntunen-Backman K., Korpela R., et al. Long-term safety and impact on infection rates of postnatal probiotic and prebiotic (synbiotic) treatment: randomized, double-blind, placebo-controlled trial. Pediatrics 2008; 122: 8–12

[176] Alvarez S., Medici M., Vintini E., Oliver G., de Ruiz Holgado A.P., Perdigon G. Effect of the oral administration of *Propionibacterium* IgA levels and on the prevention of enteric infection in mice. Microbiol Alim Nutr 1996; 14: 237–243.

[177] Adams M.C., Lean M.L., Hitchick N.C., Beagley K.W. The efficacy of *Propionibacterium jensenii* 702 to stimulate a cell-mediated response to orally administered soluble *Mycobacterium tuberculosis* antigens using a mouse model. Lait 2005; 85: 75-84.

[178] Kaneko T. A novel bifidogenic growth stimulator produced by *Propionibacterium freudenreichii*. Biosci Microflora 1999; 18: 73-80.

[179] Warminska-Radyko I., Laniewska-Moroz L., Babuchowski A. Possibilities for stimulation of *Bifidobacterium* growth by propionibacteria. Lait 2002; 82: 113-121.

[180] Roland N, Bougle D., Lebeurrier F., Arhan P., Maubois J. *Propionibacterium freudenreichii* stimulates the growth of *Bifidobacterium bifidum* in vitro and increases fecal bifidobacteria in healthy human volunteers. Int Dairy J 1998; 8: 587-588.

[181] Satomi K., Kurihara H., Isawa K., Mori H., Kaneco T. Effects of culture-powder of *Propionibacterium freudenreichii* ET-3 on fecal microflora of normal adults. Biosci Biotechnol Biochem 1999; 18: 27–30.

[182] Hojo K., Yoda N., Tsuchita H., Ohtsu T., Seki K., et al. Effect of ingested culture of *Propionibacterium freudenreichii* ET-3 on fecal microflora and stool frequency in healthy females. Biosci Microflora 2002; 21: 115–120.

[183] Yamazaki S., Kano K., Ikeda T., Isawa K., Kaneko T. Role of 2-amino-3-carboxy-1,4-naphthoquinone, a strong growth stimulator for bifidobacteria, as an electron transfer mediator for NAD(P)(+) regeneration in *Bifidobacterium longum*. Biochim Biophys Acta-General Subjects 1999; 1428: 241–250.

[184] Seki K., Nakao H., Umino H., Isshiki H., Yoda N., et al. Effects of fermented milk whey containing novel bifidogenic growth stimulator produced by *Propionibacterium* on fecal bacteria, putrefactive metabolite, defecation frequency and fecal properties in senile volunteers needed serious nursing-care taking enteral nutrition by tube feeding, properties in senile volunteers needed serious nursing-care taking enteral nutrition by tube feeding. J Intestinal Microbiol 2004; 18: 107-115.

[185] Collado M.C., Meriluoto J., Salminen S. In vitro analysis of probiotic strain combinations to inhibit pathogen adhesion to human intestinal mucus. Food Res Int 2007; 40: 629-636.

[186] Hatakka K., Ahola A.J., Yli-Knuuttila H., Richardson M., Poussa T., et al. Probiotics reduce the prevalence of oral candida in the elderly--a randomized controlled trial. J Dent Res 2007; 86: 125-130.

[187] Myllyluoma E., Kajander K., Mikkola H., Kyronpalo S., Rasmussen M., et al. Probiotic intervention decreases serum gastrin-17 in *Helicobacter pylori* infection. Dig Liver Dis 2007; 39: 516-523.

[188] Sarkar S., Misra A.K. Effect of feeding Propiono-Acido-Bifido (PAB) milk on the nutritional status and excretory pattern in rats and children. Milchwissenschaft 1998; 53: 666–668.

[189] Sidorchuk I., Bondarenko, V.M. Selection of a biologically active mutant of *Propionibacterium shermanii* and the possibility of its use in complex therapy of enteral dysbacteriosis. J Hyg Epidemiol Microbiol Immunol 1984; 28: 331-338.

[190] Okada Y., Tsuzuki Y., Miyazaki J., Matsuzaki K., Hokari R., et al. *Propionibacterium freudenreichii* component 1.4-dihydroxy-2-naphthoic acid (DHNA) attenuates dextran sodium sulphate induced colitis by modulation of bacterial flora and lymphocyte homing. Gut 2006; 55: 681-688.

[191] Suzuki A., Mitsuyama K., Koga H., Tomiyasu N., Masuda J., et al. Bifidogenic growth stimulator for the treatment of active ulcerative colitis: a pilot study. Nutrition 2006; 22: 76-81.

[192] Uchida M, Mogami O. Milk whey culture with *Propionibacterium freudenreichii* ET-3 is effective on the colitis induced by 2,4,6- trinitrobenzene sulfonic acid in rats. J Pharmacol Sci 2005; 99(4): 329-34.

[193] Mitsuyama K., Masuda J., Yamasaki H., Kuwaki K., Kitazaki S., et al. Treatment of ulcerative colitis with milk whey culture with *Propionibacterium freudenreichii*. J Intestinal Microbiol 2007; 21: 143-147.

[194] Michel C., Roland N., Lecannu G., Herve C., Avice J.C., et al. Colonic infusion with *Propionibacterium acidipropionici* reduces severity of chemically induced colitis in rats. Lait 2005; 85: 99-111.

[195] Kajander K., Myllyluoma E., Rajilic-Stojanovic M., Kyronpalo S., Rasmussen M., et al. Clinical trial: multispecies probiotic supplementation alleviates the symptoms of irritable bowel syndrome and stabilizes intestinal microbiota. Aliment Pharmacol Ther 2008; 27: 48-57.

[196] Sherman P.M. Probiotics and lactose maldigestion. Can J Gastroenterol 2004; 18: 81-82.

[197] Zarate G., Perez Chaia A. Oliver G. Some Characteristics of Practical Relevance of the b-Galactosidase from Potential Probiotic Strains of *Propionibacterium acidipropionici*. Anaerobe 2002; 8: 259-267.

[198] Somkuti G.A., Johnson T.L. Cholesterol uptake by *Propionibacterium freudenreichii*. Curr Microbiol 1990; 20: 305-309.

[199] Vorobjeva L.I., Khodjaev E.Y., Vorobjeva, N.V. Propionic acid bacteria as probiotics. Microb Ecol Health Dis 2008; 20: 109-112.

[200] Commane D., Hughes R., Shortt C., Rowland I. The potential mechanisms involved in the anti-carcinogenic action of probiotics. Mutat Res 2005; 591: 276-289.

[201] Perez Chaia A., Zárate G., Oliver G. The probiotic properties of propionibacteria. Lait 1999; 79: 175-185.

[202] Ouwehand A.C., Lagstrom H., Suomalainen T., Salminen S. Effect of probiotics on constipation, fecal azoreductase activity and fecal mucin content in the elderly. Ann Nutr Metab 2002; 46: 159-162.

[203] Hatakka K., Holma R., El-Nezami H., Suomalainen T., Kuisma M., et al. The influence of *Lactobacillus rhamnosus* LC705 together with *Propionibacterium freudenreichii* ssp. *shermanii* JS on potentially carcinogenic bacterial activity in human colon. Int J Food Microbiol 2008; 128: 406-410.

[204] Jan G., Belzacq A.S., Haouzi D., Rouault A., Metivier D., et al. Propionibacteria induce apoptosis of colorectal carcinoma cells via short-chain fatty acids acting on mitochondria. Cell Death Differ 2002; 9: 179-188.

[205] Lan A., Lagadic-Gossmann D., Lemaire C., Brenner C., Jan G. Acidic extracellular pH shifts colorectal cancer cell death from apoptosis to necrosis upon exposure to propionate and acetate, major end-products of the human probiotic propionibacteria. Apoptosis 2007; 12: 573-591.

[206] Orrhage K., Sillerstrom E., Gustafsson J., Nord C.E., Rafter J. Binding of mutagenic heterocyclic amines by intestinal and lactic acid bacteria. Mutat Res 1994; 311: 239-248.

[207] Knasmüller S., Steinkellner H., Hirschl A.M., Rabot S., Nobis E.C., Kassie F. Impact of bacteria in dairy products and of the intestinal microflora on the genotoxic and carcinogenic effects of heterocyclic aromatic amines. Mutat Res 2001; 480–481:129–138.

[208] Nowak A., Libudzisz Z. Ability of probiotic *Lactobacillus casei* DN 114001 to bind or/and metabolise heterocyclic aromatic amines in vitro. Eur J Nutr 2009; 48(7):419-27.

[209] Sreekumar O., Hosono A. The heterocyclic amine binding receptors of *Lactobacillus gasseri* cells, Mutat Res 1998; 421: 65–72.

[210] El-Nezami H.S., Chrevatidis A., Auriola S., Salminen S., Mykkanen H. Removal of common *Fusarium* toxins in vitro by strains of *Lactobacillus* and *Propionibacterium*. Food Addit Contam 2002; 19: 680-686.

[211] Gratz S., Mykkanen H., El-Nezami H. Aflatoxin B1 binding by a mixture of *Lactobacillus* and *Propionibacterium*: in vitro versus ex vivo. J Food Prot 2005; 68: 2470-2474.

[212] Niderkorn V., Boudra H., Morgavi D.P. Binding of *Fusarium* mycotoxins by fermentative bacteria in vitro. J Appl Microbiol 2006; 101: 849-856.

[213] El-Nezami H., Mykkanen H., Kankaanpaa P., Suomalainen T., Salminen S., Ahokas J. Ability of a mixture of *Lactobacillus* and *Propionibacterium* to influence the faecal aflatoxin content in healthy Egyptian volunteers:a pilot clinical study. Biosci Microflora 2000; 19: 41-45.

[214] El-Nezami H.S., Polychronaki N.N., Ma J., Zhu H., Ling W., et al. Probiotic supplementation reduces a biomarker for increased risk of liver cancer in young men from Southern China. Am J Clin Nutr 2006; 83: 1199-1203.

[215] Lee Y.K., El-Nezami H., Haskard C.A., Gratz S., Puong K.Y., et al. Kinetics of adsorption and desorption of aflatoxin B1 by viable and nonviable bacteria. J Food Prot 2003; 66: 426-430.

[216] Gratz S., Mykkanen H., Ouwehand A. C., Juvonen R., Salminen S., El-Nezami H. Intestinal mucus alters the ability of probiotic bacteria to bind aflatoxin B1 in vitro. Appl Environ Microbiol 2004; 70: 6306–6308.

[217] Haskard C., Binnion C., Ahokas J. Factors affecting the sequestration of aflatoxin by *Lactobacillus rhamnosus* strain GG. Chem Biol Interact 2000; 128:39–49.

[218] Tuomola E.M., Ouwehand A. C., Salminen S.J. Chemical, physical and enzymatic pretreatments of probiotic lactobacilli alter their adhesion to human intestinal mucus glycoproteins. Int. J Food Microbiol 2000; 60: 75–81.

[219] Halttunen T., Collado M.C., El-Nezami H., Meriluoto J., Salminen S. Combining strains of lactic acid bacteria may reduce their toxin and heavy metal removal efficiency from aqueous solution. Lett Appl Microbiol 2008; 46: 160-165.

[220] Ibrahim F., Halttunen T., Tahvonen R., Salminen S. Probiotic bacteria as potential detoxification tools: assessing their heavy metal binding isotherms. Can J Microbiol 2006; 52: 877-885.

[221] Sharon N., Lis H. Lectins-proteins with a sweet tooth: functions in cell recognition. Essays Biochem 1995; 30: 59-75.

[222] De Mejía E.G., Prisecaru V.I. Lectins as bioactive plant proteins: a potential in cancer treatment. Crit Rev Food Sci Nutr 2005; 45(6): 425-445.

[223] Vasconcelos I.M., Oliveira J.T. Antinutritional properties of plant lectins. Toxicon 2004; 44(4): 385-403.

[224] Nachbar M.S., Oppenheim J.D. Lectins in the United States diet: a survey of lectins in commonly consumed foods and a review of the literature. Am J Clin Nutr 1980; 33(11): 2338-2345.

[225] Lorenzsonn V., Olsen W.A. In vivo responses of rat intestinal epithelium to intraluminal dietary lectins. Gastroenterology 1982; 82(5): 838-848.

[226] Ayyagari R., Raghunath M., Rao B.S. Early effects and the possible mechanism of the effect of Concanavalin A (con A) and *Phaseolus vulgaris* lectin (PHA-P) on intestinal absorption of calcium and sucrose. Plant Foods Hum Nutr 1993; 43(1): 63-70.

[227] Ryder S.D., Smith J.A., Rhodes E.G., Parker N., Rhodes J.M. Proliferative responses of HT29 and Caco2 human colorectal cancer cells to a panel of lectins. Gastroenterology 1994; 106(1): 85-93.

[228] Kiss R., Camby I., Duckworth C., De Decker R., Salmon I., et al. In vitro influence of *Phaseolus vulgaris*, *Griffonia simplicifolia*, concanavalin A, wheat germ, and peanut agglutinins on HCT-15, LoVo, and SW837 human colorectal cancer cell growth. Gut 1997; 40(2): 253-261.

[229] Ryder S.D., Jacyna M.R., Levi A.J., Rizzi P.M., Rhodes J.M. Peanut ingestion increases rectal proliferation in individuals with mucosal expression of peanut lectin receptor. Gastroenterology 1998; 114(1), 44-49.

[230] Ramadass B., Dokladny K., Moseley P.L., Patel Y.R., Lin H.C. Sucrose co-administration reduces the toxic effect of lectin on gut permeability and intestinal bacterial colonization. Dig Dis Sci 2010; 55(10): 2778-2784.

[231] Evans R.C., Fea, S., Ashby D., Hackett A., Williams E., et al. Diet and colorectal cancer: an investigation of the lectin/galactose hypothesis. Gastroenterology 2002; 122(7): 1784-1792.

[232] Zárate, G., Perez-Chaia A. Dairy bacteria remove in vitro dietary lectins with toxic effects on colonic cells. J Appl Microbiol 2009; 106(3): 1050-1057.

[233] Allsop J., Work E. Cell walls of *Propionibacterium* species: fractionation and composition. Biochem J 1963, 87: 512-519.

Chapter 10

Bacteria with Probiotic Capabilities Isolated from the Digestive Tract of the Ornamental Fish *Pterophyllum scalare*

María del Carmen Monroy Dosta, Talía Castro Barrera, Francisco J. Fernández Perrino, Lino Mayorga Reyes, Héctor Herrera Gutiérrez and Saúl Cortés Suárez

Additional information is available at the end of the chapter

1. Introduction

Aquaculture has made significant advances in recent years in the production of a wide range of aquatic organisms, both for human consumption and as ornamental species (Balcazar et al., 2006; Kesarcodi-Watson et al., 2008). One of the most successful freshwater ornamental species is *Pterophyllum scalare* (angelfish), a cichlid native to the Amazon that has adapted throughout the world and has great economic potential; it is one of the most in-demand species on the market (Agudelo;2005; Soriano and Hernández, 2002; Zilberga et al., 2004). This species is grown in intensive and semi-intensive systems, where its nutritional requirements are met with artificial diets. However, due to growth conditions such as high seeding densities and limited amounts of water, the organisms are subjected to constant stress, which translates into low growth rates and diseases (Auró & Ocampo, 1999; Verjan, 2002; Akinbowale et al., 2006). Therefore, there is an ongoing search for alternatives, such as the use of nutritional supplements, to prevent the rise of diseases and improve production. One interesting strategy focuses on the use of probiotics microorganisms that promote the welfare of the host they inhabit by improving its digestion and immune response as well as by inhibiting the growth of pathogenic microorganisms (Riquelme et al., 2000; Verschuere et al.,2000; Planas et al.,2006; Wang & Xu, 2006; Vine et al., 2006; Wang, 2007; Gatesoupe, 2007).

The presence of probiotic bacteria in the digestive tracts of fish is subject to several factors such as their ability to adhere to the surface of the intestinal epithelium and the production of substances that antagonise pathogenic microorganisms (Boris et al., 1997; Del Re et al., 2000; Reid et al., 1988; Balcázar, 2002;). Difficulties involved in the study of in vivo bacterial colonisation have led to the development of new *in vitro* techniques, such as sweeping electron microscopy and molecular analyses (PCR, FISH and DAPI). The objective of this work was to isolate and identify by the isolation of 16Sr DNA, bacteria with probiotic capabilities from the digestive tract of *Pterophyllum scalare* and evaluate their ability to adhere to the epithelium intestinal using immunohistochemical techniques and bacteriological analysis.

2. Materials and methods

2.1. Isolation of microorganisms of digestive tract de *Pterophyllum scalare*

A batch of 200 healthy young fish (15 cm in length) of *P. scalare* (angel fish) was obtained from a production center in Xochimilco, Mexico City. The fish were introduced to a growth tank equipped to hold them during an acclimation period of 15 days under the same growth conditions of the production center: 28°C, pH 7, 5 mg/L dissolved oxygen and 0.3 ppm of nitrates and nitrites. Once the acclimation period had passed, the fish were starved for 24 hours. Next, 20 fish were randomly taken and dissected with a cut above the lateral line from the operculum to the base of the caudal fin. The digestive tracts of the fish were extracted and homogenised in 90 mL of sterile saline solution. They were diluted ten-fold and inoculated in 0.1 mL aliquots onto MSR, BHI and TCBS agar plates in triplicate. The plates were incubated at 35°C for 24 h. After the incubation was done counting colony forming units for each dilution (CFU / mL), was characterized colony morphology and subsequent reseeding strains were purified. Immediately was performed Gram staining to observe cell morphology using an Olympus microscope SZX12. Additional biochemical tests were performed (mobility, cytochrome C, glucose fermentation oxide, catalase, Voges Proskauer and indole) prior to molecular identification by DNA isolation 16Rs.

2.2. Tests to characterise a microorganism as probiotic

2.2.1. Resistance to acidic pH

To show the resistance of the bacteria to acidic pH, the gastric barrier was simulated by placing the isolated microorganisms in acidic growth media with pH values of 1.5, 2.5 and 3.0, and the strains that did not survive these stress conditions were discarded.

2.2.2. Growth in bile salts

To perform the growth in bile salts test, three 150 mL Erlenmeyer flasks were each filled with 100 mL of MRS broth plus 0.1%, 0.5% or 1.0% fresh bile. The flasks were inoculated with 1 mL of the microorganism strains that survived the acidic conditions and were incubated at 37°C for 3 h. The viability of the culture in MRS (Oxoid) broth medium was used as a control.

2.2.3. In vitro antagonistic capability

The strains that yielded positive results in the previous studies were used in vitro inhibition tests. For this experiment, was used the pathogen *Aeromonas hydrophila* ATCC356554A and was seeded in triplicate onto BHI agar plates, which were incubated for 24 h at 30°C. Next, using the well diffusion method, 70 µL of a suspension of the beneficial strains isolated in sterile water was added, with concentration of CFU 10^7 (colony forming units per mL). The plates were incubated for 24 h at 30ºC, after which we observed the formation of inhibition halos. The strains that showed halos larger than 2 mm were considered positive.

2.3. Molecular identification of bacteria with the isolation of 16Sr DNA

2.3.1. DNA Isolation

The Wizard Genomic DNA Purification Kit (Promega™ Madison, U.S A) was used to extract genomic DNA for the molecular identification of the bacteria that showed probiotic capabilities, following the manufacturer's instructions.

To determine the purity and integrity of the genomic DNA of interest, samples were subjected to electrophoresis in a 1% agarose gel.

2.3.2. Polymerase Chain Reaction (PCR)

PCR was performed with the isolated genomic DNA of the bacteria that showed probiotic capabilities using the universal primers 9F (5′-GAGTTTGATCCTGGCTCAG-3′) and E939R (5′- CTTGTGCGGGCCCCCGTCAATTC-3′) in a Biometra® TGradient thermocycler under the following conditions: pre-incubation at 95°C for 10 minutes; 30 cycles of denaturation 124 at 95°C for 30 seconds, hybridisation at 55°C for 30 seconds and elongation at 72°C for 1 minute; and refrigeration at 4°C. The PCR products were purified with the QIAquick PCR Purification Kit (Qiagen), following the manufacturer's instructions. Finally, the genetic sequence of each strain was determined and compared to sequences in the GenBank database using the similarity search program BLAST.

2.4. Determination of the location and permanence of the probiotic bacteria in the digestive tract of *P.scalare*

The fish were fed with the isolated probiotic bacterial strains to establish the strains' adhesion capabilities. The genomic DNA analysis indicated that these microorganisms were three different strains of the *Bacillus* genus, which were assigned the labels *Bsp1*, *Bsp2* and *Bsp3*.

2.4.1. Preparation of the probiotic strains

A sample of each bacillus was taken with a bacteriological loop, and each sample was seeded into 500 mL of TSA broth and incubated at 30°C for 48 h or until there was a starting concentration of 107 CFU/mL. A Jenway 6400® Spectrophotometer with a 620-nm wavelength was used to measure the required bacterial concentration, and CFU/mL counts were performed. The relationship between the values obtained with spectrophotometry and the number of CFU/mL was determined according to the method established by Gullian (2001).

2.4.2. Feeding the fish with Artemia enriched with the isolated bacteria

Four fish tanks (60L) were prepared with 20 fish each and were kept at 28°C and pH 7, with 5 mg/L of dissolved oxygen and a 0.2 ppm nitrite concentration. The fish were fed daily for 60 days with *Artemia franciscana* adults (50 *Artemia* per fish) enriched with 2 x 107 CFU/mL of each of the probiotic strains.

The fish were distributed in each of the four tanks arranged in the following way. Tank 1 was used as a control in which the fish were fed with *Artemia* adults without probiotics. The fish in tanks 2, 3 and 4 were fed with *Artemia* enriched with the *Bsp1*, *Bsp2* and *Bsp3* strains, respective,, each treatment was performed in triplicate. Food residues and faeces were removed from the fish tanks to maintain the quality of the water, and the physicochemical parameters were monitored (temperature, pH, dissolved oxygen, nitrites and nitrates) using a Hach DR/850 colourimeter.

2.4.3. Incorporation of the probiotic strains into Artemia franciscana adults

To incorporate the bacteria into the fish, 50 *Artemia franciscana* adults were placed in 200 mL of 149 sterile water that had been inoculated with 3 mL of the bacterial strains, to a concentration of 1×10^7 CFU/mL, for 30 min. After, an Olympus ZX12 stereo microscope was used to verify that the digestive tract of *Artemia* was completely filled with the bacteria. Next, the sample was passed through a light sieve with a 2.0-mm grid aperture size, and *Artemia* were fed to the fish.

2.4.4. Bacteriological analysis of the GIT of P. scalare during feeding in probiotics

The location and viability of the probiotics within the digestive tract of the fish were evaluated by analyzing bacteriological a portion of the GIT every 15 days for the 60 days of the administration of bacteria in the diet, using the methods of Riquelme et al. (2000).

2.4.5. Analysis of the faecal matter samples

After discontinuing the bacillus-containing feed, a bacteriological analysis of the faeces was performed to establish the permanence time of the bacteria in the digestive tract. Each week, 10 to 50 mg of faecal matter from the fish was sampled, and the presence of the administered strains was determined by quantifying them with the seeding of decimal dilutions into specific culture media (Thitaram et al., 2005). Twenty-four hours after incubation, the CFU were counted, and the morphology and Gram staining characteristics were corroborated for each bacterial group. All of the tests were performed in duplicate, and counting was performed during the 10 weeks following cessation of feeding with bacilli-enriched food.

A database was created in Excel that contained the bacterial count (CFU/mL) data from the microbiological analysis of the GIT and faeces, and descriptive statistics techniques, along with an analysis of variance (ANOVA), were applied to obtain the mean and standard deviation. When significant differences were found between the treatments (<0.005), the multiple means test with the Tukey method was performed with Systat 10.2 software.

2.5. Immunohistochemistry

Cross-sections of the intestinal tissue of the fish were removed for the immunohistochemistry analysis. The samples were placed in 10% formaldehyde in phosphate-buffered saline (PBS). Once the samples were fixed, they were processed using routine histology techniques and placed in paraffin, and 5μm cuts were made. The cuts were pre-treated with 3% 3-aminopropylethoxysilane (Sigma Laboratories). Next, the tissue sections were dewaxed at 60°C for 10 minutes, and three xylol washes of 5 minutes each were immediately performed. The tissue sections were soaked in 10% alcohol and washed twice with 70% alcohol, and a final wash with distilled water was performed for five minutes. An Immuno Cruz Staining System (Santa Cruz Biotechnology, USA) was used for Immunodetection, following the manufacturer's instructions. As a primary antibody, anti-*Bacillus*. (HRP) was used at a 1:20 dilution (Affinity Bioreagents, USA), and Grill's haematoxylin was applied for five seconds as a contrast medium.

2.6. Growth assessment of *P. scalare* fed probiotic strains isolated

In the laboratory, was prepared 15 aquaria (40 L) with 20 fish each, which were maintained for 15 days in a period of acclimation. Later the fish were fed daily for 60 days with *Artemia* adults (50 Artemia / fish) inoculated with 2 x 107 CFU/ mL of the isolated bacteria. The fish were distributed in each of the aquaria arranged as follows: the treatment 1 is assigned as a control, in this; the fish were fed *Artemia* adults without probiotics, treatment 2 to 4 were fed with enriched *Artemia* with *Bsp1*, *Bsp2* y *Bsp* respectively and treatment 5 fish fed with a combination of these. There were three replicates per treatment. To evaluate the growth of the fish were taken every 15 days biometric parameters (length, height, width and weight). A biometric data tests were applied descriptive statistics for the mean and standard deviation are also performed an analysis of variance (ANOVA). When significant differences were found between treatments (<O.OO5) was tested multiple mean comparison by Tukey method, with the program Systat 10.2. Also we calculated condition factor (Km), for which we used the following equation:

$$\text{Condition Factor Km} = 100 \, (W) / L^3$$

3. Results

3.1. Bacterial isolation

A total of 108 strains were isolated from the digestive tract of *P. scalare*, only 20 of which grew in an acidic pH in the presence of bile salts.

3.2. *In vitro* inhibition activity

Only 20 of the strains resisted the acidic pH and bile salts conditions, and 3 showed the ability to inhibit *Aeromonas hydrophila*. However, no significant differences were observed between the three strains because in all cases, inhibition halos with mean values between 19 and 24 mm were formed (Figure 1a and b).

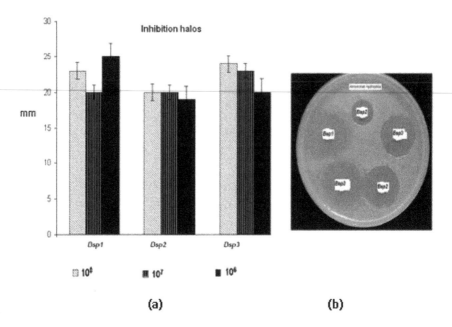

(a) **(b)**

Figure 1. *In vitro* inhibition halos of *A. hydrophila* with the *Bsp1, Bsp2* and *Bsp3* strains, 10 with mean values between 19 and 24 mm.

3.3. Molecular identification of the isolated probiotic strains of *P. scalare*

The genomic DNA sequence obtained from strain 1 was composed of 885 bp (Figure 2) and coincided with 22 types of *Bacillus sp.* and one type of *Acetobacter pasteurianus*, all with 99% sequence homology. Strain 2 yielded a sequence of 860 bp, which coincided with 51 types of *Bacillus sp.* and *Acetobacter pasteurianus*, all with 99% homology. The 900 bp sequence of strain 3 matched 100% with the synthetic construct of *Bacillus sp.* clone and showed 84% agreement with *B. weihenstephanensis*. Therefore, the three strains could only be assigned with certainty at the genus level to *Bacillus* and were labelled *Bsp1, Bsp2* and *Bsp3* (Figure 3).

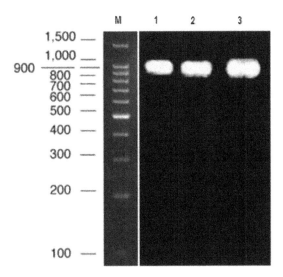

Figure 2. Comparison of the PCR product bands with the 9F and E939F universal primers from the three strains to the 100 bp molecular marker from Promega™ (M). Line 1 *Bsp1*, Line 2 *Bsp2*; Line 3 *Bsp3*.

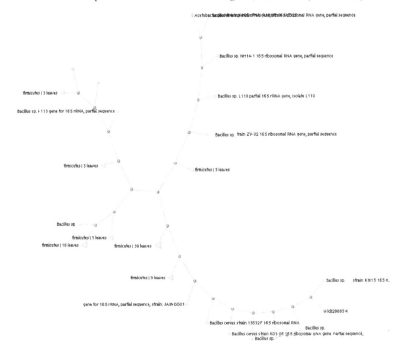

Figure 3. Phylogenetic tree of the *B. sp3* strain. Euclidean distance O.75

3.4. Colonisation and permanence of *Bacillus sp.* strains in the epithelial tissue of *P. scalare*

3.4.1. Bacteriological analysis of the digestive tract of P. scalare

The bacteriological analysis of the digestive tract of the fish during feeding with the different strains of *Bacillus* indicated that the three strains colonised the digestive tract of *P. scalare*, which was visible when we isolated the characteristic morphotypes of the bacteria supplied in the TSA media. Over the course of the experiment, it was established that the *Bsp2* strain showed the highest mean CFU/mL values (Figure 4).

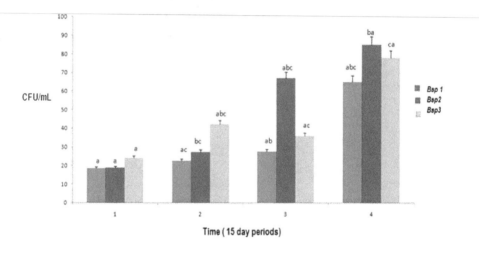

*Different letters show significant differences between the groups at each time point (p<0.05).

Figure 4. CFU/mL counts of the probiotic bacteria in the digestive tract of *P. scalare* over 60 days (four 15-day periods).

3.4.2. Bacteriological analysis of the faeces

During the bacteriological analysis of the faeces, it was established that the *Bsp3* strain had a high degree of colonisation and competition in the digestive tract of *P. scalare* because mean counts above 120 CFU/mL were obtained up to the sixth week. After concluding the feeding tests, the *Bsp3* strain was observed up to the tenth week, whereas the *Bsp1* and *Bsp2* strains had CFU/mL counts with mean values of 70 and 30, respectively, in the sixth week. From the eighth weeks on, no colonies characteristic to these strains were obtained, and bacterial growth of a different morphotype was observed (Figure 5).

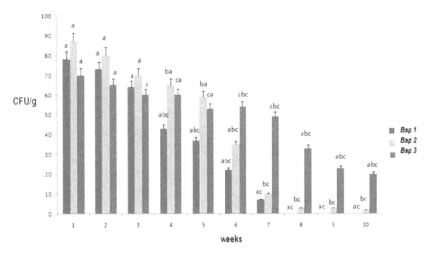

* Different letters show significant differences between groups at each time (p <0.05)

Figure 5. Counts of CFU/mL of faeces of *P. scalare*, ten weeks after discontinuing feeding of fish

3.5. Immunohistochemical analysis

In the figure 6a and b, shows the presence of the probiotics supplied to the fish. Was observed in histological cuts labeled with *Bacillus* antibodies in the intestinal lumen and on the edges of the microvilli to positive marking, a dark filter was used in these images.

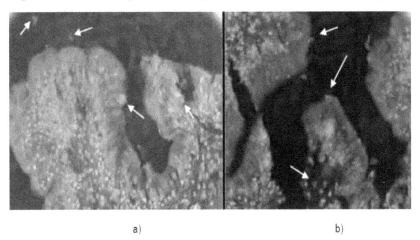

a)   b)

* The arrow indicates the Immunolabelling positive. To highlight marking, a dark filter was used in these images.

Figure 6. 6a and b. Location of probiotics in transverse sections of digestive tract marked with antibodies to *Bacillus*, in the microvilli and in the gut lumen.

3.6. Survival and growth of *P. scalare*

3.6.1. The survival of fish fed the probiotic strains was 100% compared with 80% survival of fish fed without probiotic.

3.6.1.1. Total length

The analysis of variance for total length indicated that there are significant differences between treatments (F = 15,656, df = 4, P <0.005). When making multiple mean comparison by Tukey test, it was found that treatment of fish fed *Bsp3* achieve the highest total length (4.5 cm), while fish in the control group received only a length of 3 cm (Figure 7).

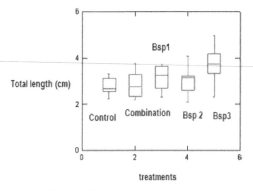

Figure 7. Comparison of the total length of fish between treatments.

3.6.1.2. Width

In regard to width of the fish we observed no significant differences between treatments fed with probiotics which reached values of 1.10 and 1.25 cm, however if there are differences with the control values obtained as 0.63cm (Figure 8).

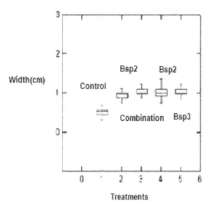

Figure 8. Comparison of the width of the fish between treatments.

3.6.1.3. *Weight*

With regard to weight, the analysis of variance indicated significant differences between treatments (F = 17,394, df = 4, P <0.001). In the analysis of multiple means by Tukey's method shows that the treatment provides greater weight is *Bsp3*, with an average weight of 1.90 g, while the combination and the control group provided weights below 1 g (Figure 9).

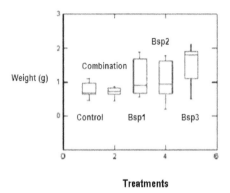

Treatments

Figure 9. Comparison of the variation in weight of fish with different treatments.

3.6.2. *Condition Factor (Km)*

The results of the Condition Factor indicate that fish fed *Bsp2, Bsp3* strains, and the combination, get better a weight - length relationship to obtain values above the initial Km compared to fish fed *Bsp1* strain and the control, that values were below the initial km (Figure 10).

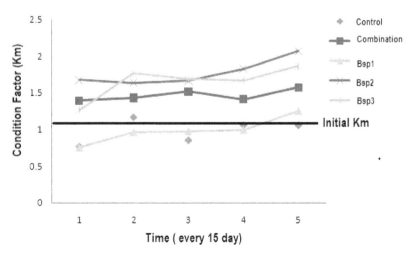

Figure 10. Condition factor of fish fed the different probiotic strains

4. Discussion

The results obtained from the molecular analysis place the three bacterial strains isolated in this work in the Bacillus genus. Although there have been studies on the use of bacteria from this genus as probiotics, there are no reports of its isolation from the digestive tract of fish, with the exception of the work of Gullian et al., (2004) in which the presence of this genus in shrimp (*Penneus vannamei*), is mentioned.

The use of universal primers such as 9F and E939R of 16S rDNA proved to 278 be adequate to amplify the 16S rDNA of the unknown strains. These results agree with those of Heyndrickx et al. (2004) and Rodicio & Mendoza (2004). The analysis of the 16S rDNA sequence of the different phylogenetic groups revealed the presence of one or more characteristic sequences, which are denoted signature oligonucleotides: short, specific sequences that are found in all (or most) of the members of a particular phylogenetic group and are never (or only on occasion) present in other groups (including the closest ones). However, despite the certain inclusion of the three stains in the *Bacillus genus*, not a single one could be identified at the species level, due to variations that were found in their sequences with respect to the sequences of known species. This identification difficulty is in agreement with the results reported by Woo et al. (2008), who explain that this variation can occur when isolating 16S rDNA because when two different bacterial species share almost all of their 16S rDNA sequence, this technique is not able to distinguish between the two; only the genus can be determined with certainty. These results imply that these could be previously unidentified species because there is no report of their isolation in samples from the digestive tract of fish. In the present study, the bacteriological analysis showed that the three probiotics were capable of colonising the digestive tract. However, there were differences in the number of cells from the 30th day of the experiment, where the number of strain *Bsp3* cells was higher than the others; however, at 45 days, the *Bsp2* strain had higher counts, averaging 65 CFU/mL and dominating both of the other two strains until the end of the experiment. These higher counts indicate that the *Bsp2* strain was better to colonize the digestive tract of the fish ($p< 0.05$) and will thrive as long as this probiotic is provided. Studies performed with aquatic organisms have also shown that, when supplying different strains of probiotics, even if they all colonise, there will always be one strain that dominates or varies its number of cells over time (Gildberg et al., 1997; Ringo and Vadstein, 1998;Ringo & Olsen., 1999; Rengpipat et al., 2000; Nikoskelainen et al., 2003; Gullian *et al.*, 2004; Macey & Coyne, 2006;). When testing the persistence of probiotics in the digestive tract of the fish, the *Bps3* strain maintained a higher cell count up to the tenth week after suspending the food-containing probiotics. The permanence of the probiotics in the faeces evidenced the great colonizing power of the digestive tract of the fish in contrast with other aquatic organisms, such as the *Abalone* mollusc, which show a marked decrease in probiotic cells during the first and second days after ceasing probiotic feed and show low amounts of these cells ($p<0.05$) in their faeces 15 days later (Macey & Coyne, 2006).

The immunodetection tests performed confirmed the presence and location of the *Bacillus* bacteria added to the fish food (*Artemia*), displaying positive markings in the microvilli and in the intestinal lumen of the front part of the angelfish intestine. Makridis et al. (2001) also showed with immunohistochemical techniques that there was Vibrio in the lumen and in the microvilli of the intestinal tube of *Hippoglossus hippoglossus* (sheer) fish larvae up to 10 days later after providing the bacteria, which were also bioencapsulated in *Artemia*. According to the results obtained in the growth of fish fed with the probiotic bacteria isolated in this study, we observed that the use of food fish was higher in treatments in which they contain added probiotic strains, especially with Bs3 strain in which the fish were much higher growth in total length, weight and width (with almost 50% increase compared to the control group and the combination of probiotic strains). These results agree with the study by Ghosh et al., (2008), which reported significant differences in the growth of ornamental fish species *Poecilia reticulata*, *Poecilia sphenops*, *Xiphophorus maculatus* and *Xiphophorus hellieri*, after being fed with feed enriched *Bacillus sp* for a period of 60 days, compared with a control treatment without probiotic.

5. Conclusion

The genetic sequence of probióticos strains isolated from *P scalare* only allowed us locate these bacteria within the genus Bacillus, because it was not possible to identify the specie, due to the variations found in the sequences of the three strains with respect to the sequences of species known until today.

The three strains of Bacillus (*Bsp1, Bsp2* and *Bsp3*) survived the gastric barrier of the intestine and had high colonization of the intestinal epithelium as well as the ability to inhibit *Aeromonas hydrophila in vitro.*

The Bacillus *Bsp3* promoted better growth in *P scalare:* total length, width and weight with almost 50% compared with control fish.

The results of this work show that the three strains used are capable of colonizing the digestive tract of angelfish. The *Bsp2* strain has the greatest capacity, although the Bsp3 strain remains longest. Thus, it could be proposed to ornamental fish producers, specifically those that grow angelfish, to use mixed *Bsp2* and *Bsp3* strains to achieve better results and indicate them the time required to provide the food probiotics again.

Although other studies have reported that the combination of probiotics provides better results in terms of growth, but in this study the combination did not give better results than those obtained with single strain.

Author details

María del Carmen Monroy Dosta, Talía Castro Barrera, Francisco J. Fernández Perrino,
Lino Mayorga Reyes, Héctor Herrera Gutiérrez and Saúl Cortés Suárez
Universidad Autónoma Metropolitana, México, D. F.

6. References

Agudelo, G.D.A.A., (2005). Establishing of a *Pterophyllum scalare* (angel or scaly fish) producing center. *La Salle Research Journal.* 2(2), 26-30.

Auró, A & Ocampo, C.L. (1999). Diagnóstico del estrés en peces. *Revista Veterinaria México* 30:337-344

Akinbowale, O.L., Peng, H., Barton, M.D. (2006) Antimicrobial resistance in bacteria isolated from aquaculture sources in Australia. *J Appl Microbiol* 100:1103–1113. doi:10.1111/j.1365-2672.2006.02812.x.

Balcazar, J.L. (2002). Uso de probióticos en acuicultura: Aspectos generales. I Congreso Iberoamericano Virtual de Acuicultura, CIVA 2002.

Balcázar, J.L., de Blas, I., Ruiz-Zarzuela, I., Cunningham, D., Vendrell, D., Múzquiz, J.L., (2006). The role of probiotics in aquaculture. *Vet. Microbiol.* 114, 173–186.

Boris, S., Suárez, J.E., Barbés, C. (1997). Characterization of the aggregation 339 promoting factor from 340 *Lactobacillus gasseri*, a vaginal isolate. J. App. Microbiol. 83, 413–420.

Del Re, B., Sgorbati, B., Miglioli, M., Palenzona, D. (2000). Adhesion,self-aggregation and hydrophobicity of 13 strains of *Bifidobacterium longum.* *Lett. Appl. Microbiol.* 31, 438–442.

Gatesoupe, F.J. (2007). Live yeasts in the gut: natural occurrence, dietary introduction, and their effects on fish health and development. *Aquaculture* 267, 20–30.

Ghosh, S., Sinha, A. & Sahu, C. (2008). Dietary probiotic supplementation in growth and health of live-bearing ornamental fishes. *Aquaculture. Nutrition.* 14, 289–299.

Gildberg, A., Mikkelsen, H., Sandaker, E., Ringø, E. (1997). Probiotic effect of lactic acid bacteria in the feed on growth and survival of fry of Atlantic cod (*Gadus morhua*). *Hydrobiologia* 352, 279-285.

Gullian, M. (2001). Study of the immune stimulus effect of prebiotic bacteria associated with the *Pennaeus vannamei* culture. Master of Science Thesis, ESPOL, Department of Ocean Engineering and Maritime Science. Guayaquil, Ecuador.

Gullian, M., Thompson, F., Rodríguez, J.(2004). Selection of probiotic bacteria and study of their inmune stimulus effect in *Pennaeus vannamei. Aquaculture.* 233, 1-14.

Heyndrickx, M., Scheldeman, P., Forsyth, G., Lebbe, L., Rodriguez-Diaz, M., Logan, N., De Vos, A.P. (2005). *Bacillus ruris* sp. nov., from dairy farms International *Journal of Systematic and Evolutionary Microbiology.* 55: 2551-2554

Kesarcodi-Watson, A., Kaspar, H., Lategan, M.J., Gibson, L.(2008). Probiotics in aquaculture: The need, principles and mechanisms of action and screening processes. *Aquaculture* 274, 1–14

Makridis, P., Ø. Bergh., J. Skjermo & O. Vadstein. (2001). Addition of bacteria bioencapsulated in *Artemia* metanauplii to a rearing system for halibut larvae. *Aquaculture International*, 9: 225-235.

Macey, B.M., Coyne, V.E. (2006). Colonization of the gastrointestinal tract of the farmed South African abalone *Haliotis midae* by the probionts *Vibrio midae* SY9, *Cryptococcus* sp. SS1, and *Debaryomyces hansenii* AY1. *Marine Biotechnology* 8:246–259

Nikoskelainen, S., Ouwehand, A., Bylund, G., Salminen, S., Lilius, E.M. (2003). 369 Immune enhancement in rainbow trout (*Oncorhynchus mykiss*) by potential probiotic bacteria (*Lactobacillus rhamnosus*). *Fish Shellfish Immunol.* 15, 443–452.

Planas, M., Pérez-Lorenzo, M., Hjelm, M., Gram, L., Fiksdal, I.U., Øivind, B., Pintado, J. (2006). Probiotic effect in vivo of Roseobacter strain 27-4 against Vibrio(Listonella) anguillarum infections in turbot (Scophthalmus maximus L.) larvae. *Aquaculture* 255, 323–333.

Reid, G., McGroarty, J.A., Angotti, R., Cook, R.L. (1988). Lactobacillus inhibitor production against *Escherichia coli* and coaggregation ability with uropathogens. *Can. J Microbiol.* 34, 344–351.

Rengpipat, S., Rukpratanpom, S., Piyatiratitivorakul,S., Menasaveta, P. (2000). Immunity enhancement in black tiger shrimp (*Pennaeus monodon*) by a probiotic bacterium (*Bacillus SII*). *Aquaculture.* 191, 271-288.

Riquelme, C., Araya, R., Vergora, N., Rojas, A., Guaita, M., Condia, M. (2000). Potential probiotic strains in the culture of Chilean scallop *Argopecten purpuratus* (Lamarck, 1819). *Aquaculture.* 154, 17–26.

Ringø, E., Vadstein, O. (1998). Colonization of *Vibrio pelagius* and *Aeromonas caviae* in early developing turbot (*Scophthalmus maximus* L.) larvae. *Journal of Applied Microbiology* 84, 227-233.

Ringo, E., Olsen, R.E. (1999). The effect of diet on aerobic bacterial flora associated with intestine of Artic charr (*Salvelinus alpinus* L.). *Journal of Applied Microbiology* 86, 22–28.

Rodicio, M.R., Mendoza, M.C. (2004). Identificación bacteriana mediante secuenciación del ARNr 16S: fundamento, metodología y aplicaciones en microbiología clínica. *Enfermedades Infecciosas y Microbiología Clínica.* 22:238-45 p.

Soriano, S.M.B., Hernández, O.D. (2002). Growth rate of the *Pterophyllum scalare* angelfish (Perciforms:cichidae) under laboratory conditions. *Acta Universitaria.* 12(2), 28-33.

Thitaram, S.N., C.H. Chung, D.F. Day, A. Hinton, J.S. Bailey and G.R. Siragusa, (2005). Isomaltooligosaccharide increases cecal bifidobacterium population in young broiler chickens. *Poult. Sci.*, 84: 998-1003.

Verján, G.(2002). Micobacteriosis en peces ornamentales. *Rev. Med. Vet. Zoot.*, 49: 51-58

Verschuere, L., Rombaut, G., Sorgeloos, P., Verstraete, W. (2000). Probiotic bacteria as biological agents in aquaculture. *Microbiol. Mole. Biol. Rev.* 64(4), 655-671.

Vine, N.G., Leukes, W.D., Kaiser, H. (2006). Probiotics in marine larviculture. *FEMS Microbiol. Rev.* 30, 404–427.

Wang, Y.B.& Xu, Z.R. (2006). Effect of probiotics for common carp (Cyprinus carpio) based on growth performance and digestive enzyme activities. *Anim. Feed Sci. Technol.* 127, 283–292.

Wang, Y.B.(2007). Effect of probiotics on growth performance and digestive enzyme activity of the shrimp Penaeus vannamei. *Aquaculture* 269, 259–264.

Woo, P.C., Ng, K.H., Lau, S.K., Yip, K.T., Fung, A.M., Leung, K.W. (2008). Usefulness of the MicroSeq 500 16S Ribosomal DNA-Based Bacterial Identification System for Identification of Clinically Significant Bacterial 410 Isolates with Ambiguous Biochemical Profiles. *Journal of Clinical Microbiology.* 41: 1996-2001

Zilberga, D., Ofira, R., Rabinskib, T., Diamantc, A. (2004). Morphological and genetic characterization of swimbladder non-inflation in angelfish *Pterophyllum scalare* (Cichlidae). *Aquaculture*. 230, 13–27.

Chapter 11

Efficiency of Probiotics in Farm Animals

Etleva Delia, Myqerem Tafaj and Klaus Männer

Additional information is available at the end of the chapter

1. Introduction

The first concept of probiotics was originally developed by [38]. He suggested that ingested bacteria could have a positive influence on the normal microbial flora of the intestinal tract. Probiotics are considered as growth and health stimulators and are used extensively in animal feeding, especially in pig and poultry production.

Probiotics have been defined also by [6] as *"a live microbial feed supplement which beneficially affects the host animal by improving its intestinal balance"*. There is a relatively large volume of literature that supports the use of probiotics to prevent or treat intestinal disorders. Currently, the best studied probiotics are the lactic acid bacteria, particularly *Lactobacillus sp* and *Bifidobacterium sp*.

Therefore, an intensive research work is carrying out in this topic from many researcher groups in different countries. Many years later, probiotics were determined as: viable microbial feed supplements, which are believed to stimulate growth and the health as well as to modify the ecology of the intestine in a beneficial manner for the host [3], [34], [54]. Probiotics should lead to beneficial effects for the host animal due to an improvement of the intestinal microbial balance [12] or of the properties of the indigenous micro-flora [21]. There are also many mechanisms by probiotics enhance intestinal health, including stimulation of immunity, competition for limited nutrients, inhibition of epithelial and mucosal adherence, inhibition of epithelial invasion and production of antimicrobial substances [47].

Possible modes of actions are the modification of the intestinal microorganisms and the nutrient availability with response to the morphology and histology as well as the transport physiology. Significant positive effects of probiotics on performance, health, vitality, gut ecology as well digestibility are observed in many studies, although the mode of action of probiotics is not still completely explained [24], [55], [25], [4]. Efficiency probiotic on a focus of combined preparation have hardly been concluded.

2. Efficiency of probiotic in farm animals

The claims made for probiotics are many and varied but it is not always possible to provide good scientific evidence to support them. However the potential benefits that can arise from applications of the probiotic concept are shown as below:

Potential beneficial effects of probiotics for farm animals by [13].

- Greater resistance to infectious diseases
- Increased growth rate
- Improved feed conversion.
- Improved digestion.
- Better absorption of nutrients
- Provision of essential nutrients
- Improved milk yield
- Improved milk quality.
- Increased egg production.
- Improved egg quality
- Improved carcass quality and less contamination

Since probiotics are discussed as alternatives to antimicrobial growth promotors their impact on performance of farm animals is of prime interest. For authorization of microorganisms as feed additives it is also required to show significant effects on performance data [54]. By far most experiments were performed with piglets. According to a literature review by [61] no significant positive effects could be found from the hitherto results with piglets and fattening pigs. Later, the evaluation of studies conducted with raising piglets drew a different picture [11]. [61] was used the strict criteria of biostatistics and only significant effects were documented. Today, trends without statistical significance are also considered as positive effect by [54]. It is obvious that majority of the experiments show trends toward positive effects, however the significance level of p≤ 0,05 was reached only in 5% of experiments. Due to the complexity of the intestine, individual variations of animals to probiotic inclusion may be the rule and not the exception. Considering this concept, the range between no effect and significant effects seem to be reasonable.

In a trial with 90 treated and 90 untreated *Bacillus cereus* –preparation weaned piglets; the probiotic treated animals gained 7% more live weight during 6 weeks after weaning with a reduced feed conversion ratio of 2.4%. Both results were not significant [25]. This point towards a high variation in the response of the individual animals to this type of feed additives [54].

With regard to the evaluation of animal performance, the same conclusion can be draw for experiments with fattening chicken carried out by [53].This is also reflected by a series of experiments with turkey, poultry under field conditions using three probiotics [34]. Again none of the effects in performance were significant, on average weight gain was improved by 1,5% (+0,1 to + 3,8) and feed conversion by –2% (-7 to –3,5). A further observation was a more pronounced effect of additive during weeks 1 to 5. However again no significance was seen in the period's week 1 plus 2 and 3 to 5, respectively [54].

Authors in [54] concluded that the inconsistency of the effectiveness of a feed additive is of course not convenient, but on the other hand comprehensible for this type of feed additive. Probiotic do not act like essential nutrients in term of a clear dose response until the requirements are met. Due to the complexity of intestine, individual variations of animals to probiotic inclusion may be the rule and not the exception. Considering this concept the range between no effect and significant effects seem to be reasonable.

3. Mode of action of probiotics

The development of probiotics for farm animals is based on the knowledge that the gut microflora is involved in resistance to disease. The gut microflora has been shown to be involved in protection against a variety of pathogens including *Escherichia coli, Salmonella Camylobacter, Clostridium* and *Rotavirus.* Hence the probiotic approach may be effective in the prevention and therapy of these infections. No attempt will be made to summarize the evidence available for all of these effects [13].

The one area where it is possible to arrive at some scientifically based conclusions is the effect that the probiotics preparations have on resistance to infections.

The stressful conditions experienced by the young animal causes changes in the composition and/or activity of the gut microflora. Probiotic supplementation seeks to repair these deficiencies and provide the type of microflora which exists in feral animals uninfluenced by modern farm rearing methods. The products available are of varying composition and efficacy but the concept is scientifically-based and intellectually sound. Under the right conditions the claims made for probiotic preparations can be realized [13].

Molecule	Defense function	References
Lysozyme	Lyses bacterial cell walls	[2], [46]
Defensins	Form pores in bacterial cell wall	[2], [42]
Mucus	Prevents bacterial adhesion made by goblet cells, a specialized epithelial cell type.	[41]
MHC class I	Presents antigen to cytotoxic T-lymphocytes	[14]
MHC Class II	Presents antigen to helper T-lymphocytes	[14]

Table 1. Defense functions of epithelial cells [37].

There are many proposed mechanisms by which probiotics may protect the host from intestinal disorders. The sum of all processes by which bacteria inhibit colonization by other strains is called colonization resistance. Much work remains to classify the mechanisms of action of particular probiotics against particular pathogens. In addition, the same probiotic may inhibit different pathogens by different mechanisms. Listed below is a brief description of mechanisms by which probiotics may protect the host against intestinal disease.

Possible mode of action of intestinal bacteria can be summarized as follows by [54]:

- Increase of desired intestinal bacteria;
- Competitive adhesion to epithelial receptors;
- Production of specific substances (bacteriocins, dipicolinic acid, bioactive peptides)
- Competition for nutrients between probiotic and undesired bacteria;
- Micro-environmental pH reduction by production of acid;
- Reduction of bacterial bile salt deconjugation;
- Passive aggregation of probiotics and pathogenic bacteria;

4. Production of inhibitory substances

Probiotic bacteria can produce a variety of substances that are inhibitory to both gram-positive and gram-negative bacteria. These inhibitory substances include organic acids, hydrogen peroxide and bacteriocins. These compounds may reduce not only the number of viable cells but may also affect bacterial metabolism or toxin production.

5. Blocking of adhesion sites

Competitive inhibition for bacterial adhesion sites on intestinal epithelial surfaces is another mechanism of action for probiotics [18]. Consequently, some probiotic strains have been chosen for their ability to adhere to epithelial cells. Gut bacteria prevent intestinal colonization by pathogenic organisms directly by competing more successfully for essential nutrients or for epithelial attachment sites [48].

6. Competition for nutrients

Competition for nutrients has been proposed as a mechanism of probiotics. Probiotics may utilize nutrients otherwise consumed by pathogenic microorganisms. However, the evidence that this occurs in vivo is lacking.

7. Degradation of toxin receptor

The postulated mechanism by which *Sacchromyces boulardii* protects animals against *C. difficile* intestinal disease is through degradation of the toxin receptor on the intestinal mucosa [5].

8. Influence on the immune system

The intestinal micro flora is an important component of host animal. A critical review of the literature indicates that probiotic supplementation of the intestinal micro flora may enhance defense, primarily by preventing colonization by pathogens and by indirect, adjuvant-like stimulation of innate and acquired immune functions [37]. The role of nonpathogenic bacteria in the development of the intestinal immune system and in protecting the host from pathogenic challenges has been studied.

Intestinal bacteria provide the host with several nutrients, including short-chain fatty acids, vitamin K, some B vitamins and amino acids [49], [67]. Intestinal bacteria also protect the host from pathogens, forming a front line of mucosal defense. The indigenous microflora induces recruitment of lamina propria immune cells, which form a second tier of defense by activation of appropriate inflammatory or immune mechanisms during infection.

Recent evidence suggests that stimulation of specific and nonspecific immunity may be another mechanism by which probiotics can protect against intestinal disease [45]. For example, per oral administration of *Lactobacillus* GG during acute rotavirus diarrhoea is associated with an enhanced immune response to rotavirus [26]. This may account for the shortened course of diarrhoea seen in treated patients. The underlying mechanisms of immune stimulation are not well understood, but specific cell wall components or cell layers may act as adjuvant and increase humoral immune responses.

Reduction of diarrhea by probiotics was studied frequently, because diarrhea is the main problem of piglets during the first weeks after weaning with utmost importance for production [54].

Probiotic	Age	Incidence of diarrhoea	Statistical significance	Literature
B. cereus	8 weeks	Reduced	+	[29]
B. cereus	Day 1-85	Reduced	+	[22]
B. cereus	Day 7-21	Reduced	+	[68]
B. cereus	Day 24-66	No effect	-	[10]
B. cereus	25 kg Live weigh	No effect	-	[27]
B. cereus	2 weeks post weaning	Reduced	+	[23]
E faecium	Day 1-70	Reduced	+	[35]
E. faecium	8 Days before/after weaning	Reduced	+	[51]
P. acidilactici	Day 5-28	Reduced	+	[9]
P. acidilactici *S. cerevisiae*	Day 5-28	Reduced	+	[9]

Table 2. Incidence of diarrhoea in piglets fed probiotic supplemented feed (Effects compared to control animals) [54].

The mucosal surface of the intestinal tract represents the largest interface between the body and its environment. An effective local immune is necessary to protect the organism against the invasion of noxious antigens and microbes [54]. No other organ of the body harbours more immune cells than the gut –associated lymphoid tissue (GALT), and a tremendous amount of antibodies is secreted into the intestinal lumen to neutralize and exclude harmful antigens. In numerous studies it has been shown that bacterial colonization influences the function of immune cells belonging to the GALT and even affects the systemic immune system [60].

Immune suppression has been observed after associating germfree rodents with defined bacterial species [69], [50]. In some studies the inductions of immune suppressive cytokines have been implicated in the so-called "by stander suppression" [7]. Moreover, it has been shown that bacterial colonization contributes to the induction and maintenance of immunological tolerance against nutritional antigens [39]. The mechanisms underlying oral tolerance are largely unknown by [54].

The numerous studies have reported immune stimulating abilities for different bacterial species. For example, *in vitro* cytokine production of macrophages was stimulated by *Bifidobacteria* [36]. *Bifidobacterium longum* as well as several other lactic acid bacteria have been found to increase the total amount of intestinal IgA [57], [65]. *Lactobacillus casei* was reported to have immune adjuvant activity by [43] and *Lactobacillus plantarum* was shown to increase antibody production against *Escherichia coli*. Induction of cytokine profiles by lactobacilli is likely to be strain-dependent [31] and it probably also depends on the host examined, since the autochthonous flora varies between different host species. Most of the animal studies with such probiotic micro organisms have been carried out in rodents with lactic acid bacteria with the goal of designing "functional food" for human consumption. Such studies however, are not necessarily suitable or transferable for the supplementation of animal feed in industrial settings [54]. Studies using swine as model system are few but, seem to be promising.

Probiotic treatment using *Bifidobacterium lactis* HN019 reduced weanling diarrhea associated with rotavirus and *Escherichia coli* infection in a piglet model [52]. Information from studies is also available about the age-dependent development of different immune cells in the intestine of the newborn and adult pigs [62], [55], [56]. Studies on these cells require large amounts of intestinal tissue that can hardly be taken from rodents. The composition of the different immune cells in the GALT is drastically changing during the first the first few weeks of life. For instance, the proliferation rate of B cells in the Peyer's Patches shows a 15-fold increase between days 1 and 42 [56]. Very few observations have been made concerning the influence of bacteria on the development of these immune cells which are the first line of defense against Intestinal infections [54].

A group of authors [54] found a decrease in CD8+ intraepithelial lymphocytes in piglets after treatment of sows and their piglets with *Enterococcus faecium* present in the feed. Neither total IgG or IgA levels in the sera of sow and piglets was affected, nor were the amounts of total IgG or IgA in the milk of the sows influenced by the probiotic treatment. Despite these observations,while the total numbers of coliform bacteria was the same in both probiotic and control herds, there appeared to be at least a 50% reduction in the numbers of pathogenic serovars in piglets from the probiotic group although the rate of isolation of these same serovars in sows was the same for both groups. ELISA-tests to detect specific antibodies against certain pathogenic *Escherichia coli* serovars are still ongoing.

9. Other effects of probiotics

Several studies indicate that in pig's intestinal morphology and function of the epithelium may be modified by probiotics [54]. In two trials significantly longer willi were measured in the jejunum of pigs receiving diets supplemented with *Bacillus cereus* [28] and *Bacillus cereus toyoi* or *Saccharomyces boulardii* respectively [17].

The probiotic product	Composition of microorganisms	Utilization
Toyocérine	*Bacillus toyoi*	In all animals
Paciflor	*Bacillus cereus CIP 5832*	In all animals
Adjulact standart	*Enterococcus spp, Lb. lactis, Lb. helveticus, Lb. acidophilus*	Calfs, piglets
Adjulact 1000	*Lb. helveticus, Enterococcus spp*	Calfs, piglets
Adjulact 2000	*Enterococcus spp, Lb. plantarum.*	Calfs,piglets
Yea -sacc	*Saccharomyces cerevisiae*	Ruminants
Lacto-sacc	*Saccharomyces cerevisiae Lb. acidophilus Ec. faecium*	In all animals
Fermacton	*Lactobacillus spp. Ec. faecium SF68 Pediococcus spp*	In all animals
Bio-Plus Porc	*Lactobacillus spp. Ec. faecium SF68 Pediococcus spp*	Pigs
Lyobacter P₁	*Lb. plantarum. Ec. faecium Lb. rhamnosus*	In all animals
Lyobacter SFL	*Ec. faecium* SFL	In all animals
Multigerm	*Lb. plantarum. Ec. faecium Lb. acidophilus*	Pigs
Biosaf SC 47	*Saccharomyces cerevisiae* SC 47	In all animals, especially in ruminants
Bio-Plus 2B	*B. subtilis B. licheniformis*	In all animals
Enteroferm	3 kind of *Lactobacillus, Enterococcus spp, Saccharomyces*	In all animals
Degeferments	*Lb. acidophillus, Lb. lactis*	In all animals
Bacteriolact	*Lb. casei, Str. thermophilus*	Calfs, piglets, lamb

Table 3. Some probiotics used as feed additives in European countries [59]

The microstructure of the epithelium is of great functional importance for nutrient transport (absorption and secretion) as well as maintenance of transcellular and paracellular barrier functions. This structure inhibits uncontrolled passage of substances and provides a barrier against infection with intestinal bacteria. Carbohydrate structures on the mucosal surface are used for adhesion by pathogenic and non pathogenic bacteria. *In vitro* studies also indicate that some probiotics *Lactobacillus plantarum* 299v and *Lactobacillus rhamnosus GG* have the ability to inhibit adherence of attaching and effacing of pathogenic *Escherichia coli* HT 29 to intestinal epithelial cells by increasing expression of the intestinal mucins MUC2 and MUC3, [32].

A group of authors [3], [66] concluded that Intestinal mucosa from pigs which were adopted to diets containing *Bacillus cereus* or *Saccharomyces boulardii* had an increased paracellular barrier function and modified nutrient transport kinetics for glucose and amino acids. For *Lactobacillus plantarum* 299v was shown, that pretreated rats were protected against increase in intestinal permeability induced by *Escherichia coli* [33].

10. Experiments in extensive farm conditions

10.1. Material and methods

Two animal trials were carried out at the same private farm of pigs. Twenty four piglets (White x Duroc) of four litters were transferred after weaning (35 days) to flat decks and randomly allocated to 4 groups with 6 animals (3 male and 3 female). The basal diet (see Table 4 and 5) was also supplemented with 1000mg, 1500mg and 2000mg/kg of the probiotic preparation (three experiment groups) or without supplementation (control group). The diets were offered ad-libidum and animals had free access to water. The probiotic preparation included the following strains: *Lactobacillus plantarum* ATCC 4336 ($5x10^9$ CFU/kg), *Lactobacillus fermentum* DSM 20016 ($5x10^9$ CFU/kg) and *Enterococcus faecium* ATCC 19434 ($5x10^{10}$ CFU/kg) (AKRON s.r.l-Milano). During the eight weeks experimental period in the first experiment and six weeks experimental period in the second experiment, body

Diet composition (g/kg feed)		Nutrient concentration (g/kg feed)	
Maize	620	ME (MJ/kg)	12,33
Soya bean meal	280	Crude protein	196.4
Sunflower meal	50	Crude fat	28,70
Fish meal	10	Crude fibre	42,90
Limestone	15	Calcium	10,77
Monocalcium phosphate	15	Phosphorus	6,50
Vitamin -mineral premix[a]	5	Lysine	11,30
L-Lysine	5	Methionine+Cystine	6,70

Table 4. Diet composition and calculated nutrient concentration on the first experiment.
[a] Contents in 1 kg: 1,200,000 IE vit. A, 120,000 IE vit. D₃, 4000 mg vit. E, 200 mg vit. B₁, 600 mg Vit. B₂, 2500 mg Niacin, 400 mg Vit. B₆, 4500 µg Vit. B₁₂, 20,000 µg Biotin, 1800 mg Pantothenic acid, 160 g Na, 50 g Mg,10,000 mg Zn, 7500 mg Fe, 7500 mg Mn, 150 mg J, 70 mg Co and 40 mg Se.

Diet composition (g/kg feed)		Nutrient concentration (g/kg feed)	
Maize	630	ME (MJ/kg)	12,90
Soya bean meal	320	Crude protein	197,1
Fish meal	10	Crude fat	28,08
Limestone	10	Crude fibre	35,94
Monocalcium phosphate	15	Calcium	8,60
Vitamin-mineral premix	10	Phosphorus	6,72
L-Lysine	5	Lysine	10,65

Table 5. Diet composition and calculated nutrient concentration on the second experiment.

weight (BW), daily weight gain (DWG) and feed conversion ratio (FCR), kg feed/kg body weight gain were measured weekly. Data are presented as arithmetic means with standard deviations (Mean ± SD). One-way analysis of variance and Student's t-test ($P < 0.05$) were performed to test the differences between levels of the probiotic in the diet.

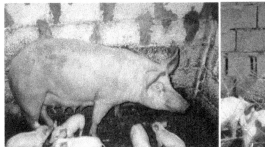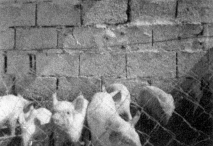

Figure 1. Piglets in the first and second experiments, in extensive farm condition.

10.2. Results and discussions

Parameters		Probiotic Dose (mg/kg feed)			
		0	1000	1500	2000
Production	n[1]				
Initial BW, kg	6	5.3 ± 0.65	5.4 ± 0.77	5.6 ± 0.37	5.1 ± 0.17
Fourth weeks[4]		12.59 ± 2.63	14.20 ± 1.62[a]	13.93 ± 0.82	10.97 ± 0.93[b]
Eighth weeks		19.89 ± 2.05	23.00 ± 2.73[a]	22.26 ± 2.42	18.84 ± 1.43[b]
DWG, g [2]		260.7 ± 33.8	314.3 ± 62.9[a]	297.6 ± 71.6	245.4 ± 46.5[b]
FCR [3]		3.01 ± 0.68	2.61 ± 0.25	2.67 ± 0.32	2.94 ± 0.42

Table 6. Effects of probiotic preparation on performance parameters in the first experiment (Mean ± SD).
[1] Number of animals/every group
[2] DWG for whole experimental period.
[3] FCR for whole experimental period.
[4] Significant differences, indicated with different superscripts.

Parameters		Probiotic Dose (mg/kg feed)			
		0	1000	1500	2000
Production	n[1]				
Initial BW, kg	6	4.8 ± 0.65	5.1 ± 0.77	5.0 ± 0.37	4.9 ± 0.17
Sixth weeks		16.37 ± 3.76	17.37 ± 4.06	16.98 ± 3.98	16.25 ± 3.45
DWG, g[2]		275.6 ± 46.7	292.3 ± 57.3	285.4 ± 51.8	270.4 ± 43.7
FCR [3]		3.20 ± 0.76	2.80 ± 0.48	2.87 ± 0.57	2.93 ± 0.68

Table 7. Effects of probiotic preparation on performance parameters in the second experiment (Mean ± SD).

In last ten years, most of the experiments were performed with piglets. According to the literature review, in many trials showed positive effects of probiotics on weaned piglets and also there were no significant effects of growing and finishing pigs. In the first trial the body weight gain was improved with graded levels (1000 and 1500 mg/kg feed) of the probiotic preparation respectively 15% to 11%, compare to control group. In the fourth and eighth weeks of this trial, a significant difference was documented. The body weight gain, on the second experiment was improved with graded levels (1000-1500 mg/kg feed) of the probiotic preparation from 3% to 6%, compare to control group, without significance. The FCR (kg feed/kg weight gain) in the first trial was improved with graded levels by up to 13.3%, 11.3% and 0.4% compare to control group and in the second trial respectively 12.5%, 10.4% and 8.5% compare to control group. The tendency for increasing of probiotic dose has not positive effects on performance parameters. Because of the low dose-response between 1000 and 1500 mg/kg feed, the level of 1000 mg/kg feed seems to be the optimal dose [64].

According to [20] on the experiments with weaned pigs and growing-finishing swine, used 1g/kg *Lactobacillus acidophilus*, which contains 4×10^6 viable cells per gram. Supplementation of the diet with 1g/kg *Lactobacillus acidophilus* on weaned pigs did not improve daily gain, feed intake or feed efficiency. Daily weight gain and feed intake of pigs, treated with 500 mg/kg *Lactobacillus acidophilus* showed non significant trends.

Reduction of diarrhoea by probiotics and vitality of piglets is one of the second topics in this study, because diarrhoea is the main problem for weaned piglets, especially during the first week after weaning. After two weeks of probiotic supplementation, we showed a reduction of diarrhoea on three treated groups. Reduction of diarrhoea by probiotic supplementation was study frequently by many scientist groups. Some of the trials showed significant effects, but the others have collected not significant data. A group of authors [29], [22], [68], [23] have used the same probiotic *Bacillus cereus* in different age of piglets, respectively 8 weeks piglets, 1-85 day after birth, 7-21 day after birth and 2 weeks post weaning. They showed statistical significance of diarrhoea reduction. [10] showed non significant effects, while they used *Bacillus cereus* in pigs 24-66 days of life.

11. Experiment in intensive farm condition

11.1. Material and methods

The animal trials were carried out at the experimental station of the Institute of Animal Nutrition of the Free University of Berlin, Germany. Thirty two piglets (White x Duroc) of three litters were transferred after weaning (28 days) to flat-decks and randomly allocated to 4 groups with 8 animals (4 male and 4 female). The basal diet was either supplemented with 1000, 1500 and 2000 mg/kg of the probiotic preparation or without supplementation (control).

The diets were offered ad libitum and animals had free access to water. The probiotic preparation included the following strains: *Lactobacillus plantarum* ATCC 14917 1×10^{11} CFU/kg, *Lactobacillus fermentum* DSM 20016 1×10^{11} CFU/kg and *Enterococcus faecium* ATCC 19434 1×10^{11} CFU/kg. During the six weeks period body weight (BW), daily weight gain (DWG) and feed conversion ratio (FCR), kg feed/kg body weight gain were measured weekly. Three piglets from each trial group were euthanized one week after probiotic administration by intracardial injection of T61 (Fa. Hoechst) after sedation with Stresnil*. Immediately after death, the abdomen was opened and ligatures were applied to collect digesta samples for pH measurement in defined segments of the duodenum, jejunum, ileum, caecum and colon. This operation was finished between 12-14 hours after death.

Diet composition (g/kg feed)		Nutrient concentration (g/kg feed)	
Maize	620	ME (MJ/kg)	12.82
Soybean meal	275	Crude protein	197.8
Soya oil	50	Crude fat	34.3
Fish meal	30	Crude fibre	31.4
Limestone	10	Calcium	9.10
Monocalcium phosphate	15	Posphorus	7.68
Vitamin -mineral premix[a]	12	Lysine	11.77
L-Lysine	10	Methionine+Cystine	7.64
Methionine+cystine	10	Threonine	8.04
Threonine	10	Tryptophane	2.37
Tryptophane	3		

Table 8. Diet composition and calculated nutrient concentration.
[a] Contents in 1 kg: 1,200,000 IE vit. A, 120,000 IE vit. D3, 4000 mg vit. E, 200 mg vit. B1, 600 mg Vit. B2, 2500 mg Niacin, 400 mg Vit. B6, 4500 µg Vit. B12, 20,000 µg Biotin, 1800 mg Pantothenic acid, 160 g Na, 50 g Mg,10,000 mg Zn, 7500 mg Fe, 7500 mg Mn, 150 mg J, 70 mg Co and 40 mg Se.

For determination of intestinal bacteria, the "Selective Media" method was used (CATC-agar (Citrat Acid Tween Carbonate - agar base) for *Enterococci spp*, MRS-agar (*Lactobacillus* agar acc to Man Rogosa and Sharp) for *Lactobacilli spp* and Mac Conkey for *Enterobacteria spp*). The colony of *aerobe and anaerobe* micro organisms by visual numbering were measured on agar plate.

The apparent nutrient digestibility was determined by the indicator method during the last week of the experiment using chromium (III) oxide (0.5%).

$$\text{Coeficient of digestibility} = 100 - \left(\frac{\% \text{ e indicator in feed x \% e nutrient in faeces}}{\% \text{ e indicator in faeces x \% e nutrient in feed}} \times 100 \right)$$

Data are presented as arithmetic means with standard deviations (Mean ± SD). One-way analysis of variance and Student's t-test ($P < 0.05$) were performed to test the differences between levels of the probiotic in the diet.

12. The methodology for determination of microbiological charge of faeces

Microbiological analyzes of faeces were performed in two periods:

- Week 1-3
- Week 5-7

In the first period, such analysis aim to consistently follow microbiological changes due to the "probiotics" effect.

In the second period, such analysis aim to compare the microbiological changes in the beginning and in the end of the experiment, as well as to judge on the duration of the "probiotics" effect after its termination.

Microbiological analyses were carried out of as follows:

3-4 hours after the feed, fresh faeces was collected in plastic boxes. Faeces of all boxes were gathered and placed in a separate box. 1 g of faeces was taken for each box, in three parallel tests A, A_1, A_2.

9 ml Ringer solution was added to it, and the following dilutions were prepared:

10^{-1}-10^{-9}, MRS for identification of *Lactobacillus spp*

10^{-4}-10^{-8}, CATC for identification of *Enterococcus spp*

10^{-3}-10^{-8}, McK for identification of *Enterobacteriaceae*

Its cultivation in Agar plates and incubation at a temperature of 37^0C was conducted within 24 hours.

13. The physiological and microbiological parameters of intestinal mucosa and digesta

A week after administration of probiotics, a total of 12 piglets were slaughtered, 3 piglets for every group.

The slaughtering of pigs a week after administration of probiotics aimed at:

- monitoring of the changes occurring in the pH digesta in the intestines.
- monitoring of all microbiological changes in digesta and mucosa, reflecting *Lactobacillus spp*, *Enterococcus spp* and *Escherichia coli* microbiological load as well as the total number of anaerobic bacteria in the jejunum, ileum, caecum and colon.

The preparation of samples for microbiological analysis was carried out as follows:

A 2x10cm area from all parts of intestine and colon is taken. Then, it is washed away with 0.9% NaCl solution, is measured its length, is thorn with a fine scalpel, is weighed and finally is placed in plastic tubes. Since jejunum is relatively long, it is divided into three parts for more convenience: jejunum 1, jejunum 2 and jejunum 3.

Measuring and weighing was done for the following parts:

Duodenum	Ileum
Jejunum 1	Caecum
Jejunum 2	Colon
Jejunum 3	

Microbiological load was estimated at:

Middle of jejunum, ileum, caecum, beginning of colon

14. The determination of anaerobic bacteria (*Lactobacillus spp*). Method of samples in ice

15 ml digesta is taken, is squeezed, and after is being cast into sterile plastic tubes and it is placed in ice.

0.5 g of this digesta is taken, 500 ml Ringer solution is added, and then is placed on ice.

Dilutions are prepared by mixing what is taken from both beakers up to 100µl.

20µl is taken by pipette and is dripped in Agar plates prepared based on the following dilutions:

MRS: 10^{-6} to 10^{-10} **Columbia - Blut:** 10^{-6} to 10^{-10}

15. Methods of samples in ice

Parts of the intestines are cut and placed in 50ml tubes together Ringer solution. Later solution is shaken and changed until no more digesta remains. The prepared solution is put into a bottle and placed in ice. Intestine is placed on a plate, mucosa is thorn and mixed. 0.5 g mucosa is taken; 500µl Ringer solution is added and placed on ice.

Dilutions are prepares as in the first case and are placed on ice.

20µl is taken by pipette and transferred to Agar plates prepared according to the following dilutions:

MRS: 10^{-5} to 10^{-9} **Columbia –Blut:** 10^{-5} to 10^{-10}

16. The determination of aerobic bacteria (*Enterobacteriaceae* and *Enterococcus spp*)

Digesta dilutions are prepared as above. 20µl solution is taken and transferred to Agar plates prepared according to the following dilutions:

Mac Conkey: 10^{-6} to 10^{-10} **CATC :** 10^{-3} to 10^{-7}

Mucosa dilutions are prepared. 20µl solution is taken and transferred to Agar plates prepared according to the following dilutions:

Mac Conkey : 10^{-3} to 10^{-7} **CATC :** 10^{-2} to 10^{-6}

Microbiological load was estimated: Middle of jejunum, ileum, caecum, beginning of colon

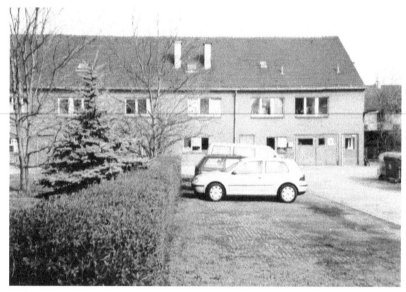

Figure 2. Institute of Animal Nutrition, Free University, Berlin

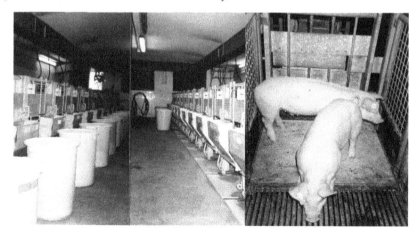

Figure 3. The animal trial at the experimental station of the Institute of Animal Nutrition.

17. Data about probiotic *"Seberini suini"*

17.1. Microbiological composition of probiotic

Lactobacillus plantarum   ATCC 14917 (LMG – S 16691) cfu 1x 10^{11}
Lactobacillus fermentum   DSM 20016 (LMG- S 16517) cfu 1x 10^{11}
Enterococcus faecium   ATCC 19434 (LMG- S 16690) cfu 1x 10^{11}

Composition of the probiotic "Seb Suini"

Lactobacillus plantarum	25 %
Enterococcus faecium	10 %
Lactobacillus fermentum	15 %
Micronized soya extraction meal	50 %

Chemical compositon %	Amino acids g/kg
Dry matter 88	Lysine 17
Crude protein 35	Leucine 17
Crude fat 1	Threonine 11
Crude fibre 5	Arginine 10
Crude ash 28	Tryptophan 3
	Izoleucine 11
	Hystidine 6
	Glycine 9
	Cystine 2
	Valine 13

Table 9. Chemical composition of the probiotic "Seb Suini" used in the experiment.

18. Physical -chemical characteristics of the probiotic

Smell	tipical, not bad
Apparent densities after shaking	0,45 kg/liter.
Point of degradability	> 250⁰C
Density	450 gr/liter
Water solubility	non digestible, hydrodispersible.
Granulometry	90% e grimcave kalojnë sitën 200 micron.
Value of pH	6,5 (10 gr on 100 ml in temperature 20⁰C)

Microbiological characteristics

Total not lactic flora	maximum 5 x 10^3 UFC/gr
Enterobacteriaceae	absent
Coliformes	absent
Enterococcus	maximum 5 x 10^2 UFC/gr
Yeasts and moulds	maximum 1 x 10^2 UFC/gr

According to the analyzes made in the Institute of Soil Chemistry, "Universitá Cattolica del Sacro Cuore"- Piacenza, results heavy metal contain

Pb	<0,6	ppm
Cd	94	ppm
Ni	11	ppm
Cr	15	ppm
As	1, 18	ppm
Hg	112	ppm

It does not contain Alfa-toxine B_1, B_2, G_1, G_2, Zearalenone, Ocratoxine, Fumosine B_1,

Deossinivalenolo   122,0g / Kg tq

19. Results and discussions

Parameters		Probiotic Dose (mg/kg feed)			
		Control	1000	1500	2000
Production	n^1				
-Initial BW, kg	8	5.6 ± 1.11	5.5 ± 1.07	5.6 ± 1.17	5.6 ± 1.02
-BW 6th week [2]	5	19.5 ± 5.10	19.8 ± 5.83	23.1 ± 3.17	22.3 ± 7.01
Feed intake, kg		24.5 ± 7.49	25.4 ± 6.44	29.79 ± 5.42	30.4 ± 7.47
DWG, g [3]		325 ± 153	341 ± 128	427 ± 71	436 ± 123
FCR [4]		1.79 ± 0.48	1.78 ± 0.31	1.65 ± 0.05	1.66 ± 0.15

Table 10. Effects of probiotic preparation on performance parameters (Mean ± SD).
[1] Number of animals, (8 piglets/ every group, at the beginning of the experiment)
[2] Number of animals, (5 piglets/every group, one week after probiotic supplementation). n = 4 at treatment 1500 mg/kg in 6th week.
[3] DWG for whole experimental period.
[4] FCR for whole experimental period.

The body weight gain was improved with graded levels of the probiotic preparation from 4.9 up to 31.7%. Caused by the high coefficient of variation the differences were not significant. The FCR (kg feed/kg weight gain) was improved with graded levels by 0.6 up to 7.3%. The differences were not significant. Because of the low dose-response between 1500 and 2000 mg/kg feed, the level of 1500 mg/kg feed seems to be the optimal dose.

The same results showed [30] on the experiments with weaned piglets, used LFP-Lactobacillus-Fermentation-Product. This probiotic contents Lactobacillus bulgaricus, Lactobacillus casei, Streptococcus thermophilus, produced in Quebec, Canada. The basal diet was supplemented with 100 mg LFP/kg feed.

The feed intake and the daily weight gain (DWG) were increased respectivly 11.8% and 10.4%, compared with the control group. The feed conversion ratio (FCR) was in the same level.

Two authors [19] used the same probiotic LFP (*Lactobacillus-fermentation-product*) on the weaned piglets. Pigs fed a diet with 0.36 ml/kg LFP required nearly 10% less feed per unit of weight gain than the control group. Also the incidence of scouring decreased (P< 0.05) in pigs fed with different levels of LFP. Overall improvement occurred up through the addition of 0.36 ml/kg LFP with no additional benefit from greater amounts. Another group of authors [44] showed the effects of microbial feed additives on performance of starter and growing-finishing pigs. One of the experimental group with weaned piglets was fed with 750 mg *Lactobacillus acidophilus*/kg feed. The second experimental group was supplemented with 1250 mg *Streptococcus faecium*/kg feed.

The addition of *Lactobacillus acidophilus* to the feed of young pigs improved average daily weight gain by 9.7 % and the feed conversion ratio by 21.4%, whereas the addition of *Streptococcus faecium* decreased average daily weight gain. The addition of acid lactic improved feed conversion, suggesting that lactic acid as a metabolite produced during fermentation might be the reason for the improvement in performance. The probiotics had no effect on growing-finishing pigs.

In a trial with 90 untreated and 90 treated (*Bacillus cereus*-preparation) weaned piglets, the probiotic treated animals gained 7% more live weight during 6 weeks after weaning with a reduced feed conversion ratio of 2.4%. However, both results were not significant. This points towards a high variation in the response of the individual animals to this type of feed additives [23].

Parameters	N^1	Probiotic Dose (mg/kg feed)			
		Control	1000	1500	2000
Digestibility [2] (in %)	5				
Dry matter		76.4 ± 6.90	73.2 ± 10.39	67.2 ± 2.22	75.7 ± 9.52
Crude fat		75.1 ± 5.48	71.2 ± 2.60	69.0 ± 9.11	70.0 ± 3.77
Crude fibre		51.1 ± 7.82	54.5 ± 7.48	52.3 ± 5.79	56.4 ± 2.31
Digesta pH	3				
Duodenum		5.54 ± 0.96	5.74 ± 0.68	5.87 ± 0.83	6.51 ± 0.77
Jejunum		6.24 ± 0.38	6.17 ± 0.66	6.29 ± 0.51	6.56 ± 0.85
Ileum[3]		7.05 ± 0.43[a]	6.43 ± 0.77[b]	6.41 ± 0.16[b]	5.25 ± 0.12[c]
Caecum		5.62 ± 0.13	5.65 ± 0.20	5.79 ± 0.39	5.55 ± 0.09
Colon		5.87 ± 0.27	6.19 ± 0.38	6.27 ± 0.37	6.18 ± 0.43

Table 11. Effects of probiotic preparation on apparent nutrient digestibility and digesta pH of defined intestinal segments (Mean ± SD).
[1] Number of animals.
[2] Crude nutrients were determined by Weende scheme.
[3] Significant differences, indicated with different superscripts.

Feeding probiotic preparation slightly increased the crude fiber digestibility compared to the control group in the range of 3.4%, 1.2% and 5.4% at supplementations with 1000, 1500 and 2000 mg/kg feed, respectively. With graded levels of the probiotic preparation pH of the chyme of ileum and caecum was slightly decreased, in contrast the pH of duodenum and jejunum was slightly increased [63]. The low effect of pH was agreement with digestibility results. The pH results in the duodenum and jejunum is in contrast to former results reported by [35]. This is possibly caused by the combination of different strains used in this study.

Two authors [19] supplemented the diets of growing pigs with LFP preparation (Lactobacillus Fermentation Produced) and observed that a supplementation of 0.72 mg LFP/kg feed increased the crude fibber digestibility with 14.2% compared to the control group (P< 0.05).

These authors assumed that the rate of passage of feed through the digestive tract was decreased by feeding LFP, which allowed more time for digestion of crude fiber. Also the urinary nitrogen excretion was greater than faecal excretion but both combined were less then intake, thus resulting in a positive nitrogen balance. In total, the digestibility of dry matter was decreased 0.4% and the digestibility of crude protein did not change, compared to the control. Another author [58] showed the influence of Lactobacillus acidophilus in broïler chicks on growth, feed conversion and crude fat digestibility. The addition of Lactobacillus acidophilus in broïler chicks diet decreased the digestibility of crude fat.

| | | | Probiotic Dose (mg/kg feed) | | |
		Control	1000	1500	2000
1st week of trial	Lactobacilli spp.	95	120	150	170
	Enterococci spp.	0.01	0.94	1.12	1.23
	Escherichia coli.	10	10	32	2
6th weeks of trial	Lactobacilli spp.	683 ± 584	223 ± 191	345 ± 403	767 ± 306
	Enterococci spp.	0.018 ± 0.031	0.1 ± 0.131	0.011 ± 0.01	0.028 ± 0.02
	Escherichia coli.	2.35 ± 3.60	15 ± 21.8	0.05 ± 0	0.083 ± 0.057

Table 12. The effect of probiotic preparation on the microbial composition of faeces (CFU*10^6/g wet weight) (Mean ± SD).
* Four faeces samples/every group were collected/every week, during the experimental period.

The effect of probiotic preparation on the microbial composition of faeces was examined early, one week after supplementation, because the first week after weaning is critical period for tends to shift the balance of the gut microflora away from beneficial bacteria towards pathogenic bacteria. One week after weaning piglets fed with the probiotic preparation showed increased the concentration of Lactobacilli spp. and Enterococci spp. compared to the control treatment. Feeding 2000 mg probiotic preparation/kg feed induced a reduction of Escherichia coli. At the end of the experiment piglets fed with 1500 and 2000 mg probiotic preparation/kg feed had reduced Escherichia coli compared to the control. These results indicate that the probiotic preparation may be less suppressive to the Escherichia coli. [40]

observed the similar microbial changes in the faeces of weaned piglets, fed with the same combined probiotic preparation.

			Probiotic Dose (mg/kg feed)		
		Control	1000	1500	2000
Jejunum	*Anaerobe bacteria.*	13.92 ±14.15	12.22 ± 12.45	8.75 ± 8.60	12.98 ± 13.07
	Lactobacilli spp.	10.24 ± 10.44	12.58 ± 12.78	8.36 ± 8.38	11.60 ± 11.55
	Enterococci spp.	7.02 ± 6.98	8.03 ± 8.22	7.00 ± 7.19	7.01 ± 6.97
	Escherichia coli.	7.57 ± 7.74	8.60 ± 8.72	6.00 ± 0.00	7.90 ± 8.02
Ileum	*Anaerobe bacteria.*	13.17 ± 13.36	13.21 ± 13.20	13.21 ± 13.20	12.60 ± 12.72
	Lactobacilli spp.	12.87 ± 13.11	12.69 ± 12.73	12.72 ± 12.95	13.68 ± 13.89
	Enterococci spp.	6.00 ± 0.00	8.82 ± 9.06	7.33 ± 7.55	7.02 ± 7.22
	Escherichia coli.	8.17 ± 8.17	11.00 ± 11.23	12.01 ± 12.25	12.05 ± 12.23
Caecum	*Anaerobe bacteria.*	13.90 ± 13.85	12.69 ± 12.84	13.75 ± 13.87	13.98 ±14.12
	Lactobacilli spp.	13.28 ± 13.48	12.60 ± 12.84	13.43 ± 13.65	13.83 ± 14.05
	Enterococci spp.	6.86 ± 7.04	10.00 ± 10.23	7.80 ± 8.03	6.84 ± 6.70
	Escherichia coli.	12.69 ± 12.93	10.00 ± 10.23	10.82 ± 11.06	10.86 ± 11.04
Colon	*Anaerobe bacteria.*	14.72 ± 14.92	13.04 ± 13.06	13.95 ± 14.18	13.93 ± 14.15
	Lactobacilli spp.	12.55 ± 12.49	13.01 ± 13.23	13.84 ± 14.08	13.92 ± 14.10
	Enterococci spp.	8.82 ± 9.06	9.00 ± 9.23	12.01 ± 12.25	9.12 ± 9.36
	Escherichia coli.	13.44 ± 13.68	11.30 ± 11.53	12.69 ± 12.93	12.39 ± 12.59

Table 13. The effect of probiotic preparation on the microbial composition of digesta, one week after probiotic supplementation. (log CFU/g wet weight), (Mean ± SD; n = 3).

The effects of the probiotic preparation on the microbial composition of the chyme showed no dose–depended effects. However there was a tendency for increasing of the concentration of *Lactobacilli* spp. and *Enterococci* spp. in the colon compared to the control.

A group of authors [1] supplemented the pig diets with a combination of *Lactobacillus fermentum* 14 and *Streptococcus salivarius* 312 for 4 days and observed a significant reduction in the *Escherichia coli* count in both the stomach and duodenum. A significant reduction of *Escherichia coli* number in the stomach was also found, when *Lactobacillus fermentum* was supplemented separate. In cases of diarrhoea caused by *Escherichia coli* the treatment as described here was not effective because the count of *Escherichia coli* in the duodenum of culture-fed pigs was still greater than 10^6/g. However, if the antibacterial effect of strain 14 could be increased some effect on scouring due to *Escherichia coli* should follow. This might be accomplished by the feeding of large numbers of organisms or by the administration in a concentrated form of the inhibitory factors produced by *Lactobacillus fermentum* strain 14. [15] showed that the application of 10^8 colony forming units (CFU) of a *Bacillus cereus* preparation/kg feed to piglets reduced counts for *Lactobacilli* spp. *Bifidobacteria, Eubacteria* and *Escherichia coli* in the duodenum and jejunum, but increased respective CFU in the ileum, caecum and colon.

Two authors [35] showed a significant reduction of *Escherichia coli* CFU in the small intestine of piglets was also noted when an *Enterococcus faecium* preparation was applied. However, at the same time *Lactobacilli spp.* and *Enterococci spp.* counts increased as a trend and statistically significant, respectively [24].

The results of studies on the ability of probiotic bacteria to reduce the colonization of pathogenic bacteria are ambiguous. Challenge studies with piglets and *Escherichia coli* O141:K85 showed no influence on clinical symptoms, mortality or excretion of hemolytic *Escherichia coli* [8]. A group of authors [24] showed that the colonization with mucosa associated *Enterobacteria spp.* was reduced when a probiotic *Bacillus cereus* preparation was supplemented.

The probiotic had no influence on the occurrence of pathogenic *Escherichia coli* as measured with a PCR assay [16]. These results point to the fact that hygienic conditions in scientific institutes may sometimes be too favorable to investigate effects of pathogenic bacteria without challenge trials [54].

These and the other studies imply that probiotics are able to reduce/enhance specific bacterial groups, but the reduction of total bacterial cell numbers as recorded for antibiotics is probably not a probiotic mode of action. In order to understand the casual relationships which lead to the observed improvements in weight gain and feed conversion or general health of animals, possible interactions between bacteria in the intestine and host animal must be studied. Of special significance are interactions between the metabolism of the host and metabolic activity of intestinal bacterial populations [54].

20. Conclusions

The supplementation of the combined probiotic preparation induced slightly the performance data. In extensive farm condition, a significant difference of daily weight gain (DWG) was documented four weeks after probiotic supplementation. A positive effect of the probiotic on feed conversion ratio (FCR), kg feed/kg weight gain and vitality was observed, also. We recommend the level of 1000mg/kg feed combined probiotic as the optimal dose.

Combined probiotic preparation induced slightly the performance data in intensive farm condition, also. However the differences were not significant. Feeding probiotic preparation slightly increased the crude fibre digestibility in all treated groups. With graded levels of the probiotic preparation pH of the chyme of ileum and caecum was slightly decreased, in contrast the pH of duodenum and jejunum was slightly increased. The probiotic preparation showed increased the concentration of *Lactobacilli spp.* and *Enterococci spp.* compared to the control. The results indicate that the probiotic preparation may be less suppressive to the *Escherichia coli.* The effects of the probiotic preparation on the microbial composition of the chyme showed no dose–depended effects. However there was a tendency for increasing of the concentration of *Lactobacilli spp.* and *Enterococci spp.* in the colon compared to the control. Possibly this was due to the combined probiotic preparation. At the end, we recommend the level of 1500 mg/kg feed combined probiotic as the optimal dose.

* Approved by competent authority according to Council Directive 86/609/EEC of 24 November1986 on the approximation of laws, regulations and administrative provisions of the Member States, regarding the protection of animals used for experimental and other scientific purposes.

Author details

Etleva Delia and Myqerem Tafaj
Faculty of Agriculture and Environment, Agricultural University of Tirana, Albania

Klaus Männer
Institut fur Tierernährung, Freie Universität Berlin, Germany

Acknowledgement

The authors are grateful to Dr. K. Schäffer and all technicians stuff for technical assistance. Research stay of Dr. E. Delia in Institut für Tierernährung, Freie Universität, Berlin, Germany was financial supported by Deutsche Gesellschaft für Technische Zusammenarbeit (GTZ) and Tempus Phare Project "Animal Science Albania" AC_JEP-14123-1999.

21. References

[1] Barrow P.A, Brooker B.E, Fuller R, Newport M.J (1980) The attachment of bacteria to the gastric epithelium of the pigs and its importance in the microecology of the intestine. J. Appl. Bacteriol. 48: 147-154.

[2] Bernet-Camard M.F, Coconnier M.H, Haudault S, Servin A.L (1996) Differentiation - associated antimicrobial functions in human colon adenocarcinoma cell lines. Exp. Cell. Res, 226: 80-89.

[3] Breves G, Walter C, Burmeister M, Shröder B (2000) In vitro studies on the effects of *Saccharomyces boulardii* and *Bacillus cereus* var. *toyoi* on nutrient transport in pig jejunum. J. Anim. Physiol and Anim Nutrition. 84: 9-20.

[4] Brooks P.H, Beal J.D, Dmeckova V, Niven S. (2003) Probiotics for pigs and beyond. In: Van Vooren and B. Rochet. Role of probiotics in animal nutrition and their link to the demands of Europian consumers, ID-Lelystad, 49-59.

[5] Castagliuolo I, Riegler M.F, Valenick L, LaMont J.T, Pothoulakis C (1999) *Saccharomyces boulardii* protease inhibits the effects of *Clostridium difficile* toxins A and B in human colonic mucosa. Infect. Immun. 67: 302–307.

[6] Collins M.D, Gibson G.R (1999) Probiotics, prebiotics and synbiotics: approaches for modulating the microbial ecology of the gut. Am. J. Clin Nutr. 69 (Suppl):1052S-1057S.

[7] Dahlman-Hoglund A, Hanson L.A, Ahlstedt S (1997) Induction of oral tolerance with effects on numbers of IgE-carrying mast cells and on bystander suppression in young rats. Clinical Experimental Immunology 108:128-137.

[8] De Cupere F, Deprez P, Demeulenaere D, Muylle E (1992) Evaluation of the effect of 3 probiotics on experimental *Escherichia coli* enterotoxaemia in weaned piglets. J. Vet. Med. Bulletin. 39: 277-284.

[9] Durst L, Feldner M, Gedek B, Eckel B (1998) Bakterien als Probiotikum in der Sauenfütterung und der Ferkelaufzucht. Kraftfutter 9: 356-364.

[10] Eidelsburger U, Kirchgessner M, Roth F.X (1992) Zum Einfluss von Fumarsäure, Salzsäure, Natriumformiat, Tylosin und Toyocerin auf tagliche Zunahmen, Futteraufnahme, Futterverwertung und Verdaulichkeit: 11. Mitt. Journal of Animal Physiologie and Animal Nutrition. 68, 82-92.

[11] Freitag M, Hensche H-U, Schulte-Sienbeck H, Reichelt B, (1998) Kritische Betrachtung des Einsatzes von Leistungsförderern in der Tierernährung. Forschungsberichte der Universität Paderborn, Nr. 8.

[12] Fuller R (1989) Probiotics in man and animals. J. Appl. Bacteriol. 66: 365-378.

[13] Fuller R (1999) Probiotics for farm animals. Probiotics: A critical Review.

[14] Gaskins H.R (1996) Immunological aspects of host microbiota interactions at the intestinal epithelium. Gastrointestinal microbiology, 2: 537-587.

[15] Gedek K, Kirchgessner M, Wiehler S, Bott A, Eidelsburger U, Roth F.X. (1993) Zur Nutritiven Wirksamkeit von *Bacillus cereus* als probiotikum in der ferkelaufzucht. Archiv Anim. Nut. 44: 215-226.

[16] Goebel S, Vahjen W, Jadamus A, Simon O (2000) PCR assay for detection of porcine pathogenic *Escherichia coli* virulence factors in the gastrointestinal tract of piglets fed a spore forming probiotic. Proc. 9th Society for Nutrition and Physiology. 64.

[17] Goerke B (2000) Untersuchungen zur Schleimhautmorphologie im Dünn-und Dickdarm nach oraler Applikation von *Saccharomyces boulardii* und *Bacillus cereus var.toyoi* beim Schwein. Doctor Thesis, Tierärztliche Hochschule Hannover, Germany.

[18] Goldin B.R, Gorbach S.L, Saxelin M, Barakat S, Gualtieri L, Salminen S (1992) Survival of *Lactobacillus* species (strain GG) in human gastrointestinal tract. Dig. Dis. Sci. 37: 121–128.

[19] Hale O.M, Newton K.I (1979) Effetcs of a nonviable *Lactobacillus species fermentation product* on performance of pigs. J. Anim. Sci. ;48(4):770-775

[20] Harper A.F, Kornegay E.T, Brayant K.L, Thoman H.R (1983) Efficacy of virginiamycin and a commercially-available *Lactobacillus* probiotic in swine diets. Anim Feed Sci Technol, 8: 69-76.

[21] Havernaar R, Ten Brink B, Huis in't Veld J.H.J (1992) Selection of strains for probiotic use. In: Probiotics. The scientific basis. R.Fuller (Ed.). Chapman& Hall, London, 209-224.

[22] Iben Ch Leibetseder J (1989) Untersuchung der leistungsfördernden Wirkung von Toyocerin in der Ferkelaufzucht. Wien. Tierärztliche Monatsschrift 76: 363-366.

[23] Jadamus A (2001) Untersuchungen zur Wirksamkeit und Wirkungsweise des sporenbildenden *Bacillus cereus* var. *toyoi* im Verdauungstrakt von Broilern und Ferkel. Degree Dissertation, Free University, Berlin

[24] Jadamus A, Vahjen W, Simon O (2000) Influence of the probiotic bacterial strain, *Bacillus cereus var. toyoi* on the development of selected microbial groups adhering to intestinal mucosal tissues of piglets. J. Anim. Feed Sci.;9: 347-362.

[25] Jadamus A, Vahjen W, Simon O (2001) Growth behaviour of a spore forming probiotic strain in the gastrointestinal tract of broiler chicken and piglets. Archiv of Anim. Nut. 54: 1-17.

[26] Kaila M, Isolauri E, Soppi E, Virtanen E, Laine S, Arvilommi H (1992) Enhancement of the circulating antibody secreting cell response in human diarrhea by a human *Lactobacillus* strain. Pediatr. Res. 32: 141–144.

[27] Kirchgessner M, Roth R.X, Eidelsburger U, Gedek B (1993) Zur nutritiven Wirksamkeit von *Bacillus cereus* als probiotikum in der Ferkelaufzucht. 1 mittelung Einfluss auf Wachstumsparameter und gastrointestinales Milieu. Archives of Animal Nutrition 44: 111-121.

[28] Klein U, Schmidts H.L (1997) Zum Einfluss des Bioregulators Paciflor auf die Morphologie der Dünndarmmukosa beim Schwein. Proceedings of the Society for Nutrition and Physiology 6:41.

[29] Kyriakis S.C, Tsiloyiannis V.K, Vlemmas J, Sarris K, Tsinas A.C, Alexopoulos C, Jansegers L (1999) The effect of probiotic LSP 122 on the control of post-weaning diarrhea syndrome of piglets. Research Veterinary Science 67, 223-228.

[30] Lessard M, Brisson G.J, (1987) Effect of *Lactobacillus Fermentation Product* on growth immune response and fecal enzyme activity in weaned pigs. Can. J. Anim. Sci. 67: 509-516.

[31] Maassen, C.B., van Holten-Neelen, C., Balk, F., den Bak-Glashouwer, M. J., Leer, R. J., Laman, J.D., Boersma, W.J. and Claassen, E (2000): Strain-dependent induction of cytokine profiles in the gut by orally administered Lactobacillus strains. Vaccine 18, 2613-2623.

[32] Mack D.R, Michael S, Wei S, McDougall L, Holligsworth M.A (1999) Probiotics inhibits enteropathogenic E. coli adherence in vitro by inducing intestinal mucin gene expression. American Journal of Physiology 276: G941-G950.

[33] Mangell P, Nejdfors P, Wang M, Ahrne S, Westrom B, Thorlacius I, Jeppsson B (2002) *Lactobacillus plantarum* 299v inhibits Escherichia coli induced intestinal permeability. Digestive Disease Science 47: 511-516.

[34] Männer K, Jadamus A, Vahjen W, Frackenpohl U, Simon O (2002) Effekte probiotischer Zusätze auf Leistungsparameter und intestinale Mikroflora. Proc. 7. Tagung, Schweine und Geflügelernährung;78-80.

[35] Männer K, Spieler A (1997) Probiotics in piglets, an alternative to traditional growth promoters. Microecology and Therapy 26: 243-256.

[36] Marin M.L, Lee J.H, Murtha J, Ustunol Z, Petka J.J (1997) Differential cytokine production in clonal macrophage and T-cell lines cultured with bifidobacteria. Journal of Dairy Science 80, 2713-2720.

[37] McCraken Vance J, Gaskins H Rex (1999) Probiotics and the immune system. Probiotics: A critical review. 85-111.

[38] Metchnikoff E (1907) The prolongation of life. Heinemann, London, UK.

[39] Moreau M.C, Corthier G (1988) Effect of gastrointestinal microflora on induction and maintenance of oral tolerance to ovalbumin in C3H/HeJ mice. Infection and Immunity, 56: 2766-2768.

[40] Morelli L (1995) Variations of *Coliformes* and *Lactobacilli spp* content in liquid or soft faeces belonging at swines treaties and not treaties. Published by AKRON-firm, Milano. on the mucosal IgA response of mice to dietary antigens. Bioscience Biotechnology Biochemistry 62: 10-15.

[41] Neutra M.R, Forstner J.F (1987) Gastrointestinal mucus: Synthesis, secretion and function 975-1009. In L.R. Johnson (ed), Physiology of the gastrointestinal tract, 2nd edition. Raven Press, New York.

[42] Oullette A.J, Selsted M.E (1996) Paneth cell defensins: Endogenous peptide components of intestinal host defense. FASEB journal 10: 1280-1289.

[43] Perdigon G, Alvarez S, de Ruiz P, Holgado A (1991) Immunoadjuvant activity of oral *Lactobacillus casei*: influence of dose on the secretory immune response and protective capacity in intestinal infections. Journal of Dairy Research 58, 485-496.

[44] Pollmann D.S, Danielson D.M, Peo E.R (1980) Effects of microbial feed additives on performace of starter and growing-finishing pigs. J. Anim. Sci. 51(3): 577-581.

[45] Pouwels P.H, Leer R.J, Boersma W.J (1996) The potential of *Lactobacillus* as a carrier for oral immunization: development and preliminary characterization of vector systems for targeted delivery of antigens. J. Biotechnol. 44: 183–192.

[46] Qu X.D, Lloyd K.C, Walsh J.H, Lehrer R.I (1996) Secretion of type II phospholipase A and cryptdin by rat small intestinal Paneth cells. Infect. Immun. 64: 5161-5165.

[47] Rolfe D.R (2000) The role of probiotic cultures in the control of gastrointestinal health. Symposium: Probiotic bacteria: Implications for Human Health.

[48] Rolfe R (1996) Colonization resistance. In R I Mackie, B A White and R E Isaacson (ed), Gastrointestinal microbiology. Gastrointestinal microbes and host interactions. Chapman and Hall. New York. 2: 501-536.

[49] Savage, D. C. (1986) Gastrointestinal micro flora in mammalian nutrition. Ann. Rev. Nutr, 6: 155-178.

[50] Scharek L, Hartmann L, Heinevette R.L, Blaut M (2000) *Bifidobacterium adolescentis* modulates the specific immune response to another human gut bacterium, *Bacteroides thetaiotaomicron*, in gnotobiotic rats. Immunobiology 202, 429-441.

[51] Scumm H, Pohl R, Willeke H (1990) Ergebnisse des Einsatzes von Suiferm bei Absatzferkeln mit Durchfällen zur Aufrechterhaltung und Wiederherstellung der gesunden Darmflora. Tierärztliche Umschau 45: 402-411.

[52] Shu Q, Qu F, Gill H.S (2001) Probiotic treatment using *Bifidobacterium lactis* HNO19 reduces weanling diarrhea associated lymphoid tissue in neonatal swine. Immunological Methods 241, 185-199.

[53] Simon O, Jadamus A, Vahjen W (2001) Probiotic feed additives–effectiveness and expected modes of action. J. Anim. Sci. 10 Supp 11: 51-67

[54] Simon O, Vahjen W, Scharek L (2003) Microorganisms as Feed Additive-Probiotics. Proc. 9 th International Symposium on Digestive Physiology in Pigs, Banff, Canada; Vol 1: 295-318.

[55] Solano-Aguilar G.I, Vengroski K.G, Beshah E, Lunney J.K (2000) Isolation and purification of lymphocyte subset from gut-associated lymphoid tissue in neonatal swine. Immunological Methods 241: 185-199.

[56] Stokes C:R, Bailey M, Wilson A.D (1994) Immunolofy of the porcine gastrointestinal tract. Veterinary Immunology and Immunopathology 43: 143-150.

[57] Takahashi T, Nakagawa E, Nara T, Yajima T, Kuwata T (1998) Effects of orally ingested *Bifidobacterium longum*

[58] Tortuer OF (1973) Influence of implantation of *Lactobacillus acidophilus* in chicks on the growth, feed conversion, malabsorption of fats syndrome and intestinal flora. Poult. Sci. 2: 197-203.

[59] Tournut J (1989) Les probiotique en élevage: applications. Revue Scientifique et Technique de l'Office International des Epizooties, 8: 533-549.

[60] Travnicek J, Mandel L, Trebichavsky I, Talafantova M (1989) Immunological state of adult germfree miniature Minnesota pigs. Folia Microbiologia. 34, 157-164.

[61] Tuschy D (1986) Verwendung von' Probiotika' als Leistungsförderer in der Tierernährung. Übersichten Tierernährung 14, 157-178.

[62] Vega-Lopez M.A, Arenas-Contreras G, Bailey M, Gonzalez-Pozos S, Stokes C.R, Ortega M.G, Mondragon-Flores R (2001) Development of intraepithelial cells in the porcine small intestine. Dev Immunology 8, 147-158.

[63] Veizaj E, Tafaj M, Männer K (2008) The effect of the combined probiotic preparation on growth performance, digestibility and microbial composition of faeces of weaned piglets. Agricultura, 5: 37-41.

[64] Veizaj-Delia E, Piu Th. Lekaj P, Tafaj M (2010) Using combined probiotic to improve growth performance of weaned piglets on extensive farm conditions. Livestock Science, 134, Issues 1-3, 249-251.

[65] Vitini E, Alvarez S, Medina M, Medici M, de Budeguer M.V, Perdigon G (2001) Gut mucosal immunostimulation by lactic acid bacteria. Biocell 24, 223-232.

[66] Winckler C, Schröder B, Breves G (1998) Effects of *Saccharomyces boulardii*, *Bacillus cereus var. caron* and *Bacillus cereus var. toyoi* on epithelial transport functions in pig jejunum. Zeitschrift für Gastroenterologiy (Suppl. 1) 30-37.

[67] Wostmann B.S (1996) Nutrition. In B.S. Wostmann (ed), Germfree and gnotobiotic animal models. CRC Press, Boca Raton Fl, 71-87.

[68] Zani J.K, Weykamp da Cruz F, Freitas dos Santos A, Gil-Turnes C (1998) Effect of probiotic CenBiot on the control of diarrhoea and feed efficiency in pigs. Journal of Applied Microbiology 84, 68-71.

[69] Zimmerman G, Bollinger R, McDonald J.C, (1970) Possible production of immunosuppression in the host by exposure to microorganisms: observations in germfree rats. Surgery Forum. 21: 236-238.

Permissions

The contributors of this book come from diverse backgrounds, making this book a truly international effort. This book will bring forth new frontiers with its revolutionizing research information and detailed analysis of the nascent developments around the world.

We would like to thank Prof. Dr. Everlon Cid Rigobelo, for lending his expertise to make the book truly unique. He has played a crucial role in the development of this book. Without his invaluable contribution this book wouldn't have been possible. He has made vital efforts to compile up to date information on the varied aspects of this subject to make this book a valuable addition to the collection of many professionals and students.

This book was conceptualized with the vision of imparting up-to-date information and advanced data in this field. To ensure the same, a matchless editorial board was set up. Every individual on the board went through rigorous rounds of assessment to prove their worth. After which they invested a large part of their time researching and compiling the most relevant data for our readers. Conferences and sessions were held from time to time between the editorial board and the contributing authors to present the data in the most comprehensible form. The editorial team has worked tirelessly to provide valuable and valid information to help people across the globe.

Every chapter published in this book has been scrutinized by our experts. Their significance has been extensively debated. The topics covered herein carry significant findings which will fuel the growth of the discipline. They may even be implemented as practical applications or may be referred to as a beginning point for another development. Chapters in this book were first published by InTech; hereby published with permission under the Creative Commons Attribution License or equivalent.

The editorial board has been involved in producing this book since its inception. They have spent rigorous hours researching and exploring the diverse topics which have resulted in the successful publishing of this book. They have passed on their knowledge of decades through this book. To expedite this challenging task, the publisher supported the team at every step. A small team of assistant editors was also appointed to further simplify the editing procedure and attain best results for the readers.

Our editorial team has been hand-picked from every corner of the world. Their multi-ethnicity adds dynamic inputs to the discussions which result in innovative outcomes. These outcomes are then further discussed with the researchers and contributors who give their valuable feedback and opinion regarding the same. The feedback is then collaborated with the researches and they are edited in a comprehensive manner to aid the understanding of the subject.

Apart from the editorial board, the designing team has also invested a significant amount of their time in understanding the subject and creating the most relevant covers. They scrutinized every image to scout for the most suitable representation of the subject and create an appropriate cover for the book.

The publishing team has been involved in this book since its early stages. They were actively engaged in every process, be it collecting the data, connecting with the contributors or procuring relevant information. The team has been an ardent support to the editorial, designing and production team. Their endless efforts to recruit the best for this project, has resulted in the accomplishment of this book. They are a veteran in the field of academics and their pool of knowledge is as vast as their experience in printing. Their expertise and guidance has proved useful at every step. Their uncompromising quality standards have made this book an exceptional effort. Their encouragement from time to time has been an inspiration for everyone.

The publisher and the editorial board hope that this book will prove to be a valuable piece of knowledge for researchers, students, practitioners and scholars across the globe.

List of Contributors

Renata Ernlund Freitas de Macedo
School of Agricultural Sciences and Veterinary Medicine, Pontifical Catholic University of Parana, Sao Jose dos Pinhais, Parana, Brazil

Sérgio Bertelli Pflanzer and Carolina Lugnani Gomes
Food Technology Department, Faculty of Food Engineer, State University of Campinas, Campinas, Sao Paulo, Brazil

Rafael Vieira de Azevedo
State University of Norte Fluminense Darcy Ribeiro, Center for Agricultural Science and Technology, Campos dos Goytacazes, Rio de Janeiro, Brazil

Luís Gustavo Tavares Braga
State University of Santa Cruz, Department of Agricultural and Environmental Sciences, Ilhéus, Bahia, Brazil

Yunior Acosta Aragón
Biomin Holding GmbH, Herzogenburg, Austria

Everlon Cid Rigobelo and Fernando Antonio de Ávila
UNESP Animal Science Faculty of Dracena, UNESP Department of Veterinary Pathology, Brazil

José Maurício Schneedorf
Biochemistry Laboratory, Exact Sciences Institute, Federal University of Alfenas, MG, Brazil

Oscar M. Laudanno
Gastroenterologia Experimental, School of Medicina, Rosario UNR, Argentina

Frédérique Chaucheyras-Durand
Lallemand Animal Nutrition, Blagnac, France
INRA UR 454 Microbiologie, Saint-Genès Champanelle, France

Eric Chevaux
Lallemand Animal Nutrition, Blagnac, France

Cécile Martin
INRA UMR 1213 Herbivores, Saint-Genès Champanelle, France

Evelyne Forano
INRA UR 454 Microbiologie, Saint-Genès Champanelle, France

Luciana Kazue Otutumi and Marcelo Biondaro Góis
Universidade Paranaense, Brazil

Elis Regina de Moraes Garcia
Universidade Estadual do Mato Grosso do Sul, Brazil

Maria Marta Loddi
Universidade Estadual de Ponta Grossa, Brazil

Gabriela Zárate
Centro de Referencias para Lactobacilos (CERELA)-CONICET, San Miguel de Tucumán, Argentina

María del Carmen Monroy Dosta, Talía Castro Barrera, Francisco J. Fernández Perrino, Lino Mayorga Reyes, Héctor Herrera Gutiérrez and Saúl Cortés Suárez
Universidad Autónoma Metropolitana, México, D. F.

Etleva Delia and Myqerem Tafaj
Faculty of Agriculture and Environment, Agricultural University of Tirana, Albania

Klaus Männer
Institut fur Tierernährung, Freie Universität Berlin, Germany